Atlas of Head and Neck Robotic Surgery

Ziv Gil • Moran Amit
Michael E. Kupferman
Editors

Atlas of Head and Neck Robotic Surgery

Springer

Editors
Ziv Gil
Israel Institute of Technology
The Head and Neck Center
Rambam Healthcare Campus
Haifa, Israel

Michael E. Kupferman
Department of Head and Neck Surgery
MD Anderson Cancer Center
Houston, TX, USA

Moran Amit
Israel Institute of Technology
The Head and Neck Center
Rambam Healthcare Campus
Haifa, Israel

Department of Head and Neck Surgery
Houston, TX, USA

ISBN 978-3-319-49576-7 ISBN 978-3-319-49578-1 (eBook)
DOI 10.1007/978-3-319-49578-1

Library of Congress Control Number: 2017943536

Printed on acid-free paper

This Springer imprint is published by Springer Nature
The registered company is Springer International Publishing AG
The registered company address is: Gewerbestrasse 11, 6330 Cham, Switzerland

To my children Ada, Izhar, Yanai and Elisheva that their spirit is carried within me.

Ziv Gil

For my parents, who tried, and my wife, Heli.

Moran Amit

For my wife, Debra, and our children Asaph, Gabrielle and Jacob.

Michael E. Kupferman

Biography

Professor Gil is a Barbara S. Goodman Endowed Investigator (ICRF) and the chairman of the Department of Otolaryngology—Head and Neck Surgery, Rambam Healthcare Campus, Israel Institute of Technology. He holds an MD/PhD degree in biophysics and neuroscience and is also the head of the Applied Cancer Research Laboratory and a member of the Rappaport Research Institute and the Clinical Research Institute at Rambam. He received his training at Memorial Sloan Kettering Cancer Center and the University of Pittsburgh Medical Center. He received awards from the Israeli Parliament, NY Head and Neck Society, Israeli Cancer Society, and Folks Foundation and multiple international research grants. He is the author of three books and 200 scientific publications and book chapters. Dr. Gil established new techniques in skull base and robotic surgery. He serves on the editorial boards of multiple journals including *Otolaryngology—Head and Neck Surgery, Journal of Neurological Surgery, Head and Neck*, and more. In 2014 he established the first comprehensive Head and Neck Center in Israel.

Moran Amit, MD/PhD, in cancer biology and immunology, completed his training in head and neck surgery at the University of Texas MD Anderson Cancer Center, Houston, Texas, USA. Dr. Amit's clinical focus is on robotic head and neck surgery (especially trans-oral robotic approaches to the oropharynx and parapharyngeal space, TORS) and functional rehabilitation of head and neck cancer patients. Dr. Amit is a co-founder of the Adenoid Cystic Carcinoma International Study (AXIS) Group and a board member of the International Consortium for Outcome Research (ICOR) in Head and Neck Cancer. He is a board member of the The European academy of tumor immunology and a member of the American Association for cancer research and the International Papillomavirus Society. Dr. Amit has published extensively in the areas of oral cavity, skull base, and salivary gland cancer. He received awards from the Chief Officer, Medical Corps, Israel Defense Forces, American Head and Neck Society, Israeli Cancer Society, and multiple international research grants for his research on tumor immunology and resistance to treatment. Dr. Amit is a Barbara S. Goodman Endowed Investigator (ICRF).

Dr. Michael Kupferman is an Associate Professor of Head and Neck Surgery at the University of Texas MD Anderson Cancer Center. He is an internationally-recognized expert in Head and Neck Oncology, with expertise in the surgical management of pediatric head and neck cancer and skull base tumors. His clinical practice focuses on upper aerodigestive tract cancers, melanoma, salivary gland and skull base tumors, as well as robotic surgery of the head and neck. Dr. Kupferman is also the medical director of the Voice Center at MD Anderson, and is the leader for clinical trials exploring the role of transoral robotic surgery for head and neck cancer. Dr. Kupferman is also a physician executive in the MD Anderson Cancer Network, where he leads the development, management and growth of clinical oncology programs across the Cancer Network. He obtained his medical degree from the University of Pennsylvania School of Medicine and completed residency in Otolaryngology—Head and Neck Surgery at the Hospital of the University of Pennsylvania. He also completed a combined clinical and research fellowship in advanced Head and Neck Surgical Oncology at MD Anderson Cancer Center. He has published over 125 peer-reviewed manuscripts and book chapters, and his laboratory research in the mechanisms of metastasis has been funded by the National Institutes of Health, American College of Surgeons, American Head and Neck Society, AAO and numerous private foundations.

Contents

Robotics in Surgery

1

Moran Amit, Shorook Na'ara, and Ziv Gil

1.1 Introduction

Over the last two decades, robotic-assisted surgery has revolutionized minimally invasive surgery in multiple surgical specialties. The first robotic surgery system, the PUMA 560, was developed in 1985 to provide greater precision in performing image-guided intracranial biopsies. Further refinement in the early 1990s led to ROBODOC, which was the first robotic system to receive FDA approval for arthroscopic hip surgery in 1994 [1]. Interest in medical robots led to collaborative efforts between the National Aeronautics and Space Administration (NASA) and Stanford Research Institute (SRI) in the early 1980s, to develop telepresence surgery, the virtual placement of a remotely located surgeon in the operative field.

Experience with minimally invasive laparoscopic procedures has helped surgeons understand the limitations of rigid equipment and two-dimensional views. This has resulted in the development of semirigid robotic equipment with three-dimensional views for the operative setting. Combining these tools with telepresence surgery led to the development of the Automated Endoscopic System for Optimal Positioning (AESOP), a robotic arm (controlled by a surgeon's voice commands) that manipulates an endoscopic camera [2]. The first robotic system that enabled surgery over a large distance consisted of two separate subsystems, i.e., "surgeon-side" and "patient-side" (ZEUS, Computer Motion, California). The operator site was located in New York and the animals were in Strasbourg. The two sites were connected through a high-speed terrestrial optical-fiber network that transports data through dedicated connections using asynchronous transfer mode (ATM) technology [3].

Shortly thereafter, Intuitive Systems (Sunnyvale, CA) released the SRI Telepresence Surgery System that was recently updated to the current da Vinci Surgical System, the most common robotic system in use today [4].

In short, the current da Vinci system functions as a master-slave robot, with the surgeon manipulating instruments connected by a cable network to the robotic cart. The system comprises three arms (one for the 12 mm 0° or 30° camera and two accommodate 8 mm and 5 mm instruments). The camera not only enables magnification but also three-dimensional viewing of the surgical field.

M. Amit, MD, PhD • S. Na'ara, MD
Z. Gil, MD, PhD (✉)
The Head and Neck Center, Department of Otolaryngology Head and Neck Surgery, The Laboratory for Applied Cancer Research, Rambam Healthcare Campus, Clinical Research Institute at Rambam, Rappaport Institute of Medicine and Research, The Technion, Israel Institute of Technology, Haifa 66036, Israel
e-mail: ziv@baseofskull.org; g_ziv@rambam.health.gov.il

Z. Gil et al. (eds.), *Atlas of Head and Neck Robotic Surgery*, DOI 10.1007/978-3-319-49578-1_1

Robot-assisted surgery enables excellent visualization and the capacity to manipulate and resect tumors due to the six degrees of freedom offered by the robotic arms and by the camera.

1.2 Applications in Fields Other Than Otolaryngology

Robot-assisted surgery is currently utilized in almost every surgical field. In general surgery, there is an abundance of reports on its use in cholecystectomy, Heller myotomy, Nissen fundoplication, bowel resection with reanastomosis, splenectomy, and Whipple and hepatobiliary surgery [5]. These reports endorse the benefits of stable visualization and improved dexterity of the robotic arms with suturing and dissection. Cardiothoracic surgeons used robotic surgery first in 1998 to perform coronary revascularization procedures and mitral valve replacements [6]. Numerous additional case series have since been published, describing esophagectomy, lung resection, tumor resections, atrial fibrillation ablations, and congenital cardiac anomalies. Results have been encouraging, with evidence demonstrating fewer blood transfusions, shorter hospital stays, faster returns to preoperative function levels, and improved quality of life compared to patient series of sternotomy [7]. Multiple pediatric surgery robotic-assisted procedures include tracheoesophageal fistula repair, cholecystectomy, Nissen fundoplication, Morgagni's hernia repair, Kasai portoenterostomy, and congenital diaphragmatic hernia repair.

Gynecologists utilize robotic surgery in hysterectomies, myomectomies, and tubal reanastomoses and achieve similarly positive results as in laparoscopic and open procedures. However, a recent Cochrane review showed an uncertain benefit for robotic surgery in gynecology because it is unclear if it affects rates of complications [8]. Oncologic outcomes were similar to laparoscopic and open methods. The setup time for both exposure and docking of the robotic arms is longer with robot-assisted surgery but may be associated with a shorter hospital stay following hysterectomy. In addition, gynecologic surgeons observed another major disadvantage; the lack of haptic feedback, which is a virtual tactile feedback technology that provides mechanical feedback to the surgeon. Currently, in the United States, robotic-assisted hysterectomy is mainly used for benign conditions and has been shown to be more expensive than conventional laparoscopic hysterectomy, with no difference in overall rates of complications [9].

The development of robotic technology has paved the way for the performance of highly complex procedures such as transplant surgery, in a minimally invasive fashion. The first fully robotic kidney transplantations were performed in the late 2000s. The use of the robotic-assisted approach has enabled transplantation of kidneys with minimal complications and has significantly shortened the recovery period. This has made possible kidney transplantation in obese patients, who were frequently denied access to transplantation.

The field of urologic surgery has perhaps seen the greatest incorporation of robotic surgery: To date, more than two-thirds of prostatectomies are performed with robotic assistance [10]. Positive margin status and PSA levels achieved by the robotic technique are comparable to those achieved by open procedures [11]. However, surgeons noted significantly lower blood loss and transfusion rates, less pain, and shorter hospital stays for robotic techniques than open prostatectomies; erectile and urinary functional outcomes were found to be equivalent among open, laparoscopic, and robotic prostatectomies [12].

1.3 Evolution of Robotic Applications in Otolaryngology

The first TORS procedure was reported in Washington by McLeod et al. only a little more than one decade ago [13]. Since then, surgeons have laid infrastructure for its use, and it has been successfully incorporated into routine practice in the field of otolaryngology. Incorporation of robotic-assisted surgery in otolaryngology can be attributed to three main driving forces: (1) technological advancements that improved visualization and instrumentation, (2) fast learning curve, and (3) better understanding of head and neck cancer biology while exploring organ conservation treatment protocols.

Traditionally, surgical removal of oropharyngeal cancer required mandibulotomy with or without free flap reconstruction in most cases. Unfortunately, this approach results in significant morbidity. Mandibulotomy patients often require tracheotomies and feeding tubes. In addition, postoperative recovery, including rehabilitation, might further be slowed by adjuvant chemotherapy and/or radiation [14]. The pendulum started to shift in the late 1980s when multiple institutions investigated alternative treatment protocols based on organ preservation. The VA trial and RTOG 91-11 showed that survival rates following chemotherapy and radiation protocols were equivalent to those for patients who underwent surgery followed by radiation. By preserving the functional laryngopharyngeal complex, these protocols became the standard of care in the treatment of squamous cell carcinoma of the larynx [15, 16]. Alongside the highly conformal radiation delivery techniques (e.g., IMRT), molecular targeted therapies (e.g., cetuximab) were successfully introduced and represent an evolutionary advancement in head and neck cancer management. Nonetheless, survival and quality of life are still poor for some patients [17].

Over the last decade, we encountered an increase in oropharyngeal squamous cell carcinoma (OPSCC) caused by the human papilloma virus (HPV). HPV was recognized as a powerful prognostic biomarker for responsiveness to radiotherapy; however, HPV-positive patients tend to be younger, and thus the potential is greater for long-term sequelae from radiation, such as radiation-induced malignancy [18]. The development of successful minimally invasive surgical techniques has assisted in achieving sound oncological resection with local control and possibly sparing patients from undergoing concurrent chemoradiation.

First attempts to control OPSCC with minimally invasive techniques in the modern radiotherapy era used transoral laser microsurgery (TLM). While no randomized trials have compared surgery and radiation, small series from various institutions have shown success at achieving local control by using TLM as the primary modality for OPSCC [19]. However, rigid narrow field exposure through laryngoscopes is very limited and challenging to maneuver within the complex anatomy of the oropharynx.

Robotic surgery overcomes some of these limitations and provides a unique advantage by introducing angled optics and instrumentation with multiple degrees of rotation, which allows access to the entire upper aerodigestive tract surface. In addition, superior optics enable a precise three-dimensional assessment of resection margins, less collateral tissue damage, and an excellent view of the surgical bed.

1.4 Feasibility

Robotic-assisted salivary gland excision and neck dissection in a porcine model were the first applications of robotics in otolaryngology, as documented at Stanford University in 2003 [20]. Among the advantages claimed were the elimination of hand tremor and superior visualization without tactile sensation. Next, Hockstein and O'Malley reported gaining wide access to the laryngopharynx using mouth gag retractors in an airway mannequin and cadaver [21]. Later, Weinstein performed a supraglottic laryngectomy in a canine model [21]. The authors reported increased exposure with the mouth gag, yielding adjustable visualization of the larynx [22]. The final step before attempts on live human surgery was the technological increment achieved by coupling of 5-mm instruments and other mouth retractors to the robotic system at Cleveland Clinic by Solares [23]. The latter incorporated the CO2 laser with the robotic arm for robotic-assisted supraglottic laryngectomy and demonstrated the importance of evaluating variable patient factors such as oral opening and neck extension.

Weinstein and O'Malley first reported the efficacy of robotic-assisted head and neck surgery. They described a series of patients with early-stage, base of tongue squamous cell carcinomas who underwent complete en bloc resection of their tumors with negative margins. No immediate complications were noted, and patients were able to return to a full diet within 6 weeks of surgery [24]. With the feasibility of TORS established in OPSCC, institutions have begun recruiting patients for clinical trials such as ECOG3311 and RTOG1221 to assess treatment de-escalation of HPV+ patients with surgery and surgical intensification of treatment in HPV patients. Currently, robotic-assisted surgery has a wide range of applications in otorhinolaryngology. These include transoral surgery for sleep disorders, malignant and benign tumor resection from the upper aerodigestive tract, and skull base surgery. In addition, various approaches have been utilized for neck surgery, i.e., the transaxillary approach for thyroid and parathyroid surgery, and the retroauricular approach for neck dissection, congenital lesion resection, and salivary gland surgery. Table 1.1 summarizes published applications of robotic-assisted surgery in otorhinolaryngology.

Table 1.1. Published applications of robotic-assisted surgery in otorhinolaryngology

Approach	Site	Pathology	Number of published cases	References
TORS	Oral cavity	Malignancies	8	[25–27]
	Oropharynx: base of tongue and tonsils	Malignancies	1,337	[24–36]
		Benign lesions	19	[13, 37–39]
		OSA	726	[40–50]
	Hypopharynx	Malignancies	21	[26, 27, 51–53]
	Larynx: supraglottis and glottis	Malignancies	63	[23, 25–27, 34, 51, 54–56]
		Congenital malformations and benign lesions	6	[57, 58]
	Parapharyngeal space	Benign and malignant tumors	45	[59–67]
Transaxillary approach	Thyroid	PTC and benign nodules	2,074	[68–79]
	Parathyroid	Parathyroid adenoma and hyperplasia	15	[78–81]
Thoracoscopic approach	Mediastinal parathyroid	Parathyroid adenoma and hyperplasia	10	[82–87]
Retroauricular/postauricular approach	Thyroid	PTC	4	[88]
	Neck dissection		19	[27, 89]
	Branchial cleft cyst		3	[90]
	Submandibular gland		13	[91]
	TGDC		1	[92]
Modified facelift	Neck dissection		44	[27, 93]

TORS transoral robotic surgery, *OSA* obstructive sleep apnea, *PTC* papillary thyroid carcinoma, *TGDC* thyroglossal duct cyst

1.5 Oncologic and Functional Outcomes

The effectiveness of a therapeutic modality appears to be strongly inversely related to the number of clinical trials that investigate the modality. While most head and neck cancers are surgically treated, only few clinical trials isolate any given surgical question.

Long-term survival outcomes of TORS are not currently available. Still, several institutions have published promising small cohort short-term data. A phase I study of 27 patients with early-stage tonsillar squamous cell carcinoma undergoing TORS revealed a 92 % negative margin rate. Population-based analysis revealed that TORS is associated with a lower rate of positive margins than non-robotic surgery and that high-volume centers have the lowest rates of positive margins and unplanned readmissions [28]. After achieving resection with negative margins, adjuvant treatment may be administered. However, even if the patient requires adjuvant therapy, the toxicity from the lower dose of radiation, with possible sparing of concurrent chemoradiation, tends to be significantly less following adequate robotic surgery and to result in better functional outcomes [94]. In addition, most patients do not need a tracheotomy or extended hospitalization.

From a functional standpoint, many clinical studies have shown improved post-TORS swallowing function compared with other surgical modalities and compared with primary chemoradiation therapy, along with shorter hospital stay and faster recovery, as well as a more efficient return to work after completion of therapy [29]. Most patients after TORS for OPSCC maintain full oral feeding and eventually acceptable to normal physiological swallowing. In a negligible minority of patients, elective temporary tracheotomy (1–2 weeks) is performed at the discretion of the surgeon, based on the estimated risk of postoperative upper airway obstruction due to mucosal swelling and the risk of postoperative bleeding. Faster recovery means that adjuvant therapy, if indicated, may start sooner, which improves locoregional control [30, 31].

Favorable oncological and functional outcomes of TORS, which permit resection of the tumor en bloc while preserving patients' swallowing ability, led the FDA to approve, in December 2009, TORS for use in selected benign and malignant tumors of the head and neck. Using TORS, a mandibulotomy and/or pharyngotomy is avoided. As evidence accumulates regarding survival implications of HPV status in patients undergoing primary surgical therapy, TORS may play a significant role in the application of surgery to escalate or de-escalate first-line treatment for select patients with OPSCC.

1.6 Cost

High costs are a significant concern and a potential disadvantage of the implementation of a robotic program solely for TORS. With an initial cost of 1.5 million US dollars and annual maintenance fees of 100,000 US dollars, most programs rely on sharing the robotic facility with other departments. Disposable equipment such as graspers, cautery arms, and other surgical instruments total approximately 200 dollars per case. A nationwide cross-sectional analysis of more than 9,000 patients showed that after controlling for all other variables, TORS patients had lower rates of gastrostomy tube placement and tracheotomy tube placement, shorter length of hospitalization (mean, −1.5 days), and lower hospital-related costs (mean, −$4,285) [95].

1.7 Training

Naturally, as the popularity of robotic surgery is growing, practitioners are seeking training and certification in this area. The pitfall of such market-driven health care is the possibility that adverse outcomes may decrease positive results of surgery when less-experienced surgeons perform oncologic resections simply because TORS is a new and marketable procedure [96]. Intuitive surgical provides a training curriculum on their website, which includes didactic lectures on the da Vinci console, cadaver dissections, and live case observation. Nearly 1,500 surgical clips of TORS can be viewed on YouTube, and representatives for the company provide surgeon tutoring during practitioners' initial procedures.

Robust outcomes data are not yet available, but potentially, robot-assisted surgery will become a standardized integral part of treatment protocols such as the National Comprehensive Cancer Network (NCCN). Once integrated, the implementation of a standardized curriculum for robotic surgery into residency and fellowship education will be vital. Current data indicate that the performance of simple tasks such as grasping inanimate objects and suturing on latex is highly intuitive, and introducing residents to basic robotic surgical skills eases their transition to live patient cases [97]. As a result, many training programs now provide cadaver dissection courses using the robot as part of their training. Training is discussed in more depth in Chapter 4.

1.8 Future Directions

To date, available data on head and neck robotic surgery, mainly TORS, indicate that it is a safe efficacious procedure for benign conditions such as obstructive sleep apnea. As stated, current efforts are being directed to implement TORS in oncology treatment protocols. Attempts are also being made to extend the applications of robot-assisted surgery and to use TORS in innovative ways and in other areas in the head and neck. An example is the field of skull base surgery, which requires precise motions with a steady hand. Surgeons have illustrated an approach to the midline and anterior skull base using two trocars inserted transcervically and placing the camera head in the oral cavity [98]. Anterior skull base and sella were accessed and dissected via bilateral Caldwell Luc incisions and maxillary antrostomies [99].

Robotic-assisted surgery is also being utilized in reconstructive surgery [100]. Microvascular anastomosis in narrow and deep spaces such as the oropharynx has been shown to be fast and effective, in a tremor-free manner. TORS free flap oropharyngeal reconstruction provides improved functional recovery and avoids the need for long-term healing by secondary intention of the oropharyngeal defect.

As current instrumentation is bulky, rigid, and passive, access is limited to narrow 3D complex spaces such as the larynx and skull base. Approaches to such areas will become possible as finer analytical instrumentation such as flexible lasers and Doppler probes will emerge. To overcome some of these obstacles, a flexible nonlinear robot was designed based on the experience gained by the use of the da Vinci system. This robot was further customized and transformed into the Medrobotics(®) Flex(®) System (Medrobotics Corp., Raynham, MA, USA), which was developed specifically for use in surgical applications requiring nonlinear maneuverability such as transoral surgery. The Medrobotics® Flex(®) System is an operator-controlled flexible endoscope system that includes rigid chip-on-tip endoscope and computer-assisted controllers, with two external channels for use with compatible, 3.5 mm flexible instruments. In 2015, the FDA approved the use of the Flex System for transoral resections of head and neck tumors.

Conclusion

Head and neck applications of robotic surgery are an evolutionary increment in surgical capabilities. While robotic-assisted head and neck surgery confers significant advantages, its limitations should be acknowledged. Patients can benefit from en bloc removal of their tumors via minimally invasive surgery without a cervical incision while preserving function and potentially avoiding adjuvant radiation and long-term sequelae. While long-term oncologic and functional data are needed to fully validate its use, early results are promising.

References

1. Bargar WL, Bauer A, Borner M. Primary and revision total hip replacement using the Robodoc system. Clin Orthop Relat Res. 1998;354:82–91.
2. Nguyen NT, Hinojosa MW, Finley D, Stevens M, Paya M. Application of robotics in general surgery: initial experience. Am Surg. 2004;70(10):914–7.
3. Marescaux J, Leroy J, Gagner M, Rubino F, Mutter D, Vix M, et al. Transatlantic robot-assisted telesurgery. Nature. 2001;413(6854):379–80.
4. http://www.intuitivesurgical.com. Intuitive Surgical Inc.
5. Toro JP, Lin E, Patel AD. Review of robotics in foregut and bariatric surgery. Surg Endosc. 2015; 29(1):1–8.
6. Bush B, Nifong LW, Chitwood Jr WR. Robotics in cardiac surgery: past, present, and future. Rambam Maimonides Med J. 2013;4(3):e0017.
7. Rodriguez E, Chitwood WR. Robotics in cardiac surgery. Scand J Surg: SJS: Off Organ Finn Surg Soc Scand Surg Soc. 2009;98(2):120–4.
8. Liu H, Lawrie TA, Lu D, Song H, Wang L, Shi G. Robot-assisted surgery in gynaecology. Cochrane Database Syst Rev. 2014;12:CD011422.
9. Committee opinion no. 628: robotic surgery in gynecology. Obstet Gynecol. 2015;125(3):760–7.
10. Jain S, Gautam G. Robotics in urologic oncology. J Minim Access Surg. 2015;11(1):40–4.
11. Barocas DA, Salem S, Kordan Y, Herrell SD, Chang SS, Clark PE, et al. Robotic assisted laparoscopic prostatectomy versus radical retropubic prostatectomy for clinically localized prostate cancer: comparison of short-term biochemical recurrence-free survival. J Urol. 2010;183(3):990–6.
12. Eifler JB, Cookson MS. Best evidence regarding the superiority or inferiority of robot-assisted radical prostatectomy. Urol Clin N Am. 2014;41(4): 493–502.
13. McLeod IK, Melder PC. Da Vinci robot-assisted excision of a vallecular cyst: a case report. Ear Nose Throat J. 2005;84(3):170–2.
14. Oliveira CM, Nguyen HT, Ferraz AR, Watters K, Rosman B, Rahbar R. Robotic surgery in otolaryngology and head and neck surgery: a review. Minim Invasive Surg. 2012;2012:286563.
15. Forastiere AA, Goepfert H, Maor M, Pajak TF, Weber R, Morrison W, et al. Concurrent chemotherapy and radiotherapy for organ preservation in advanced laryngeal cancer. N Engl J Med. 2003;349(22):2091–8.
16. The Department of Veterans Affairs Laryngeal Cancer Study Group. Induction chemotherapy plus radiation compared with surgery plus radiation in patients with advanced laryngeal cancer. N Engl J Med. 1991;324(24):1685–90.
17. Chen AY, Halpern M. Factors predictive of survival in advanced laryngeal cancer. Arch Otolaryngol Head Neck Surg. 2007;133(12):1270–6.
18. Ang KK, Harris J, Wheeler R, Weber R, Rosenthal DI, Nguyen-Tan PF, et al. Human papillomavirus and survival of patients with oropharyngeal cancer. N Engl J Med. 2010;363(1):24–35.
19. Grant DG, Hinni ML, Salassa JR, Perry WC, Hayden RE, Casler JD. Oropharyngeal cancer: a case for single modality treatment with transoral laser microsurgery. Arch Otolaryngol Head Neck Surg. 2009;135(12):1225–30.
20. Haus BM, Kambham N, Le D, Moll FM, Gourin C, Terris DJ. Surgical robotic applications in otolaryngology. Laryngoscope. 2003;113(7):1139–44.
21. Hockstein NG, Nolan JP, O'Malley Jr BW, Woo YJ. Robotic microlaryngeal surgery: a technical feasibility study using the daVinci surgical robot and an airway mannequin. Laryngoscope. 2005;115(5): 780–5.
22. Hockstein NG, Nolan JP, O'Malley Jr BW, Woo YJ. Robot-assisted pharyngeal and laryngeal microsurgery: results of robotic cadaver dissections. Laryngoscope. 2005;115(6):1003–8.
23. Solares CA, Strome M. Transoral robot-assisted CO2 laser supraglottic laryngectomy: experimental and clinical data. Laryngoscope. 2007;117(5): 817–20.
24. O'Malley Jr BW, Weinstein GS, Snyder W, Hockstein NG. Transoral robotic surgery (TORS) for base of tongue neoplasms. Laryngoscope. 2006;116(8):1465–72.
25. Lawson G, Matar N, Remacle M, Jamart J, Bachy V. Transoral robotic surgery for the management of head and neck tumors: learning curve. Eur Arch Otorhinolaryngol: Off J Eur Fed Otorhinolaryngol Soc. 2011;268(12):1795–801.
26. Boudreaux BA, Rosenthal EL, Magnuson JS, Newman JR, Desmond RA, Clemons L, et al. Robot-assisted surgery for upper aerodigestive tract neoplasms. Arch Otolaryngol Head Neck Surg. 2009;135(4):397–401.
27. Byeon HK, Holsinger FC, Kim DH, Kim JW, Park JH, Koh YW, et al. Feasibility of robot-assisted neck dissection followed by transoral robotic surgery. Br J Oral Maxillofac Surg. 2015;53(1):68–73.
28. Chen MM, Roman SA, Kraus DH, Sosa JA, Judson BL. Transoral robotic surgery: a population-level analysis. Otolaryngol Head Neck Surg: Off J Am Acad Otolaryngol Head Neck Surg. 2014; 150(6):968–75.
29. Sinclair CF, McColloch NL, Carroll WR, Rosenthal EL, Desmond RA, Magnuson JS. Patient-perceived and objective functional outcomes following transoral robotic surgery for early oropharyngeal carcinoma. Arch Otolaryngol Head Neck Surg. 2011; 137(11):1112–6.
30. Lorincz BB, Mockelmann N, Busch CJ, Knecht R. Functional outcomes, feasibility, and safety of resection of transoral robotic surgery: single-institution series of 35 consecutive cases of transoral robotic surgery for oropharyngeal squamous cell carcinoma. Head Neck. 2015;37(11):1618–24.

31. Lee SY, Park YM, Byeon HK, Choi EC, Kim SH. Comparison of oncologic and functional outcomes after transoral robotic lateral oropharyngectomy versus conventional surgery for T1 to T3 tonsillar cancer. Head Neck. 2014;36(8):1138–45.
32. Weinstein GS, O'Malley Jr BW, Snyder W, Sherman E, Quon H. Transoral robotic surgery: radical tonsillectomy. Arch Otolaryngol Head Neck Surg. 2007;133(12):1220–6.
33. Moore EJ, Olsen KD, Kasperbauer JL. Transoral robotic surgery for oropharyngeal squamous cell carcinoma: a prospective study of feasibility and functional outcomes. Laryngoscope. 2009;119(11):2156–64.
34. Iseli TA, Kulbersh BD, Iseli CE, Carroll WR, Rosenthal EL, Magnuson JS. Functional outcomes after transoral robotic surgery for head and neck cancer. Otolaryngol Head Neck Surg: Off J Am Acad Otolaryngol Head Neck Surg. 2009;141(2):166–71.
35. Weinstein GS, O'Malley Jr BW, Cohen MA, Quon H. Transoral robotic surgery for advanced oropharyngeal carcinoma. Arch Otolaryngol Head Neck Surg. 2010;136(11):1079–85.
36. Moore EJ, Olsen KD, Martin EJ. Concurrent neck dissection and transoral robotic surgery. Laryngoscope. 2011;121(3):541–4.
37. Pellini R, Mercante G, Ruscito P, Cristalli G, Spriano G. Ectopic lingual goiter treated by transoral robotic surgery. Acta Otorhinolaryngol Ital: Organo Ufficiale Soc Ital Otorinolaringol Chir Cervicofac. 2013;33(5):343–6.
38. Leonardis RL, Duvvuri U, Mehta D. Transoral robotic-assisted lingual tonsillectomy in the pediatric population. JAMA Otolaryngol Head Neck Surg. 2013;139(10):1032–6.
39. Kimple AJ, Eliades SJ, Richmon JD. Transoral robotic resection of a lingual thyroglossal duct cyst. J Robot Surg. 2012;6(4):367–9.
40. Vicini C, Dallan I, Canzi P, Frassineti S, La Pietra MG, Montevecchi F. Transoral robotic tongue base resection in obstructive sleep apnoea-hypopnoea syndrome: a preliminary report. ORL J Otorhinolaryngol Relat Spec. 2010;72(1):22–7.
41. Vicini C, Dallan I, Canzi P, Frassineti S, Nacci A, Seccia V, et al. Transoral robotic surgery of the tongue base in obstructive sleep Apnea-Hypopnea syndrome: anatomic considerations and clinical experience. Head Neck. 2012;34(1):15–22.
42. Arora A, Chaidas K, Garas G, Amlani A, Darzi A, Kotecha B, et al. Outcome of TORS to tongue base and epiglottis in patients with OSA intolerant of conventional treatment. Sleep Breathing = Schlaf Atmung. 2015;8:636–643.
43. Chiffer RC, Schwab RJ, Keenan BT, Borek RC, Thaler ER. Volumetric MRI analysis pre- and post-transoral robotic surgery for obstructive sleep apnea. Laryngoscope. 2015;125(8):1988–95.
44. Eesa M, Montevecchi F, Hendawy E, D'Agostino G, Meccariello G, Vicini C. Swallowing outcome after TORS for sleep apnea: short- and long-term evaluation. Eur Arch Otorhinolaryngol: Off J Eur Fed Otorhinolaryngol Soc. 2015;272(6):1537–41.
45. Lin HS, Rowley JA, Badr MS, Folbe AJ, Yoo GH, Victor L, et al. Transoral robotic surgery for treatment of obstructive sleep apnea-hypopnea syndrome. Laryngoscope. 2013;123(7):1811–6.
46. Lin HS, Rowley JA, Folbe AJ, Yoo GH, Badr MS, Chen W. Transoral robotic surgery for treatment of obstructive sleep apnea: factors predicting surgical response. Laryngoscope. 2015;125(4):1013–20.
47. Glazer TA, Hoff PT, Spector ME. Transoral robotic surgery for obstructive sleep apnea: perioperative management and postoperative complications. JAMA Otolaryngol Head Neck Surg. 2014;140(12):1207–12.
48. Toh ST, Han HJ, Tay HN, Kiong KL. Transoral robotic surgery for obstructive sleep apnea in Asian patients: a Singapore sleep centre experience. JAMA Otolaryngol Head Neck Surg. 2014;140(7):624–9.
49. Vicini C, Montevecchi F, Campanini A, Dallan I, Hoff PT, Spector ME, et al. Clinical outcomes and complications associated with TORS for OSAHS: a benchmark for evaluating an emerging surgical technology in a targeted application for benign disease. ORL J Otorhinolaryngol Relat Spec. 2014;76(2):63–9.
50. Friedman M, Hamilton C, Samuelson CG, Kelley K, Taylor D, Pearson-Chauhan K, et al. Transoral robotic glossectomy for the treatment of obstructive sleep apnea-hypopnea syndrome. Otolaryngol Head Neck Surg: Off J Am Acad Otolaryngol Head Neck Surg. 2012;146(5):854–62.
51. Park YM, Lee WJ, Lee JG, Lee WS, Choi EC, Chung SM, et al. Transoral robotic surgery (TORS) in laryngeal and hypopharyngeal cancer. J Laparoendosc Adv Surg Tech A. 2009;19(3):361–8.
52. Park YM, Kim WS, Byeon HK, De Virgilio A, Jung JS, Kim SH. Feasibility of transoral robotic hypopharyngectomy for early-stage hypopharyngeal carcinoma. Oral Oncol. 2010;46(8):597–602.
53. Kucur C, Durmus K, Dziegielewski PT, Ozer E. Transoral robot-assisted carbon dioxide laser surgery for hypopharyngeal cancer. Head Neck. 2015;37(5):743–5.
54. Alon EE, Kasperbauer JL, Olsen KD, Moore EJ. Feasibility of transoral robotic-assisted supraglottic laryngectomy. Head Neck. 2012;34(2):225–9.
55. Dowthwaite S, Nichols AC, Yoo J, Smith RV, Dhaliwal S, Basmaji J, et al. Transoral robotic total laryngectomy: report of 3 cases. Head Neck. 2013;35(11):E338–42.
56. Kayhan FT, Kaya KH, Sayin I. Transoral robotic cordectomy for early glottic carcinoma. Ann Otol Rhinol Laryngol. 2012;121(8):497–502.
57. Rahbar R, Ferrari LR, Borer JG, Peters CA. Robotic surgery in the pediatric airway: application and

safety. Arch Otolaryngol Head Neck Surg. 2007;133(1):46–50. discussion
58. Muderris T, Bercin S, Sevil E, Acar B, Kiris M. Transoral robotic surgery for atypical carcinoid tumor of the larynx. J Craniofac Surg. 2013;24(6): 1996–9.
59. Chan JY, Tsang RK, Eisele DW, Richmon JD. Transoral robotic surgery of the parapharyngeal space: a case series and systematic review. Head Neck. 2015;37(2):293–8.
60. O'Malley Jr BW, Quon H, Leonhardt FD, Chalian AA, Weinstein GS. Transoral robotic surgery for parapharyngeal space tumors. ORL J Otorhinolaryngol Relat Spec. 2010;72(6):332–6.
61. De Virgilio A, Park YM, Kim WS, Byeon HK, Lee SY, Kim SH. Transoral robotic surgery for the resection of parapharyngeal tumour: our experience in ten patients. Clin Otolaryngol: Off J ENT-UK; Off J Neth Soc Otorhinolaryngol Cervicofac Surg. 2012;37(6):483–8.
62. Park YM, De Virgilio A, Kim WS, Chung HP, Kim SH. Parapharyngeal space surgery via a transoral approach using a robotic surgical system: transoral robotic surgery. J Laparoendosc Adv Surg Tech A. 2013;23(3):231–6.
63. Desai SC, Sung CK, Genden EM. Transoral robotic surgery using an image guidance system. Laryngoscope. 2008;118(11):2003–5.
64. O'Malley Jr BW, Weinstein GS. Robotic skull base surgery: preclinical investigations to human clinical application. Arch Otolaryngol Head Neck Surg. 2007;133(12):1215–9.
65. Kim GG, Zanation AM. Transoral robotic surgery to resect skull base tumors via transpalatal and lateral pharyngeal approaches. Laryngoscope. 2012;122(7): 1575–8.
66. Arshad H, Durmus K, Ozer E. Transoral robotic resection of selected parapharyngeal space tumors. Eur Arch Otorhinolaryngol: Off J Eur Fed Otorhinolaryngol Soc. 2013;270(5):1737–40.
67. Amit M, Gil Z. Transoral robotic resection of parapharyngeal space tumors. Oper Tech Otolaryngol Head Neck Surg. 2014;25(3):293–8.
68. Lobe TE, Wright SK, Irish MS. Novel uses of surgical robotics in head and neck surgery. J Laparoendosc Adv Surg Tech Part A. 2005;15(6):647–52.
69. Byeon HK, Ban MJ, Lee JM, Ha JG, Kim ES, Koh YW, et al. Robot-assisted Sistrunk's operation, total thyroidectomy, and neck dissection via a transaxillary and retroauricular (TARA) approach in papillary carcinoma arising in thyroglossal duct cyst and thyroid gland. Ann Surg Oncol. 2012;19(13): 4259–61.
70. Miyano G, Lobe TE, Wright SK. Bilateral transaxillary endoscopic total thyroidectomy. J Pediatr Surg. 2008;43(2):299–303.
71. Kang SW, Jeong JJ, Yun JS, Sung TY, Lee SC, Lee YS, et al. Robot-assisted endoscopic surgery for thyroid cancer: experience with the first 100 patients. Surg Endosc. 2009;23(11):2399–406.
72. Kang SW, Lee SC, Lee SH, Lee KY, Jeong JJ, Lee YS, et al. Robotic thyroid surgery using a gasless, transaxillary approach and the da Vinci S system: the operative outcomes of 338 consecutive patients. Surgery. 2009;146(6):1048–55.
73. Lee J, Nah KY, Kim RM, Ahn YH, Soh EY, Chung WY. Differences in postoperative outcomes, function, and cosmesis: open versus robotic thyroidectomy. Surg Endosc. 2010;24(12):3186–94.
74. Lee J, Yun JH, Nam KH, Choi UJ, Chung WY, Soh EY. Perioperative clinical outcomes after robotic thyroidectomy for thyroid carcinoma: a multicenter study. Surg Endosc. 2011;25(3):906–12.
75. Tae K, Ji YB, Jeong JH, Lee SH, Jeong MA, Park CW. Robotic thyroidectomy by a gasless unilateral axillo-breast or axillary approach: our early experiences. Surg Endosc. 2011;25(1):221–8.
76. Lee KE, Rao J, Youn YK. Endoscopic thyroidectomy with the da Vinci robot system using the bilateral axillary breast approach (BABA) technique: our initial experience. Surg Laparosc Endosc Percutan Tech. 2009;19(3):e71–5.
77. Lee S, Ryu HR, Park JH, Kim KH, Kang SW, Jeong JJ, et al. Excellence in robotic thyroid surgery: a comparative study of robot-assisted versus conventional endoscopic thyroidectomy in papillary thyroid microcarcinoma patients. Ann Surg. 2011;253(6):1060–6.
78. Landry CS, Grubbs EG, Morris GS, Turner NS, Holsinger FC, Lee JE, et al. Robot assisted transaxillary surgery (RATS) for the removal of thyroid and parathyroid glands. Surgery. 2011;149(4):549–55.
79. Lee KE, Kim HY, Park WS, Choe JH, Kwon MR, Oh SK, et al. Postauricular and axillary approach endoscopic neck surgery: a new technique. World J Surg. 2009;33(4):767–72.
80. Katz L, Abdel Khalek M, Crawford B, Kandil E. Robotic-assisted transaxillary parathyroidectomy of an atypical adenoma. Minim Invasive Ther Allied Technol: MITAT: Off J Soc Minim Invasive Ther. 2012;21(3):201–5.
81. Tolley N, Arora A, Palazzo F, Garas G, Dhawan R, Cox J, et al. Robotic-assisted parathyroidectomy: a feasibility study. Otolaryngol Head Neck Surg: Off J Am Acad Otolaryngol Head Neck Surg. 2011;144(6):859–66.
82. Profanter C, Schmid T, Prommegger R, Bale R, Sauper T, Bodner J. Robot-assisted mediastinal parathyroidectomy. Surg Endosc. 2004;18(5):868–70.
83. Brunaud L, Ayav A, Bresler L, Schjott B. Da Vinci robot-assisted thoracoscopy for primary hyperparathyroidism: a new application in endocrine surgery. J Chir. 2008;145(2):165–7.
84. Chan AP, Wan IY, Wong RH, Hsin MK, Underwood MJ. Robot-assisted excision of ectopic mediastinal parathyroid adenoma. Asian Cardiovasc Thorac Ann. 2010;18(1):65–7.
85. Harvey A, Bohacek L, Neumann D, Mihaljevic T, Berber E. Robotic thoracoscopic mediastinal parathyroidectomy for persistent hyperparathyroidism:

case report and review of the literature. Surg Laparosc Endosc Percutan Tech. 2011;21(1):e24–7.
86. Ismail M, Maza S, Swierzy M, Tsilimparis N, Rogalla P, Sandrock D, et al. Resection of ectopic mediastinal parathyroid glands with the da Vinci robotic system. Br J Surg. 2010;97(3):337–43.
87. Timmerman GL, Allard B, Lovrien F, Hickey D. Hyperparathyroidism: robotic-assisted thoracoscopic resection of a supernumary anterior mediastinal parathyroid tumor. J Laparoendosc Adv Surg Tech A. 2008;18(1):76–9.
88. Byeon HK, Holsinger FC, Tufano RP, Chung HJ, Kim WS, Koh YW, et al. Robotic total thyroidectomy with modified radical neck dissection via unilateral retroauricular approach. Ann Surg Oncol. 2014;21(12):3872–5.
89. Tae K, Ji YB, Song CM, Jeong JH, Cho SH, Lee SH. Robotic selective neck dissection by a postauricular facelift approach: comparison with conventional neck dissection. Otolaryngol Head Neck Surg: Off J Am Acad Otolaryngol Head Neck Surg. 2014;150(3):394–400.
90. Song CM, Ji YB, Kim KR, Tae K. Robot-assisted excision of branchial cleft cysts using a postauricular facelift approach. Auris Nasus Larynx. 2015;42(5):424–7.
91. Lee HS, Kim D, Lee SY, Byeon HK, Kim WS, Hong HJ, et al. Robot-assisted versus endoscopic submandibular gland resection via retroauricular approach: a prospective nonrandomized study. Br J Oral Maxillofac Surg. 2014;52(2):179–84.
92. Kim CH, Byeon HK, Shin YS, Koh YW, Choi EC. Robot-assisted sistrunk's operation via a retroauricular approach for thyroglossal duct cyst. Head Neck. 2013;36:456–8.
93. Albergotti WG, Byrd JK, Nance M, Choi EC, Koh YW, Kim S, et al. Robot-assisted neck dissection through a modified facelift incision. Ann Otol Rhinol Laryngol. 2016;125(2):123–9.
94. Weinstein GS, Quon H, O'Malley Jr BW, Kim GG, Cohen MA. Selective neck dissection and deintensified postoperative radiation and chemotherapy for oropharyngeal cancer: a subset analysis of the University of Pennsylvania transoral robotic surgery trial. Laryngoscope. 2010;120(9):1749–55.
95. Richmon JD, Quon H, Gourin CG. The effect of transoral robotic surgery on short-term outcomes and cost of care after oropharyngeal cancer surgery. Laryngoscope. 2014;124(1):165–71.
96. Nickel JC. Are we being seduced by a robot? Can Urol Assoc J = J Assoc Urol Can. 2009;3(5):359–63.
97. Moles JJ, Connelly PE, Sarti EE, Baredes S. Establishing a training program for residents in robotic surgery. Laryngoscope. 2009;119(10):1927–31.
98. O'Malley Jr BW, Weinstein GS. Robotic anterior and midline skull base surgery: preclinical investigations. Int J Radiat Oncol Biol Phys. 2007;69(2 Suppl):S125–8.
99. Hanna EY, Holsinger C, DeMonte F, Kupferman M. Robotic endoscopic surgery of the skull base: a novel surgical approach. Arch Otolaryngol Head Neck Surg. 2007;133(12):1209–14.
100. Selber JC, Sarhane KA, Ibrahim AE, Holsinger FC. Transoral robotic reconstructive surgery. Semin Plast Surg. 2014;28(1):35–8.

Robotic Instrumentation, Personnel, and Operating Room Setup

2

Ryan Goepfert and Michael Kupferman

2.1 Introduction

Robotic-assisted surgery (RAS) is becoming an increasingly important tool for certain diseases treated by the otolaryngologist and head and neck surgeon. As RAS expertise evolves and its use increases, many studies are underway to evaluate RAS as a replacement or alternative to established surgical techniques known to be invasive, potentially disfiguring, and sometimes devastating in terms of functional morbidity. Transoral robotic surgery (TORS) is the prime example of evolution within this surgical field for the management of primary or recurrent benign and malignant lesions of the pharynx and larynx, in particular the oropharynx and supraglottic larynx [1–4]. RAS has been rapidly integrated into the field due to a number factors, including (1) less morbid surgical access, (2) improved visualization, and (3) enhanced surgical precision in confined anatomic spaces [5–8]. It has also been championed for its cosmetic appeal, which allows for the avoidance of a conspicuous incision, such as for transaxillary thyroidectomy/parathyroidectomy or retroauricular neck dissection [9–11]. Moreover, RAS has been described for use in free tissue reconstruction as well as in the surgical management of sleep apnea [12–14]. The focus of this chapter is to provide general guidelines for operating room setup and communication, surgical instrumentation and equipment, and the necessary expertise of surgical personnel.

R. Goepfert, MD • M. Kupferman, MD (✉)
Department of Head and Neck Surgery,
MD Anderson Cancer Center, 1515 Holcombe Blvd,
Unit 1445, Houston, TX 77030, USA
e-mail: mekupfer@mdanderson.org

2.2 Robotic Devices

Two robotic devices are currently FDA approved for use in otolaryngology-head and neck surgery, namely, the *da Vinci* Standard, S®, and Si® Surgical Systems made by Intuitive Surgical Inc. (Sunnyvale, CA) and the Flex® Robotic System made by Medrobotics Corporation (Raynham, MA), which received FDA approval in July 2015. Due to the novelty of and lack of experience with the Flex® System by these authors, the main focus of this chapter will be the *da Vinci* Si® robot though many principles of setup, communication, and personnel remain applicable between systems.

The *da Vinci* Surgical System functions as a traditional master-slave arrangement, consisting of three main components: surgeon console, patient-side cart, and vision system.

The surgeon console ("master") allows the primary surgeon an ergonomically adjustable seat with a binocular, three-dimensional view of the surgical field. The surgeon controls the robotic instruments through bimanual thumb and index or middle finger controls while preserving traditional hand-eye surgical positioning. One important difference between the

Z. Gil et al. (eds.), *Atlas of Head and Neck Robotic Surgery*, DOI 10.1007/978-3-319-49578-1_2

Standard/S® and Si® models is the capability to use a secondary console, thus allowing for participation of a co-surgeon or, more importantly, for direct supervision of a surgical trainee by the primary surgeon while preserving three-dimensional observation and immediate control of the instrumentation.

The patient-side cart (i.e., robotic arms, "slave") contains the four robotic arms that house the endoscopic camera and three potential instruments. Primarily given space limitations, TORS generally uses only two of these instruments at one time in addition to the camera. Specifics on cameras and instruments are discussed below.

The vision system contains the image processing equipment as well as a high-definition monitor for use by the surgical technician and bedside surgical assistant, which has touch-screen notation capabilities. Also housed within the vision system are the cautery generator and insufflation equipment, if needed.

The Flex® Robotic System employs a flexible endoscopic camera along with two ports for flexible instruments that are controlled in a manner analogous to transnasal endoscopic surgery. The main difference and purported advantage of this system is its flexibility, thereby providing enhanced exposure to deeper areas of the pharynx and larynx that may be more challenging to access with the current *da Vinci* system or with traditional rigid instrumentation [15, 16]. Though this system is promising, it is fledgling by comparison, and additional studies are needed to elucidate its specific use and applicability within the field.

2.3 Operating Room Arrangement and Robotic Surgery Personnel

RAS represents a fundamentally different coordination of care among members of the surgical team given distinct instrumentation, a unique technological interface between patient and surgeon, and remote communication/interaction between primary surgeon, surgical assistant and technician, and the anesthesiologist. Arrangement of the components of the surgical system and characteristics of personnel will vary according to the operating room orientation and space, though the following describes some ideal characteristics and arrangement (Fig. 2.1). All personnel should be familiar with the surgical equipment, setup, and basic troubleshooting to facilitate safe and efficient RAS. Hospitals typically require operating room staff and surgical providers involved with these procedures to complete robotic training commensurate with their position and responsibilities.

With the surgical bed in a central location, the anesthesiologist and anesthesia cart are at the foot of the patient. Similar to other surgical procedures involving the upper aerodigestive tract, the anesthesiologist plays a pivotal role and communication about anticipated challenges and/or relevant pathology. The anesthetic team should be facile with transnasal intubation and use of laser-safe endotracheal tubes, if needed. The patient-side cart can be positioned on the right or left side of the patient with the leg of the cart forming an approximate 30-degree angle with the surgical bed. Opposite the patient-side cart are the surgical technician, instrument table(s), and vision system. The circulating nurse should have easy access to surgical technician, instruments, and vision system. The surgical assistant sits at the head of the bed, should have an ergonomic view of the vision system monitor, and should be positioned to facilitate communication with the primary surgeon and transfer of instruments with the surgical technician. The primary role of the bedside surgical assistant is to ensure optimum surgical visibility through suctioning of smoke and/or blood, providing additional soft tissue retraction, and occasionally through application of external hyoid pressure. This assistant should be facile with the placement of vascular clips and also must have endoscopic skills as they are working from a monitor rather than by direct visualization. Lastly, the surgeon console should be located near the surgical assistant if operating room orientation/space allows since this provides immediate access to the patient by the primary surgeon and facilitates two-way communication (though a microphone on the surgeon console connects to a speaker on the patient-side cart for surgeon to assistant verbal communication).

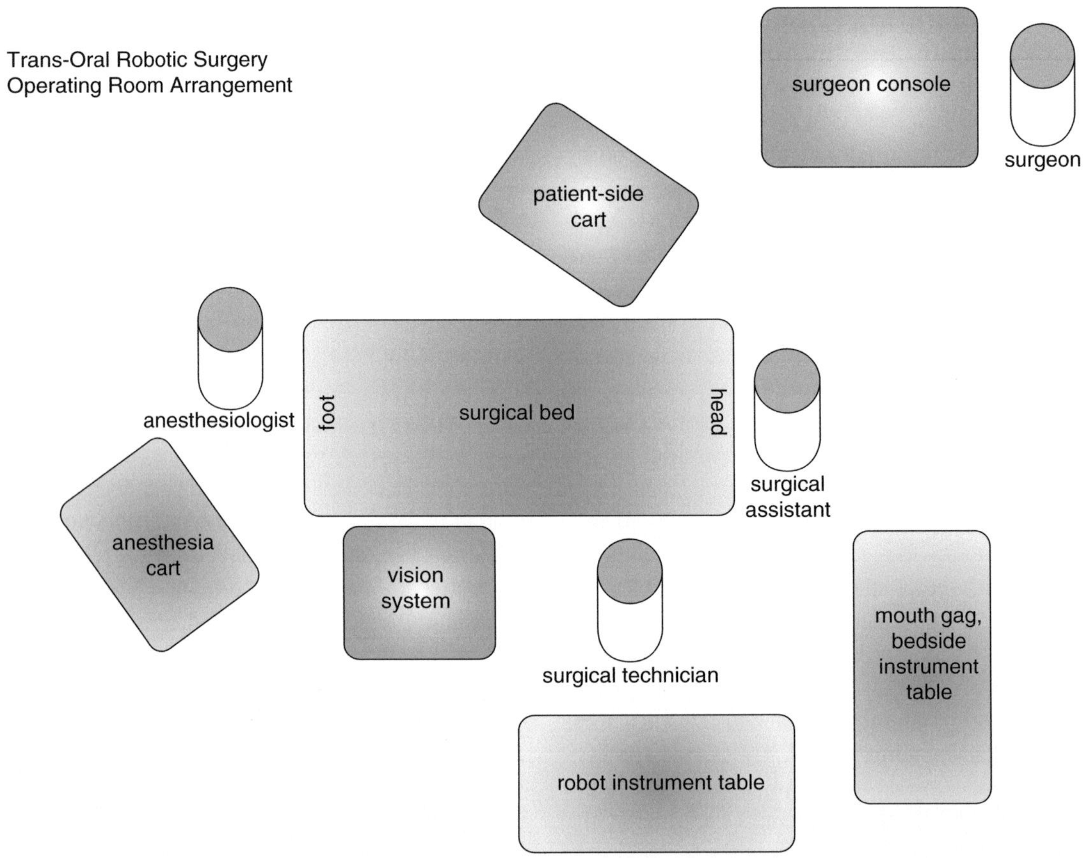

Fig. 2.1 Diagram of TORS operating room arrangement

2.4 Patient Positioning and Exposure

The patient is positioned supine and the bed is rotated 180° from the anesthesia cart. Surgical beds not equipped with the ability to slide in relation to their base should be reversed to allow space for the legs of the patient-side cart as well as those of the surgical assistant. Nasotracheal intubation through the contralateral nostril in relation to the surgical site minimizes interference of the endotracheal tube with the procedure. Induction and intubation may be completed after bed rotation for improved efficiency, though this must be carefully considered in the context of patient safety, in collaboration with the anesthesiologist. Wire-reinforced endotracheal tubes can help guard against compression with oral intubation though must be used cautiously since collapse of these tubes results in luminal narrowing that can only be ameliorated through tube replacement. The endotracheal tube should be secured with tape or via circumdental or nasoseptal suturing. The eyes should be protected with plastic shields or with tape and moist gauze as part of standard laser precautions. Careful wrapping of the patient's head with surgical towels and foam padding can further secure the endotracheal tube and protect the patient's eyes and face. If an open neck procedure is planned, the ventilator circuitry should be routed in such a way as to avoid need for subsequent additional positioning or setup.

For RAS of the upper aerodigestive tract, direct laryngoscopy may be performed after intubation to characterize anatomy of interest as well as specifics of exposure. A synthetic tooth guard should be placed to protect the upper dentition, or a moist gauze in the case of an edentulous patient. To assist with manipulation of the base of tongue during placement of the mouth gag and to maximize exposure, a nonabsorbable suture (commonly 2-0 silk) is placed through-and-through the central anterior tongue and tied with an air knot to prevent strangulation. More than one pass of the suture may be completed to minimize the chance of "cheese-wiring" the anterior tongue with traction. For superior lesions and depending on placement of the endotracheal tube, a red rubber catheter may be placed through the nose and out the mouth for soft palate retraction. With regard to additional patient positioning to maximize exposure, a shoulder roll or flexion of the head of bed may be beneficial.

Several different retractors have been developed for exposure of the oropharynx, supraglottis, hypopharynx, and glottic larynx (see Chap. 6 in this book). The Crowe-Davis and Dingman mouth gags provide suitable access to the upper oropharynx including the tonsils and soft palate. The Crowe-Davis is perhaps the oldest and simplest of these devices, commonly being used in non-robotic tonsillectomy. The Dingman mouth gag is similar though it includes the ability to laterally retract the patient's lips. For lesions in the base of tongue and beyond the FK (Feyh-Kastenbauer), retractor employs longer tongue blades of different lengths and shapes and allows for additional degrees of manipulation of the extension and angulation of the blade (Fig. 2.2). The Flex® retractor is a more recently developed system that combines several advantages of each to achieve great versatility. A surgical headlight is helpful during placement of the retractor. Suspension of the retractor should ideally be accomplished through a support directly attached to the surgical bed as opposed to the patient's chest or a Mayo stand. This, combined with lowering the surgical bed, minimizes the chance of collision or interference between the retraction apparatus and the patient-side cart.

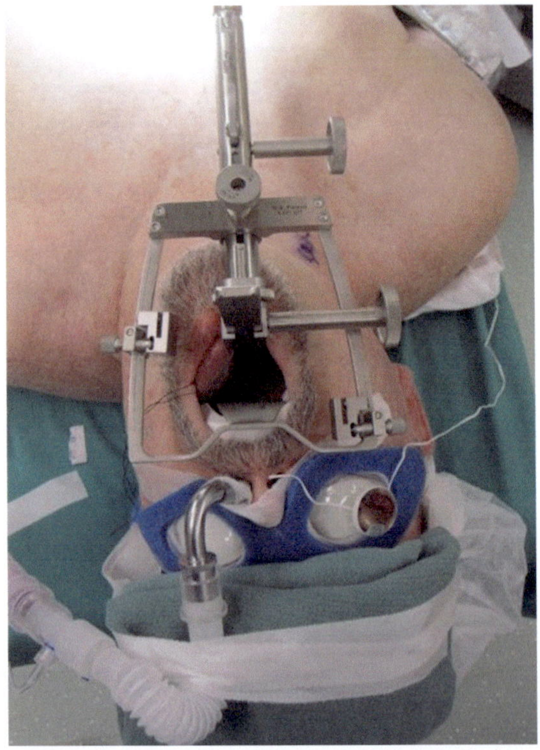

Fig. 2.2 Obtaining initial operative exposure of right oropharynx using the Feyh-Kastenbauer (FK) retractor. Note contralateral nasotracheal intubation and ventilator circuitry, silk tongue suture, tooth guard, eye protection, and head wrap

2.5 Robotic and Surgical Assistant Instrumentation

Once the mouth gag is engaged, the surgical team should take note of the time as portions of the tongue are now ischemic from retraction. Using the *da Vinci* system, the 12 mm endoscopic camera is used for TORS, specifically the 0-degree camera for the soft palate and palatine tonsils and the 30-degree camera for the lower pharynx and larynx. The camera is placed in the central position at a depth that allows adequate visualization but ensures maneuverability of the laterally placed instruments. The *da Vinci* Surgical Systems employ EndoWrist® instruments that feature seven degrees of freedom and 90 degrees of articulation as well as motion scaling and tremor reduction. The two most commonly used instruments in TORS are the 5 mm permanent (monopolar) cautery spatula and the 5 mm Maryland dissector (Fig. 2.2). The authors have found the 8 mm Cadiere forceps to be particularly effective for gentle grasping and retracting, with minimal tissue injury, and utilize this instrument for nearly all TORS (Fig. 2.2). The cautery should be placed ipsilateral to the area of dissection, while the dissector should be contralateral to improve retraction and avoid crossing of the instrument arms (Fig. 2.3). Taken together, the instruments should make a V or triangular formation with respect to the central camera, and the two instrument tips should converge on the area of interest (Fig. 2.4). Additionally, aftermarket flexible CO2 lasers are available and may be particularly useful for resections involving the supraglottis and hypopharynx (Fig. 2.5) [17–19]. Regardless of which instruments are chosen, great care must be taken during their initial placement so as to avoid trauma to the oral cavity, dentition, and pharynx. Proper placement maximizes arm mobility thereby avoiding collisions, making use of the full use of the robot's mechanical and dexterous advantage, and helping to ensure a more efficient, safer surgery. Once in place, robotic arms should be assessed for adequate maneuverability and responsiveness prior to mucosal incision.

After placement of the camera and instrumentation, the surgical assistant should sit at the head of the bed, ideally in a chair with height adjustability. Using a metal or plastic Yankauer suction and Hurd retractor, the assistant helps to optimize exposure. Metal Yankauer suction has the advantage of a narrower diameter than the plastic version though one must make sure the suction tip is securely screwed in place to avoid separation and the resultant foreign body situation. Nevertheless, the curvature of these suctions can be beneficial in providing additional retraction in the base of tongue or vallecula while concurrently evacuating smoke, blood, or secretions. Laparoscopic peanuts and the paddle dissector end of the Hurd

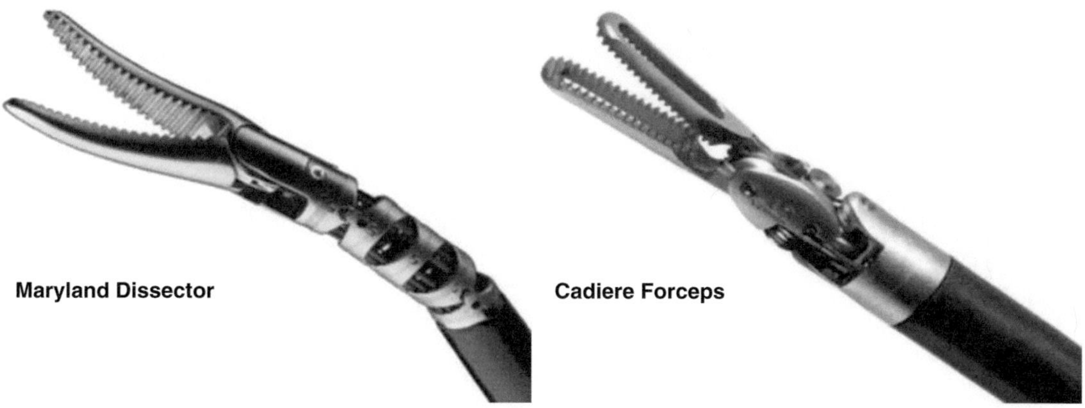

Fig. 2.3 *da Vinci* EndoWrist® instruments, Maryland dissector (*left*) and Cadiere forceps (*right*) (©2016 Intuitive Surgical, Inc. Used with permission)

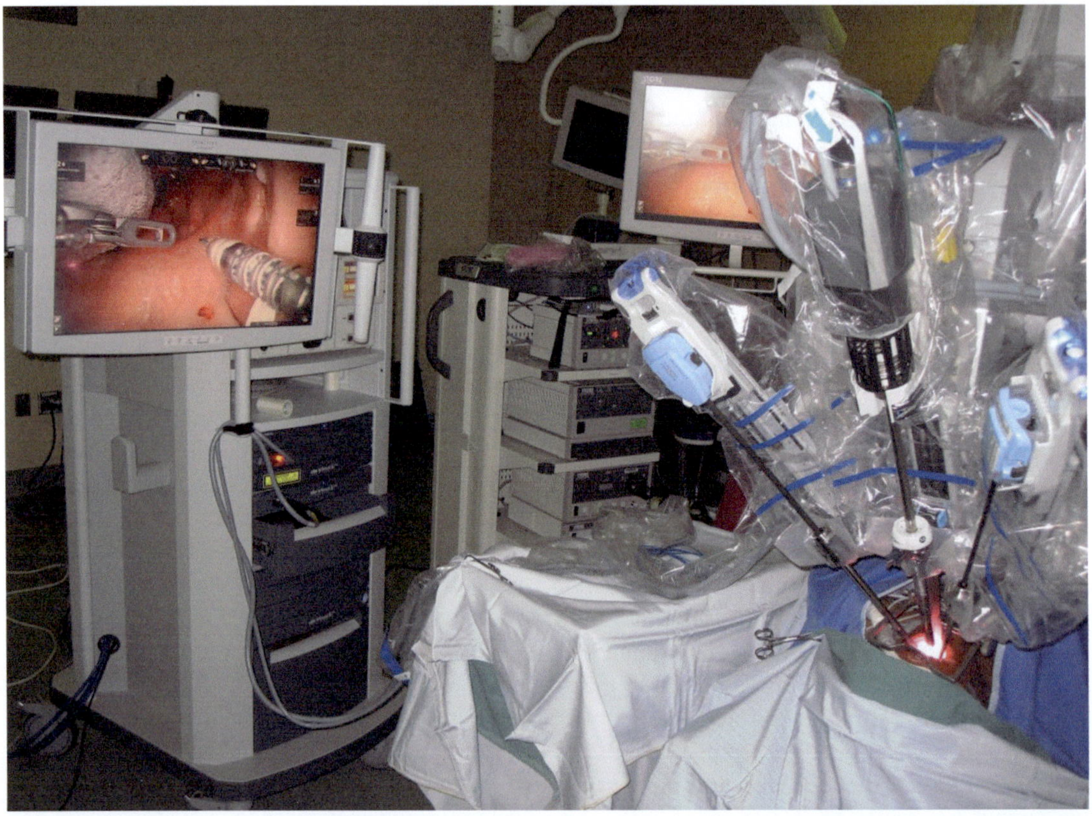

Fig. 2.4 Example of *da Vinci* robotic arm orientation and vision cart placement. Note central camera, ipsilateral monopolar cautery, and contralateral forceps placement

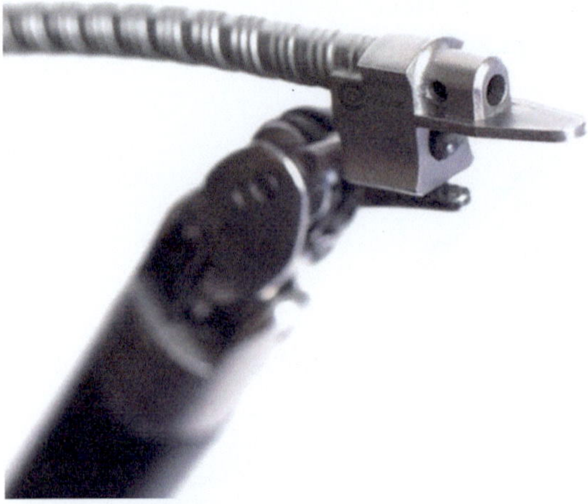

Fig. 2.5 C02 laser using BeamPath® robotic fiber and FlexGuide™ fiber conduit (OmniGuide Surgical, Lexington, MA) (©2016 OmniGuide Surgical, Inc. Used with permission)

retractor may also be of assistance in retraction. Care must be taken using non-insulated, metal instruments as these have the possibility to conduct monopolar current to other areas in the patient's oral cavity such as the lips. Use of a plastic double cheek retractor may be used in combination with specific mouth gags to guard against this possibility.

In addition to retraction, the surgical assistant must also be able to assist with hemostasis. This may require the placement of vascular clips prophylactically on prominent branches of the lingual and ascending pharyngeal arteries, or in response to inadvertent vessel transection. The 22 cm Karl Storz endoscopic clip applier is very useful given its length and low profile though some advocate for use of the automatic laparoscopic clip appliers. Also available in the surgical field should be a suction electrocautery and an extended length bipolar cautery. In the unfortunate scenario where blood obscures the lens of the robotic camera, a deft surgical assistant, equipped with a headlight, Yankauer suction or suction cautery, tonsil sponges, and even topical hemostatic matrix (such as Floseal® or Surgiflo®) can be indispensable for obtaining hemostasis until reestablishment of visualization. Lastly, regardless of whether an open procedure in the neck such as vessel ligation or neck dissection is planned, all open surgical and tracheostomy instrumentation should be immediately available.

The above scenarios provide a detailed description of the instrumentation and setup for TORS. Additional procedures such as transaxillary thyroidectomy or retroauricular neck dissection utilize an incision in a remote location with development of a soft tissue plane under direct visualization followed by placement of a self-retaining retractor to maintain the working space [11, 20–22]. Common retracting systems include the Chung and Kuppersmith retractors. Varying degrees of dissection may be completed under direct visualization prior to placement of robotic arms. A small additional incision (such as the anterior chest, peri-areolar area, or contralateral axilla) may be used to accommodate another surgical arm for retraction. In contrast to development of a broad soft tissue plane for access, CO2 insufflation has also been described for visualization in the central or lateral neck in a manner similar to the non-robotic, endoscopic approach [23]. Lastly, these procedures commonly employ extended harmonic advanced energy devices such as the 23 cm Harmonic ACE®+ shears or synthetic vascular clips such as the Hem-o-lock® system for vessel ligation.

Conclusion

Robotic surgery draws on traditional transoral and open surgical principles but represents a fundamentally different surgical approach that necessitates thoughtful operating room arrangement, algorithms for troubleshooting equipment and instrumentation, and effective communication among all members of the surgical team. These should be modified by each surgical team through their acquisition of robotic experience. With the continued pace of technological evolution in surgery, further refinements to TORS should be anticipated.

References

1. McLeod IK, Melder PC. Da Vinci robot-assisted excision of a vallecular cyst: a case report. Ear Nose Throat J. 2005;84(3):170–2.
2. O'Malley Jr BW, et al. Transoral robotic surgery (TORS) for base of tongue neoplasms. Laryngoscope. 2006;116(8):1465–72.
3. Weinstein GS, et al. Transoral robotic surgery: supraglottic partial laryngectomy. Ann Otol Rhinol Laryngol. 2007;116(1):19–23.
4. Weinstein GS, et al. Transoral robotic surgery: radical tonsillectomy. Arch Otolaryngol Head Neck Surg. 2007;133(12):1220–6.
5. Park YM, et al. Feasibility of transoral robotic hypopharyngectomy for early-stage hypopharyngeal carcinoma. Oral Oncol. 2010;46(8):597–602.
6. Kayhan FT, Kaya KH, Sayin I. Transoral robotic cordectomy for early glottic carcinoma. Ann Otol Rhinol Laryngol. 2012;121(8):497–502.
7. O'Malley Jr BW, Weinstein GS. Robotic skull base surgery: preclinical investigations to human clinical application. Arch Otolaryngol Head Neck Surg. 2007;133(12):1215–9.
8. Hanna EY, et al. Robotic endoscopic surgery of the skull base: a novel surgical approach. Arch Otolaryngol Head Neck Surg. 2007;133(12):1209–14.
9. Kang SW, et al. Robotic thyroid surgery using a gasless, transaxillary approach and the da Vinci S system: the operative outcomes of 338 consecutive patients. Surgery. 2009;146(6):1048–55.

10. Tolley N, et al. Robotic-assisted parathyroidectomy: a feasibility study. Otolaryngol Head Neck Surg. 2011;144(6):859–66.
11. Lee HS, et al. Robot-assisted Supraomohyoid neck dissection via a modified face-lift or retroauricular approach in early-stage cN0 squamous cell carcinoma of the oral cavity: a comparative study with conventional technique. Ann Surg Oncol. 2012;19(12):3871–8.
12. Mukhija VK, et al. Transoral robotic assisted free flap reconstruction. Otolaryngol Head Neck Surg. 2009; 140(1):124–5.
13. Vicini C, et al. Transoral robotic tongue base resection in obstructive sleep apnoea-hypopnoea syndrome: a preliminary report. ORL J Otorhinolaryngol Relat Spec. 2010;72(1):22–7.
14. Lee JM, et al. Transoral robot-assisted lingual tonsillectomy and uvulopalatopharyngoplasty for obstructive sleep apnea. Ann Otol Rhinol Laryngol. 2012;121(10):635–9.
15. Rivera-Serrano CM, et al. A transoral highly flexible robot: novel technology and application. Laryngoscope. 2012;122(5):1067–71.
16. Johnson PJ, et al. Demonstration of transoral surgery in cadaveric specimens with the medrobotics flex system. Laryngoscope. 2013;123(5):1168–72.
17. Solares CA, Strome M. Transoral robot-assisted CO2 laser supraglottic laryngectomy: experimental and clinical data. Laryngoscope. 2007;117(5):817–20.
18. Kucur C, et al. Transoral robot-assisted carbon dioxide laser surgery for hypopharyngeal cancer. Head Neck. 2015;37(5):743–5.
19. Desai SC, et al. Transoral robotic surgery using a carbon dioxide flexible laser for tumors of the upper aerodigestive tract. Laryngoscope. 2008;118(12): 2187–9.
20. Lee J, Chung WY. Robotic surgery for thyroid disease. Eur Thyroid J. 2013;2(2):93–101.
21. Landry CS, et al. Robot assisted transaxillary surgery (RATS) for the removal of thyroid and parathyroid glands. Surgery. 2011;149(4):549–55.
22. Kuppersmith RB, Holsinger FC. Robotic thyroid surgery: an initial experience with North American patients. Laryngoscope. 2011;121(3):521–6.
23. Lee KE, Choi JY, Youn YK. Bilateral axillo-breast approach robotic thyroidectomy. Surg Laparosc Endosc Percutan Tech. 2011;21(4):230–6.

3 Anesthetic Consideration for Robotic Transoral Surgery

Dana Baron Shahaf and Avi Weissman

Anesthesia for otolaryngologic and head and neck surgery has been described extensively in the anesthetic literature [1, 3, 4, 10, 15, 16, 19, 21]. This chapter is designated to the unique anesthetic consideration for transoral robotic techniques. Many cases require a neck dissection to be performed before or after the TORS (see elsewhere in the atlas). Hence, we will include anesthetic considerations for neck dissection as these procedures are sequential.

When planning the anesthesia approach for transoral robotic surgery (TORS), one should be ready to address the pitfalls and possible complications. Complications can be a result of robotic use [24, 28] and can be divided into intraoperative (bleeding and injury to the facial, lingual, and hypoglossal nerves; cranial nerves IX, X, and XI; and sympathetic chain) and postoperative (seroma formation, fascial edema, CSF leak, Horner's syndrome, meningitis, infections, vocal cord paralysis) [19, 25].

Anesthesia considerations for TORS are similar as in all other transoral interventions, such as tonsillectomies [5, 14, 18, 23]. Nevertheless, additional anesthetic considerations should be taken into account, the bulky structure of the robotic equipment and possible surgical complications. The patient is turned 180° away from the anesthesiologists' workstation, and a fairly large device is placed in the vicinity of the patient's head [28]. Once the robot has been positioned and engaged, the anesthesiologist is unable to readily access the patient. Thus, any lines, monitors, and patient protective devices must be placed before and should be secured to ensure no kinking or displacement. It is impossible to allow changes in patients' position or any kind of access to the patient if the robot is not detached first. Therefore, any patient management necessitates movement of the robot, which potentially could result in delay in critical treatment and might cause complications, especially in patients with comorbidity or pediatric cases (see Table 3.1) [34, 36, 39, 43, 44].

The surgery is done under general endotracheal anesthesia with standard ASA monitoring. An arterial line is advised for close tracking of blood pressure due to close proximity to brain structures [35].

Neck dissection precedes the TORS. This allows for a shorter operation time, decreased tissue manipulation, and minimized laryngopharyngeal swelling [26, 27]. General anesthesia induction is possible with propofol (2 mg/kg), fentanyl (2–3 mcg/kg), and a short-acting paralysis with succinylcholine 1 mg/kg to allow quick monitoring of the accessory nerve within 5–7 min. After nasal airway preparation with topical lidocaine lubricant and a vasoconstrictor like phenylephrine, the patient's trachea is intubated nasally. The tube is sutured to the patient's

D.B. Shahaf (✉) • A. Weissman
Department of Anesthesiology, Rambam Health Care Campus, Haifa, Israel
e-mail: dana.barons@gmail.com

Z. Gil et al. (eds.), *Atlas of Head and Neck Robotic Surgery*, DOI 10.1007/978-3-319-49578-1_3

nasal septum and reinforced with tape. Extra care should be taken to avoid any bleeding while intubating. The eyes should be secured with safety goggles and the teeth protected with a molded dental guard. Due to limited access to the patient once surgery begins, the patients' arms should be properly tucked along the sides. Appropriate padding should be applied to protect pressure points and from the relatively heavy equipment within and outside the drapes. It is also necessary to attach extensions to the arterial and intravenous (IV) lines for easier access to the patient. The intravenous fluids and infusion pumps should be placed at the feet, near the anesthesia monitors (Table 3.1) [6, 7, 26, 33, 36].

Patients who undergo major maxillofacial surgery are at risk for considerable intraoperative bleeding. Controlled hypotensive anesthesia might reduce the extent of intraoperative bleeding and can potentially improve the visual quality of the surgical field. Nevertheless, hypotension carries the risk of hypoperfusion to vital organs and is unsafe in certain patients. Thus, the reduction of blood pressure should be adjusted according to the patient's general condition, age, and coexisting diseases. Normotensive or modified hypotensive anesthesia should be used for patients with ischemic heart disease, carotid artery stenosis, disseminated vascular disease, kidney dysfunction, or severe hypertension who are scheduled to undergo a major maxillofacial operation [2].

Table 3.1 Anesthesia checklist

Monitors and lines
1. Standard ASA monitoring (pulse, ECG, ETCO2, NIBP)
2. Arterial line
Safety
1. IV patency
2. Eyes secured
3. Teeth protected
4. Arms tucked
5. Pressure points padded
6. No heavy equipment in contact with patient
7. IV fluids, infusion pumps, and anesthetic machine are placed near patient's feet
8. Appropriate extension to all lines

The second stage of the surgery, the TORS, commences when the neck dissection is completed. At this point, patients' immobility must be absolutely guaranteed by pharmacological paralysis. Rocuronium is usually used (continuous drip 0.3 mg/kg/h) if there are no contraindications. Sudden jaw closure against the robotic arms can occur and lead to devastating consequences [36, 37]. Anesthesia is usually maintained with sevoflurane 1 MAC, continuous remifentanil infusion (0.06–0.1 mcg/kg/min), and continuous rocuronium infusion (0.3 mg/kg/h). We find remifentanil very useful in blunting sympathetic response during insertion of the mouth robotic arms and for surgical resection [14]. In addition, intravenous paracetamol and/or non steroidal anti inflamatory drugs (NSAID's) should be administered if there are no contraindications [32]. A long-acting opioid can be used as well, guided by the patient's risk of postoperative sedation and airway obstruction. All patients are given dexamethasone 10 mg after induction to minimize airway swelling in response to manipulation during surgery [31]. In addition, meticulous fluid management plays an important role in reducing edema [13]. Ondansetron is administrated for postoperative nausea and vomiting treatment [11].

At the end of the surgery, a decision should be made whether the patient is a proper candidate for immediate endotracheal tube extubation [40]. Risk factors for post-extubation upper airway edema may include head and neck surgery, high BMI, excess intraoperative fluid administration, blood products transfused, and female gender [13]. Moreover, patients suffering from sleep apnea are at greater risk for postoperative airway complications; therefore, they should have close cardiopulmonary observation for 24 h period after the operation [20]. The anesthesiologist should ask himself a few crucial questions: What was the duration of the surgery? Does the patient suffer from facial edema? Was there a difficult intubation? Should we expect for late edema that might obstruct the airway? Was surgery at any proximity to the recurrent laryngeal nerve? Is there any expected damage to the vocal cords? If all these questions are negatively answered, then extubation is safe. In addition as in any surgery, some of the other extubation criteria include; the ability to follow commands, an intact gag reflex, train of four >0.9, adequate pain control, and less than 0.1 end-expiratory concentrations of inhaled anesthetics. Objective criteria include the following parameters; tidal volume, peak voluntary negative inspiratory pressure, alveolar-arterial PaO2 gradient, and dead space to tidal volume ratio [9, 17, 22, 41, 42, 45]. For successful extubation, patients should be fully awake. Commonly, we place an appropriately sized nasal airway prior to extubation. The nasal airway is generally well tolerated and left in place as long as needed. We find that this helps to maintain a fairly patent airway, especially when the patient drifts off to sleep. An appropriate dose of sugamadex is used at the end of surgery in order to reverse the rocuronium to a target train of four (TOF) >0.9 [12]. Conversely, there are centers in which patients are kept intubated for 24 h postoperative and then extubated in ICU with the presence of the surgeon after observing the resection site and the entire laryngopharyngeal mucosa [29, 30].

In the postanesthesia care unit (PACU), patients are positioned with the head up in 30–45°. Supplementary O2 is administered via nasal cannula or face mask. Pain control can be optimized with a multimodal approach: paracetamol, NSAID's, and tramadol. If needed, longer-acting opioids, such as morphine, can be used judiciously. Intravenous steroids are continued for 1–3 days to reduce airway edema [8, 38].

In summary, the main challenges for the anesthesiologist are potentially the difficult airway, prolonged surgery in the head and neck vicinity, and limited access to the patient in emergent situations. Accordingly, appropriate preparation, good knowledge of potential problems, and good communication with the surgical team are essentials for success.

References

1. Abdelmalak B, Doyle J. Anesthesia for otolaryngologic surgery. 2012. Retrieved from https://www.google.com/books?hl=en&lr=&id=VLohAwAAQBAJ&oi=fnd&pg=PR1&dq=anesthesia+forotolaryngologic+surgery&ots=QECjM1HN9I&sig=zEw9dCSI14AaaQs02-cPcY9ryoQ.
2. Barak M, Yoav L, el-Naaj IA. Hypotensive anesthesia versus normotensive anesthesia during major maxillofacial surgery: a review of the literature. Sci World J. 2015. Retrieved from http://www.hindawi.com/journals/tswj/aa/480728/.
3. Bredin S. Anaesthesia for otolaryngologic surgery. 2013. Retrieved from http://journals.lww.com/ejanaesthesiology/Abstract/2013/07000/Anaesthesia_for_otolaryngologic_surgery_.18.aspx.
4. Bryson P, Benninger M. Otolaryngology instruments 10 for the anesthesiologist. Anesth Otolaryngol. 2012. Retrieved from https://www.google.com/books?hl=en&lr=&id=oyjgcqd-mwkC&oi=fnd&pg=PA18&dq=anesthesia+forotolaryngologic+surgery&ots=cp4K7XeF1i&sig=gTUya3eZrSt5H7p10SUAsTkU5Qk.
5. Canto G, Pachêco-Pereira C. Adenotonsillectomy complications: a meta-analysis. Pediatrics. 2015. Retrieved from http://pediatrics.aappublications.org/content/early/2015/09/15/peds.2015-1283.abstract.
6. Carrau RL, Prevedello DM, de Lara D, Durmus K, Ozer E. Combined transoral robotic surgery and endoscopic endonasal approach for the resection of extensive malignancies of the skull base. Head Neck. 2013; 35(11):E351–8. http://doi.org/10.1002/hed.23238
7. Chi J, Mandel J, Weinstein G, O'Malley B. Anesthetic considerations for transoral robotic surgery. Anesthesiol Clin. 2010;28:411–22. Retrieved from http://www.sciencedirect.com/science/article/pii/S193222751000056X
8. Clemens M, Hanson S, Rao S, Truong A. Rapid awakening protocol in complex head and neck reconstruction. Head Neck. 2015. Retrieved from http://onlinelibrary.wiley.com/doi/10.1002/hed.23623/full.
9. Clemens MW, Hanson SE, Rao S, Truong A, Liu J, Yu P. Rapid awakening protocol in complex head and neck reconstruction. Head Neck. 2015;37(4):464–70. http://doi.org/10.1002/hed.23623
10. Cordovani D. Anesthesia for otolaryngologic surgery. Can J Anesth. 2014. Retrieved from http://search.proquest.com/openview/c27fdbea832a33ee80ef05fb59a0416b/1?pq-origsite=gscholar.
11. Coyle MJ, Main B, Hughes C, Craven R, Alexander R, Porter G, Thomas S. Enhanced recovery after surgery (ERAS) for head and neck oncology patients. Clin Otolaryngol Off J ENT-UK Off J Neth Soc Otorhinolaryngol Cervicofac Surg. 2016;41(2):118–26. http://doi.org/10.1111/coa.12482
12. Dalton A, Foulds L, Wallace C. Extubation and emergence. Anaesth Intensive Care Med. 2015;16(9):446–51. http://doi.org/10.1016/j.mpaic.2015.06.019
13. DeMuro J, Mongelli M, Hanna A. Perioperative upper airway edema: risk factors and management. Crit Care Shock. 2013. Retrieved from http://criticalcareshock.org/files/Perioperative-upper-airway-edema-Risk-factors-and-management.pdf.

14. Ehsan Z, Mahmoud M, Shott S. The effects of anesthesia and opioids on the upper airway: a systematic review. Laryngoscope. 2016. Retrieved from http://onlinelibrary.wiley.com/doi/10.1002/lary.25399/full.
15. Fowler N, Scharpf J. Clinical head and neck anatomy for the anesthesiologist. Anesth Otolaryngol Surg. 2012. Retrieved from https://www.google.com/books?hl=en&lr=&id=VLohAwAAQBAJ&oi=fnd&pg=PA1&dq=anesthesia+forotolaryngologic+surgery&ots=QECjM1HN9I&sig=7r_hf4VKZW9MtlVTVLeQsYz-7OE.
16. Glassenberg R. Anesthesia for Otolaryngologic Surgery. J Am Soc. 2014. Retrieved from https://anesthesiology.pubs.asahq.org/article.aspx?articleid=1936509.
17. Graboyes E, Bradley J. Prognosis and patterns of failure for the extubation of patients who remain intubated after head and neck surgery. Ann Otol. 2014. Retrieved from http://aor.sagepub.com/content/early/2014/09/03/0003489414549576.abstract.
18. Hackmann T. Anaesthesia for adenotonsillectomy. Can J Anesth/J Can. 1994. Retrieved from http://www.springerlink.com/index/P61273571112LQ42.pdf.
19. Healy D. Anesthesia for head and neck surgery. ASA refresher courses in anesthesiology. 2015. Retrieved from http://journals.lww.com/asa-refresher/Citation/2015/00000/Anesthesia_for_Head_and_Neck_Surgery.9.aspx.
20. Hoff PT, D'Agostino MA, Thaler ER. Transoral robotic surgery in benign diseases including obstructive sleep apnea: safety and feasibility. Laryngoscope. 2015;125(5):1249–53. http://doi.org/10.1002/lary.25026
21. Iseli T, Iseli C, Golden J. Outcomes of intubation in difficult airways due to head and neck pathology. ENT Ear Nose Throat J. 2012. Retrieved from http://search.ebscohost.com/login.aspx?direct=true&profile=ehost&scope=site&authtype=crawler&jrnl=01455613&AN=73279528&h=mvLYPlCF7q%2F669mCZtJK4Y892gIEpfNoJlF0cqbJpdcFjjlMgAArIQSO%2FSj6JO%2BtVa93jW6sFmGJYZ7tPSFYwQ%3D%3D&crl=c.
22. Ito K, Simons Z, Anderson C, Ito H. Postoperative extubation in head and neck surgery patients: risk factors for failure and proposal for extubation criteria. J Surg. 2014. Retrieved from https://www.infona.pl/resource/bwmeta1.element.elsevier-71bf0648-85d6-39e9-b93f-71e412fbb940.
23. Jöhr M. Anaesthesia for tonsillectomy. Curr Opin Anesthesiol. 2006. Retrieved from http://journals.lww.com/co-anesthesiology/Fulltext/2006/06000/Anaesthesia_for_tonsillectomy.7.aspx
24. Kakar PN, Das J, Roy PM, Pant V. Robotic invasion of operation theatre and associated anaesthetic issues: a review. Indian J Anaesth. 2011;55(1):18–25. http://doi.org/10.4103/0019-5049.76577
25. Khandawala P. Parapharyngeal space tumors. Int J Head Neck Surg. 2012. Retrieved from http://www.jaypeejournals.com/eJournals/ShowText.aspx?ID=2021&Type=FREE&TYP=TOP&IN=~/eJournals/images/JPLOGO.gif&IID=170&isPDF=YES.
26. Kim C, Chang J, Choi E. Robotically assisted selective neck dissection in parotid gland cancer. Laryngoscope. 2013. Retrieved from http://onlinelibrary.wiley.com/doi/10.1002/lary.23716/full.
27. Kucur C, Durmus K, Gun R, Old M. Safety and efficacy of concurrent neck dissection and transoral robotic surgery. Head Neck. 2015. Retrieved from http://onlinelibrary.wiley.com/doi/10.1002/hed.24033/abstract.
28. Lee JR. Anesthetic considerations for robotic surgery. Korean J Anesthesiol. 2014;66(1):3–11. http://doi.org/10.4097/kjae.2014.66.1.3
29. Lörincz B, Busch C. Feasibility and safety of transoral robotic surgery (TORS) for early hypopharyngeal cancer: a subset analysis of the Hamburg University TORS-trial. Eur Arch Otorhinolaryngol. 2015. Retrieved from http://link.springer.com/article/10.1007/s00405-014-3259-0.
30. Lörincz B, Möckelmann N, Busch C, Knecht R. Functional outcomes, feasibility, and safety of resection of transoral robotic surgery: single-institution series of 35 consecutive cases of transoral robotic surgery for oropharyngeal squamous cell. Head Neck. 2015. Retrieved from http://onlinelibrary.wiley.com/doi/10.1002/hed.23809/full.
31. Mahant S, Keren R, Localio R. Dexamethasone and risk of bleeding in children undergoing tonsillectomy. Otolaryngol Head Neck Surg. 2014. Retrieved from http://oto.sagepub.com/content/150/5/872.short.
32. Majumdar S, Das A. Intravenous paracetamol infusion: Superior pain management and earlier discharge from hospital in patients undergoing palliative head-neck cancer surgery. Perspect Clin Res. 2014. Retrieved from http://www.ncbi.nlm.nih.gov/pmc/articles/PMC4170535/
33. O'Malley BW, Weinstein GS, Snyder W, Hockstein NG. Transoral robotic surgery (TORS) for base of tongue neoplasms. Laryngoscope. 2006;116(8):1465–72. http://doi.org/10.1097/01.mlg.0000227184.90514.1a
34. O'Malley B, Weinstein G. Transoral robotic surgery (TORS) for base of tongue neoplasms. Laryngoscope. 2006. Retrieved from http://onlinelibrary.wiley.com/doi/10.1097/01.mlg.0000227184.90514.1a/full.
35. O'Malley B, Weinstein G. Robotic skull base surgery: preclinical investigations to human clinical application. Head Neck. 2007. Retrieved from http://archderm.jamanetwork.com/article.aspx?articleid=484916.
36. Oliveira CM, Nguyen HT, Ferraz AR, Watters K, Rosman B, Rahbar R. Robotic surgery in otolaryngology and head and neck surgery: a review. Minim Invasive Surg. 2012. http://doi.org/10.1155/2012/286563.
37. Oliveira C, Nguyen H, Ferraz A. Robotic surgery in otolaryngology and head and neck surgery: a review. Minim Invasive Surg. 2012. Retrieved from http://www.hindawi.com/journals/mis/2012/286563/abs/.
38. Rinaldi V, Pagani D, Torretta S, Pignataro L. Transoral robotic surgery in the management of head and neck tumours. Ecancermedicalscience. 2013;7:359. http://doi.org/10.3332/ecancer.2013.359
39. Schreuder HWR, Verheijen RHM. Robotic surgery. BJOG Int J Obstet Gynaecol. 2009;116(2):198–213. http://doi.org/10.1111/j.1471-0528.2008.02038.x

40. Siddiqui A, Dogar S, Lal S. Airway management and postoperative length of hospital stay in patients undergoing head and neck cancer surgery. J Anaesthesiol Clin Pharmacol. 2016. Retrieved from http://www.ncbi.nlm.nih.gov/pmc/articles/PMC4784213/.
41. Twohig E, Leader R, Shaw R, Charters P. Staged extubation to manage the airway after operations on the head and neck. Br J Oral Maxillofac Surg. 2016. Retrieved from http://www.sciencedirect.com/science/article/pii/S0266435616000899.
42. Twohig E, Shaw R. The role of staged extubation in head and neck surgery. Br J Oral Maxillofac Surg. 2015. Retrieved from http://www.bjoms.com/article/S0266-4356(15)00388-5/abstract.
43. Weinstein G, O'Malley B, Hockstein N. Transoral robotic surgery: supraglottic laryngectomy in a canine model. Laryngoscope. 2005. Retrieved from http://onlinelibrary.wiley.com/doi/10.1097/01.MLG.0000170848.76045.47/full.
44. Weinstein GS, O'Malley BW, Cohen MA, Quon H. Transoral robotic surgery for advanced oropharyngeal carcinoma. Arch Otolaryngol Head Neck Surg. 2010;136(11):1079–85. http://doi.org/10.1001/archoto.2010.191
45. Wong P, Iqbal R, Light K. Head and neck surgery in a tertiary centre: predictors of difficult airway and anaesthetic management. Proc Singapore Healthcare. 2016. Retrieved from http://psh.sagepub.com/content/25/1/19.short.

4 Robotic Surgery Training

Kunal Jain, Gregory S. Weinstein, Bert W. O'Malley Jr., and Jason G. Newman

In December of 2009, the US Food and Drug Administration approved the use of the da Vinci Surgical System for transoral robotic surgery (TORS). Prior to that, most surgeons in training or already in practice had not been exposed to the surgical robot or to the techniques for TORS. Training programs have since been created to bridge gaps in knowledge and technical skills. Over time, these programs have grown and progressed to incorporate evolving technology and surgical techniques that have accompanied the widespread adoption of TORS.

Prior to the advent of TORS, other surgical specialties including urology, general surgery, and gynecology had been using the robot for a variety of surgical procedures. These specialties have developed surgical training programs, several of which have laid the early foundations for the robotic training labs for TORS. Over the past several years, various otolaryngology departments have developed structured curricula for training head and neck surgery residents and fellows in robotic surgery [1–3].

As with other surgical training programs, a stepwise approach to skill acquisition should be taken. A well-designed robotics training program should therefore have three components: access to didactics materials, access to an inanimate or simulated robotics training environment, and a sufficient number of TORS operative cases for surgical console training [3]. Ideally, this TORS training should occur during residency or fellowship with the supervision of a TORS-experienced surgeon in a structured environment with stepwise progression. An alternate program is also discussed for head and neck surgeons in practice below (see Fig. 4.1).

K. Jain, MD (✉)
Otorhinolaryngology-Head & Neck Surgery, McGovern Medical School, University of Texas Health Science Center, Houston, USA
e-mail: Kunal.S.Jain@uth.tmc.edu

G.S. Weinstein • B.W. O'Malley Jr. • J.G. Newman, MD
Otorhinolaryngology, Head and Neck Surgery, University of Pennsylvania, Philadelphia, PA, USA

Z. Gil et al. (eds.), *Atlas of Head and Neck Robotic Surgery*, DOI 10.1007/978-3-319-49578-1_4

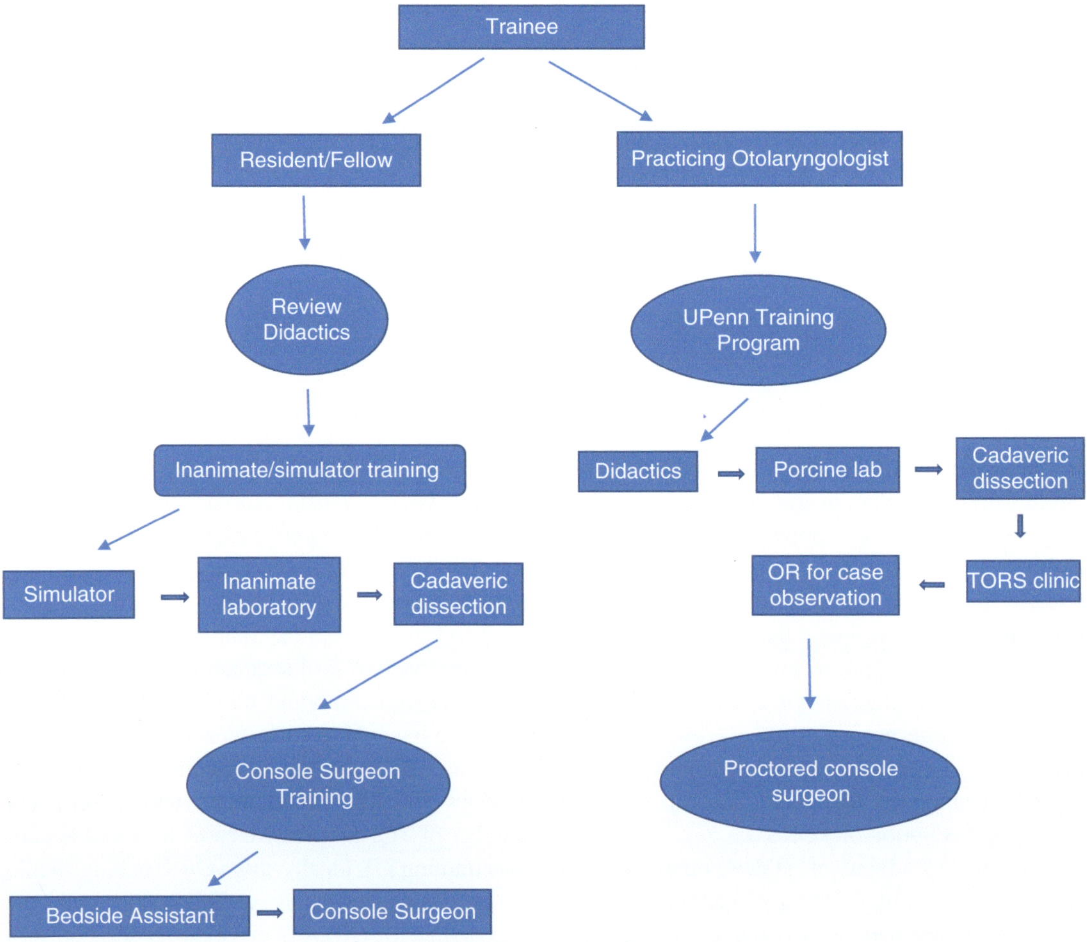

Fig. 4.1 Diagram of the pathway to robotic training

4.1 Didactics

Most otolaryngologists are not familiar with the robotic system and therefore need an introduction to the technology. There is a learning curve involved with understanding and utilizing the technology and equipment. It is important for trainees to familiarize themselves with the technology, its advantages, and limitations. Further, trainees also have to familiarize themselves with the indications for using the robot in head and neck cases. Although beyond the scope of this chapter, a thorough understanding of the indications for TORS is critical to the success of the surgical procedures. As with other surgical procedures, appropriate mentorship is of great benefit in creating a working knowledge of surgical indications.

Didactics for TORS include textbook chapters from transoral surgery books such as this one, procedure and device educational videos available online (davincisurgerycommunity.com), device manuals, and procedure guides [4, 5]. Lastly, trainees must also review head and neck surgical anatomy from a transoral approach. This requires learning "inside-out" anatomy from the transoral approach, as most head and neck surgeons are used to an "outside-in" approach from the neck. This anatomic understanding is critical for performing safe and effective TORS and for recognizing contraindications to the surgery.

4.2 Inanimate or Simulated Robotics Training Environment

The da Vinci Skills Simulator provides familiarity with the da Vinci console and the three-dimensional environment. The simulator includes a series of exercises that consist of tasks that the surgeon completes using the console controls, geared toward improving general robotic surgery skills. Studies in other specialties have shown that the da Vinci Skills Simulator scores correlate with surgeon experience and that simulator training improves robotic surgery skills [6–8]. Simulator tasks help to develop skills such as camera movement, clutching, and wrist motion skills. While the simulations are not designed for transoral robotic surgery specifically, they allow for mastering basic skills behind the console that are applicable to TORS. Additionally, simulators are widely available, easy to use for trainees, and affordable for teaching institutions.

Trainees can practice basic robotic skills in an inanimate laboratory with simple tasks using the surgical robot. The laboratory allows trainees to use the same robot used in surgery, familiarizing them with the operative setup and instrumentation. Several institutions have shown the beneficial use of the inanimate laboratory for transoral surgical training for residents [2].

The final step of inanimate training is cadaveric dissection performed with the surgical robot. This allows for teaching of the inside-out anatomy, progression of surgical steps for transoral procedures, and hands-on training of the complex and advanced maneuvers performed during TORS.

4.3 Console Surgeon Training

When learning TORS for live patients, the first step involves working as the bedside assistant. TORS is based on a four-handed technique and is dependent on a good assistant. Being an active assistant allows the trainee to learn the anesthesia techniques, equipment positioning, room setup, and patient positioning necessary for efficient implementation of TORS. This also helps the trainee learn mouth retractor placement, arm and camera positioning, and control of bleeding with clip application. Much like the rest of surgical training, an astute bedside assistant is able to anticipate the console surgeon's next step in the surgical procedure and the retraction of tissues needed. This enhances the trainee's understanding of the procedure.

The second step is as the console surgeon with the TORS mentor being either on the other teaching console, at the bedside, or actively observing using the interactive screen. This allows the mentor to step in if the trainee is struggling through a step or if there are any critical structures at risk of injury. Training behind the console adheres to a stepwise progression of experience with proficiency in the first steps being required before advancing to the next steps. Various TORS procedures have been organized into a structured curriculum from the University of Pennsylvania, which can be considered a prototype for a console surgeon training program [3].

4.4 Training for Head and Neck Surgeons in Practice

An alternate training program is used for practicing otolaryngologists. Since 2009, the only place to obtain complete TORS training for practicing otolaryngologists has been at the University of Pennsylvania.

The training program includes porcine lab training, cadaver dissection, time in clinic to learn TORS indications, and live observation of one to three cases in the operating room. Furthermore, there are didactics given by the faculty at the University of Pennsylvania during the weeklong training program and also available through the da Vinci website.

Following this training, the trainee may require assistance by experienced proctoring surgeons during their first da Vinci procedures. The number of proctored procedures is dependent on a hospital's training and credentialing requirements, and intuitive surgical has established proctoring networks for otolaryngology.

It is recommended that for the first few cases, the surgeon plan on doing relatively simple procedures such as lingual tonsillectomy or T1 tumors prior to more complicated cases. The minimum number of cases needed for competency is not established presently and is dependent on the hospital's requirements.

4.5 Learning Curve in Robotic Surgery

What should the trainee expect as he/she gains experience in TORS? One study found no differences in room setup time, operative time, and total time in the room, comparing the initial 20 TORS cases to the following 20 cases [9]. The longest study to date was a 4-year experience from the University of Alabama. The authors found that the mean operative time decreased by 47%, and hospital stay decreased from 3 to 1.4 days from the first year to the last year. There was also noted to be a decrease in postoperative bleeding and airway edema as experience was gained. However, they did not find any difference with more experience between frequency of negative margins, number of tracheostomies or feeding tubes, and number of aborted cases [10].

Minimum case numbers for establishing resident/fellow competency have not been established, and different individuals may achieve competency at different rates. The learning curve is steepest behind the console with hands-on training much like the rest of surgical training. This is aided by the dual-console system, which allows for resident and fellow training while ensuring patient safety. Currently, at the author's institution, the minimum goal for training is participation in 20 cases as a console surgeon.

Conclusion

Training in robotic surgery is a worthwhile undertaking for the experienced head and neck surgeon as well as the otolaryngologist in training. As the indications for the use of the robot expand due to advancing technology and surgical knowledge and improved outcomes, the robot will become a more common tool for the ot olaryngologist in training as well as in practice.

References

1. Moles JJ, Connelly PE, Sarti EE, Baredes S. Establishing a training program for residents in robotic surgery. Laryngoscope. 2009;119:1927–31.
2. Curry M, Malpani A, Li R, Tantillo T, Jog A, Blanco R, et al. Objective assessment in residency-based training for transoral robotic surgery. Laryngoscope. 2012;122:2184–92.
3. Sperry SM, Omalley BW, Weinstein GS. The University of Pennsylvania curriculum for training otorhinolaryngology residents in transoral robotic surgery. ORL. 2014;76:342–52.

4. www.davincisurgerycommunity.com. Accessed on 28 Jan 2016.
5. Weinstein GS, O'Malley BW. Transoral robotic surgery (TORS). San Diego: Plural Pub; 2012.
6. Hung AJ, Zehnder P, Patil MB, et al. Face, content and construct validity of a novel robotic surgery simulator. J Urol. 2011;186(3):1019–24.
7. Hung AJ, Patil MB, Zehnder P, et al. Concurrent and predictive validation of a novel robotic surgery simulator: a prospective, randomized study. J Urol. 2012;187(2):630–7.
8. Sturm LP, Windsor JA, Cosman PH, Cregan P, Hewett PJ, Maddern GJ. A systematic review of skills transfer after surgical simulation training. Ann Surg. 2008;248(2):166–79.
9. Richmon JD, Agrawal N, Pattani KM. Implementation of a TORS program in an academic medical center. Laryngoscope. 2011;121(11):2344–8.
10. White HN, Frederick J, Zimmerman T, Carroll WR, Magnuson JS. Learning curve for transoral robotic surgery: a 4-year analysis. JAMA Otolaryngol Head Neck Surg. 2013;139(6):564–7.

5 Anatomical Considerations in Transoral Robotic Approach

Abie H. Mendelsohn

5.1 Introduction

The term "inside-out anatomy" is emphasized when transoral robotic surgery (TORS) is taught within many of the head and neck robotic surgery texts. This term "inside-out" appropriately describes the new perspective to which the head and neck surgeon must adapt in order to proceed safely and efficiently. New TORS surgeons must flip their traditional anatomic relationships that were taught during open cervical dissection as these structures are now encountered from within the pharynx extending outward toward the cervical soft tissues and the skin. Each of the specific applications of TORS in the chapters to follow will discuss the stepwise progression approaching and preserving the critical neurovascular structures within each region. Specifically to be discussed include TORS lateral oropharyngectomy in Chap. 5, TORS glossectomy in Chap. 6, TORS partial laryngectomy in Chap. 7, and TORS parapharyngeal space dissection in Chap. 12. Instead of duplicating reviews of the inside-out anatomic relationships, this chapter will focus on anatomical considerations required for successful performance of TORS beyond the specifics of each anatomic subsite.

5.2 Transoral Exposure

During the early years of TORS when clinical experience was limited, most surgeons would recommend assessing each patient's candidacy under general anesthesia. However as clinical experience grows, many centers are foregoing this extra trip to the operating room and instead making the determination of TORS candidacy clinically. Initial investigations have looked into the possibility of predicting adequate transoral exposure based on combined anthropometric measures. A cadaveric study evaluated the utility of combining multiple anthropometric distances (*significant measurements included mandibular body height, hyoid-mental distance, and neck circumference*), but this study's findings need additional evaluation to understand its true clinical application [2]. Another study aiming to predict exposure utilized cephalometrics from preoperative radiology, which demonstrates improved promise of clinical applications [3]. Yet currently, no combined measurement has shown reliable prediction for achievement of adequate transoral exposure, and so, in this author's opinion, the ability to predict adequate oral exposure comes from surgical volume experience in combination with a detailed preoperative examination.

A.H. Mendelsohn, MD, FACS
Department of Head and Neck Surgery, David Geffen School of Medicine at UCLA,
Los Angeles, CA, USA
e-mail: AMendelsohn@mednet.ucla.edu

Z. Gil et al. (eds.), *Atlas of Head and Neck Robotic Surgery*, DOI 10.1007/978-3-319-49578-1_5

5.3 Trismus

The preoperative evaluation of all TORS surgical candidates includes an oral examination, during which patients open their mouths. The excursion of the mandible is thereby always assessed, but perhaps not always appreciated. In particular, subtle limitations of jaw opening or subtle signs of pain with jaw opening can easily be overlooked. The exact definition of trismus varies depending on the referenced text, but it is generally described as any degree of jaw opening restriction. Precise measurements have been suggested by a selected oral surgery textbooks [1], though this distinction is purely academic in its application to TORS patients as the presence of trismus at any level should alert the TORS surgeon.

Trismus, or the restriction of jaw opening resulting in a limited inter-incisor distance, can be due to the dysfunction of either the temporomandibular joint (TMJ) or dysfunction of the muscles controlling TMJ articulation. In either situation, trismus of any severity should be considered a contraindication for TORS. In the first situation, that of TMJ dysfunction, the resultant trismus is unlikely to be relieved under general anesthesia as a relaxation of the muscles of mastication will not affect joint ankylosis. A limited inter-incisor opening will cause an inability to successfully navigate the recessed areas of the pharynx and larynx and should be considered a contraindication based on technical grounds applicable to pharyngeal as well as laryngeal TORS procedures.

In the second cause of trismus, that of mastication muscle dysfunction or irritation also represents a contraindication for TORS. Although, irritation of the muscles of mastication can frequently be relaxed under general anesthesia, thereby providing access to the larynx and pharynx, it is the underlying pathophysiology of the trismus that should be seen as a warning sign to the TORS surgeon. As it relates to TORS, the muscle that produces trismus will be the medial pterygoid. The medial pterygoid muscle arises from the medial surface of the lateral pterygoid plate as well as from the maxillary tuberosity. It inserts onto the lingual surface of the mandible, from the angle of the mandible extending upward along the inner ramus to the level of the mandibular foramen. It acts in tandem with the masseter creating elevation, or closure, of the mandible. The irritation of this muscle is of great concern for the TORS surgeon as its involvement (even from neighboring irritation) represents unresectable tumor extent, as displayed in Fig. 5.1. Therefore, this second cause of trismus should be viewed as an oncologic contraindication as opposed to a technical contraindication of the first cause of trismus.

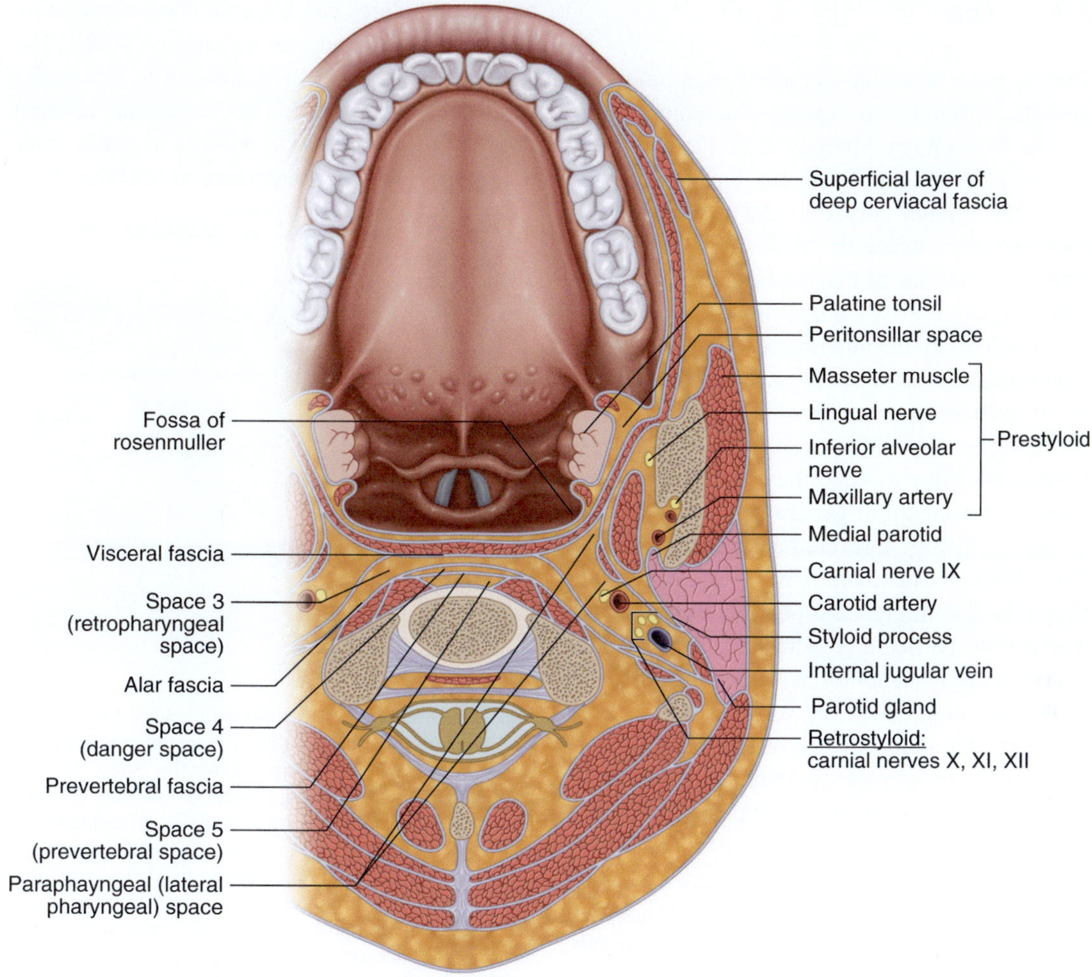

Fig. 5.1 Medial pterygoid muscle. The medial pterygoid (*yellow arrow*) is found deep to the middle pharyngeal constrictor muscle group. The middle constrictors along with the styloglossus muscle serve as the deep oncologic margin of lateral pharyngeal and glossopharyngeal tumors. If the middle constrictors are violated by tumor growth, irritation of the medial pterygoid muscle will produce trismus. This etiology of trismus should be seen as a contraindication for TORS from an oncologic standpoint

5.4 Tori

Tori, or torus in single use, are benign bony outgrowths within the oral cavity which are thought to arise from physical irritation. Tori tend to grow in distinct positions, along the hard palate and along the lingual cortex of the mandible. Tori palatinus grow typically as a single outgrowth along the midline of the hard palate and are of little consequence to the TORS surgeon. Tori mandibulares on the other hand are of substantial importance. As seen in Fig. 5.2, tori mandibulares grow from the medial, or lingual, surface of the anterior mandible in an uneven pattern. Unless extensive in size, they are rarely symptomatic and therefore generally are not elicited during the history portion of a patient evaluation. The physical examination can very often skip over this seemingly unimportant aspect of the oral cavity, particularly when an obvious exophytic pharyngeal tumor is distracting the surgeon's attention. However, a gloved finger used to palpate the inner surface of the mandible can save the TORS surgeon significant stress by identifying this significant anatomic consideration.

Tori mandibulares fill the floor of mouth space with bony outgrowths. They will therefore block the oral tongue from being translocated to within the soft movable tissue of the floor of the mouth. Aside from trismus, it is this author's opinion that tori mandibulares can have the most devastating effect on access and performance of TORS. The presence of tori is also significant as this entity can be readily excised. This author has referred patients for tori resection within the weeks leading up to TORS, or concurrent with TORS, with subsequent excellent exposure.

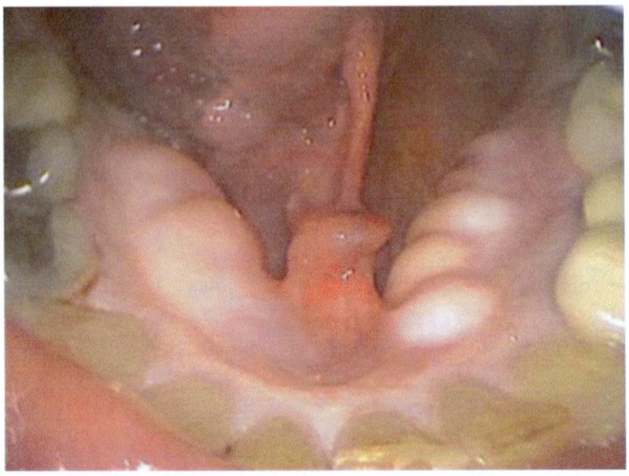

Fig. 5.2 Tori mandibulares. Intraoral photograph demonstrates the irregular bony outgrowths of tori mandibulares. These benign calcified lesions generally cause a severe limitation of anterior tongue retraction down into the floor of mouth. During the preoperative evaluation, finger palpation of the inner cortex of the mandible will readily identify the presence of these obstructive lesions which is significant as the straightforward removal of these lesions pre-TORS can provide exposure to otherwise inaccessible anatomy (protuberant submandibular ducts are seen in the midline abutting the frenulum of the tongue)

5.5 Teeth

Similar to direct laryngoscopy, edentulous patients will provide improved TORS exposure as compared to exposure of dentate patients. With most retraction systems placing the inferior fulcrum point on the upper central incisors, it is these teeth that are the most concerning for excessive length restricting exposure. However in this author's view, it is only in the most extreme cases of elongated dentition, or of dental prosthesis such as veneers, that produce a substantial effect on TORS exposure without additional confounding anatomical considerations. More commonly, large teeth will play a role in preventing successful TORS exposure when other factors are also suboptimal. The pressure placed on the upper central incisors should be discussed with patients, particularly with those patients who have placed previous investment in dental care.

Yet distinct from direct laryngoscopy, other teeth besides the upper central incisors have considerations during TORS. The TORS surgeon should take note of the presence and shape (*sharp* vs. *dull*) of the lower incisors. In all but the most accessible palatine tonsil tumor, some degree of tongue protrusion is required. By retracting the tongue out of the mouth to achieve the protrusion, the tongue will be compressed against the lower incisors which may result in ventral tongue laceration or contusion. The presence and position of the posteriormost molars will also impact the TORS approach, both maxillary and mandibular. As the robotic instruments approach through the lateral aspect of the oral cavity, patients with third molars (*wisdom teeth*) in place may offer restricted instrument movement or dental injury by the serrated neck of the instruments burring down the enamel of these teeth.

5.6 Carotid Artery

Catastrophic bleeding is the most serious intra- and postoperative complication of TORS. Special attention must be placed to understand the relationship between the laryngopharynx and the internal carotid arteries. Ideally, a distance of 2.5 cm should be between the pharyngeal mucosa and the carotid arterial wall [6]. While a medialized carotid is the general term of abnormally close relationship between the pharynx and the artery, the specific patterns of carotid aberrations include tortuosity, kinking, and coiling [5]. The overall incidence of medialized carotid arteries has been estimated between 10 % and 40%, making this anatomic anomaly quite common [4]. In the preoperative assessment, surgeons should pay close attentions to the posterior pharyngeal wall during flexible indirect laryngoscopy. At times, medialized carotid arteries may cause indentation of the posterior pharyngeal wall, as seen in Fig. 5.3, which can relay a strong pulsating motion to the pharynx. Radiologic evaluation will confirm this clinical finding and define the course of the common carotids as well as the internal and external branches. The TORS surgeon must be aware of this aberrant finding. Patients with medialized carotid arteries are unlikely to be acceptable candidates for TORS.

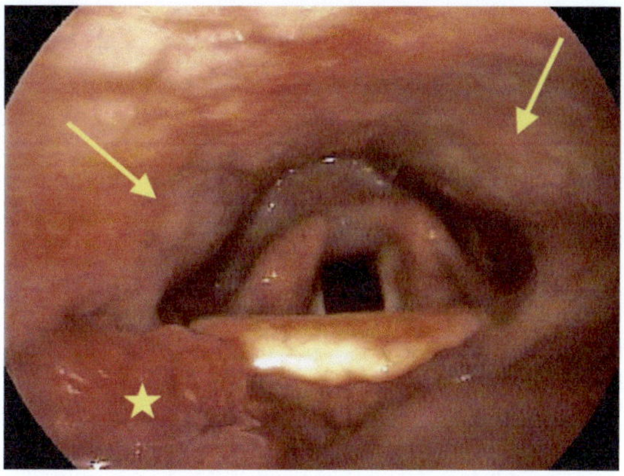

Fig. 5.3 Medialized carotid arteries. Indirect laryngoscopy from a patient undergoing evaluation for TORS resection of a right base of tongue squamous cell carcinoma (*star*). The patient was found to have bilateral pulsating fullness at the posterior pharyngeal wall (*arrows*). Imaging confirmed the presence of medialized internal carotid arteries within 3 mm of the pharynx. This close association of the carotid artery is considered a contraindication for TORS

5.7 Feeding Vessels

Similar to assessing for carotid artery anatomic variants, tumors under consideration for TORS resection should also be evaluated for feeding vessels. Prevention of intraoperative and postoperative hemorrhage is largely dependent on the correct identification of vascular structures prior to transection. Therefore, in addition to understanding the anatomic relationships of the named arterial branches of the laryngopharynx, the preoperative imaging must be carefully inspected for neovascularization. Tumors, especially those with endophytic growth patterns, can develop feeding vessels as large or even larger than named arterial branches, with an example in Fig. 5.4. These feeding vessels can many times be controlled with open proximal cervical arterial branch ligation, though their presence and significance should not be overlooked.

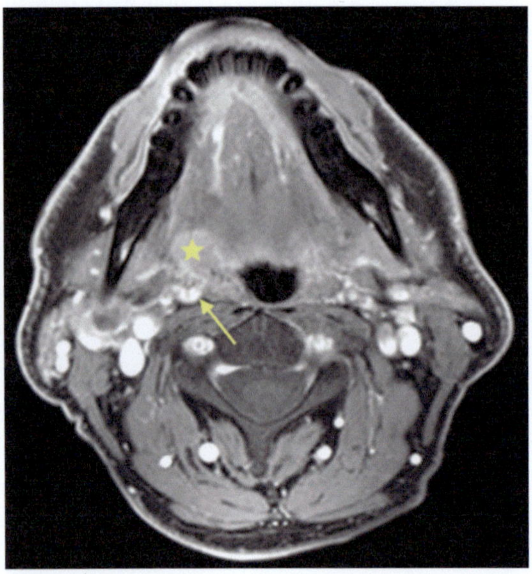

Fig. 5.4 Feeding vessels. Preoperative imaging can identify tumor-feeding vessels as large as the named cervical arterial branches. Displayed is an MRI, T1 fat-saturated post-contrast, scan of a patient with glossopharyngeal fold squamous cell carcinoma (*star*) undergoing evaluation for TORS resection. This image demonstrates a large caliber vessel (*arrow*) arising from the facial artery

5.8 Cervical Spine

The issue of patients with limited cervical spine extension is one that does not play a large role in the preoperative anatomical assessment of the TORS patient. Generally, a neutral neck position is all that is required for pharyngeal exposure. The exception to this rule is found with patients with limited chin to chest (*mentum to sternum*) distance. In such a patient, a shoulder role can be useful to provide distance between the neck of the robotic oral retractors and the anterior chest wall. Therefore, in asymptomatic patients having no history of cervical spinal surgery or pain, no additional evaluation or radiology is necessary prior to TORS.

5.9 Pediatric Patients

The application of TORS in the pediatric patient has shown increased utilization, mainly in the repair of laryngeal cleft [7, 8]. The anatomic considerations for the pediatric patient follow the same process as the adult patient, but each with increased significance as the smaller anatomic dimensions of the pediatric patient limits the available room to maneuver. One important distinction though is the more superior position of the pediatric larynx as compared with the adult larynx. This relationship brings the pediatric larynx closer to the oral cavity and therefore more accessible for robotic instrumentation. The more superior position of the pediatric larynx also allows for robotic access with standard tonsil oral retractors (i.e., Crowe-Davis) as opposed to an operative pharyngoscope (i.e., FK-WO, LARS) required for robotic access to the adult larynx.

Conclusion

We have discussed several anatomical considerations that must be assessed before successful TORS can take place. Some issues may prevent exposure and visualization such as tori, teeth, and trismus due to TMJ ankylosis. Other issues may risk patient safety and oncologic resection such as medialized carotid arteries, feeding vessels, and trismus due to medial pterygoid muscle dysfunction. In all, the TORS surgeon must have an appreciation of these factors before considering proceeding with the complexities of transoral robotic surgery.

References

1. Hupp JR, Ellis E, Tucker MR. Contemporary oral and maxillofacial surgery. 5th ed. St. Louis: Mosby Elsevier; 2008.
2. Arora A, Kotecha J, Acharya A, et al. Determination of biometric measures to evaluate patient suitability for transoral robotic surgery. Head Neck. 2015;37(9):1254–60.
3. Luginbuhl A, Baker A, Curry J, Drejet S, Miller M, Cognetti D. Preoperative cephalometric analysis to predict transoral robotic surgery exposure. J Robot Surg. 2014;8(4):313–7.
4. Pfeiffer J, Ridder GJ. A clinical classification system for aberrant internal carotid arteries. Laryngoscope. 2008;118(11):1931–6.
5. Weibel J, Fields WS. Tortuosity, coiling, and kinking of the internal carotid artery. I. Etiology and radiographic anatomy. Neurology. 1965;15:7–18.
6. Deutsch MD, Kriss VM, Willging JP. Distance between the tonsillar fossa and internal carotid artery in children. Arch Otolaryngol Head Neck Surg. 1995;121(12):1410–2.
7. Ferrell JK, Roy S, Karni RJ, Yuksel S. Applications for transoral robotic surgery in the pediatric airway. Laryngoscope. 2014;124(11):2630–5.
8. Leonardis RL, Duvvuri U, Mehta D. Transoral robotic-assisted laryngeal cleft repair in the pediatric patient. Laryngoscope. 2014;124(9):2167–9.

Retractors for Transoral Robotic Surgery

6

Emily Funk, Aaron Baker, David Goldenberg, and Neerav Goyal

6.1 Introduction

With the introduction of endoscopic and transoral robotic approaches (TORS) to lesions of the head and neck, larger surgical approaches such as a lip-split mandibulotomy, lateral pharyngotomy, or transhyoid approach can be avoided for oropharyngeal and laryngeal lesions. TORS has made significant advances over the past 10+ years and is a viable option in the surgical treatment of benign and malignant lesions of these sites. However, to be a viable alternative to open surgery, one of the major requirements of TORS is obtaining adequate exposure of the surgical site, allowing for visualization of and access to the lesion to be excised. Without this, it is not possible to place instruments through the oral cavity in a manner that safely maximizes the use of the increased dexterity. While the majority of TORS surgeons use the da Vinci robot (Intuitive Surgical, Sunnyvale, CA), more recent advances in robotic technology have brought devices to the market that are designed with the head and neck surgeon in consideration, such as the Medrobotics Flex robot (Medrobotics, Raynham, MA).

To this end, multiple retractor systems have been used and specifically designed for minimally invasive work in the oropharynx, hypopharynx, and larynx. Factors in choosing a retractor system include freedom of motion, accommodation of endotracheal tube, and safe oral retraction methods to avoid ischemic or traumatic injury. The ultimate goal of novel retraction methods is to produce a mechanism by which the operator has an adequate field of view of the surgical site, while also accommodating an endoscopic camera and robotic effector arms. This chapter will review the currently available retractors that are utilized in TORS.

6.2 Crowe-Davis and McIvor Retractors

The Crowe-Davis and McIvor retractors are the standard retractors used in tonsillectomy, the most common oropharyngeal procedure performed by otolaryngologists (Fig. 6.1). Retractor systems using blades to move the tongue out of the surgical field of view had been in place since the late 1800s. Samuel Crowe, while in training under Harvey Cushing at the Johns Hopkins Hospital, in conjunction with Dr. Cushing's anesthesiologist, Dr. Davis, developed a retractor with a self-ratcheting tongue blade that allowed for stable retraction of the tongue, with a notch for an endotracheal tube allowing for ventilation. In addition, this retractor design includes an open

E. Funk, BA • A. Baker, MD, MS
D. Goldenberg, MD (✉) • N. Goyal, MD, MPH
Division of Otolaryngology – Head and Neck Surgery, Department of Surgery, Penn State Milton S. Hershey Medical Center, Hershey, PA, USA
e-mail: dgoldenberg@hmc.psu.edu

Z. Gil et al. (eds.), *Atlas of Head and Neck Robotic Surgery*, DOI 10.1007/978-3-319-49578-1_6

lateral end, allowing for the surgeon to have increased range of motion on that side with the surgical instruments [1, 2]. The Crowe-Davis gag relies on the patient having stable and intact anterior dentition for the superior portion of the retractor to seat. In the 1940s, Robert McIvor, seeing the pitfalls of the gags available at the time, designed the McIvor atraumatic gag, using a closed loop superior contact point posterior to the canines to provide seating for the retractor [3]. This retractor is also useful in the edentulous patient by placing the "point" of the retractor in the arch of the palate, providing stable retraction on the maxillary alveolus.

With many years of experience with these standard retractors for oropharyngeal surgery, it is no surprise that the Crowe-Davis and McIvor have been adapted for use in TORS procedures involving the oropharynx, with excellent exposure of the tonsillar pillars and soft palate. Placement of the retractor is familiar to all but the most junior of otolaryngology residents and is typically simple and fast. Accessibility of the robotic instruments and camera is typically adequate for lesions located anterior to the base of tongue, although some base of tongue lesions may be accessible [4]. The open-sided design of the Crowe-Davis retractor does, ostensibly, allow for an increased lateral range of motion compared to the McIvor, without collision with the retractor.

As discussed by Weinstein and O'Malley [5], the Crowe-Davis also provides adequate exposure of the base of tongue; however, it is limited in its flexibility for these procedures, as there are few options for the tongue retraction blade and no attachments for retraction of the cheek or lateral portion of the tongue (Fig. 6.1). Again, the open lateral portion of the frame is noted as a strength, allowing for increased lateral motion of the robotic arms and camera.

Hockstein et al. [6] have described the use of the McIvor mouth gag in laryngeal procedures in a mannequin model with improved use of instruments and exposure when compared to operating through a standard Lindholm laryngoscope.

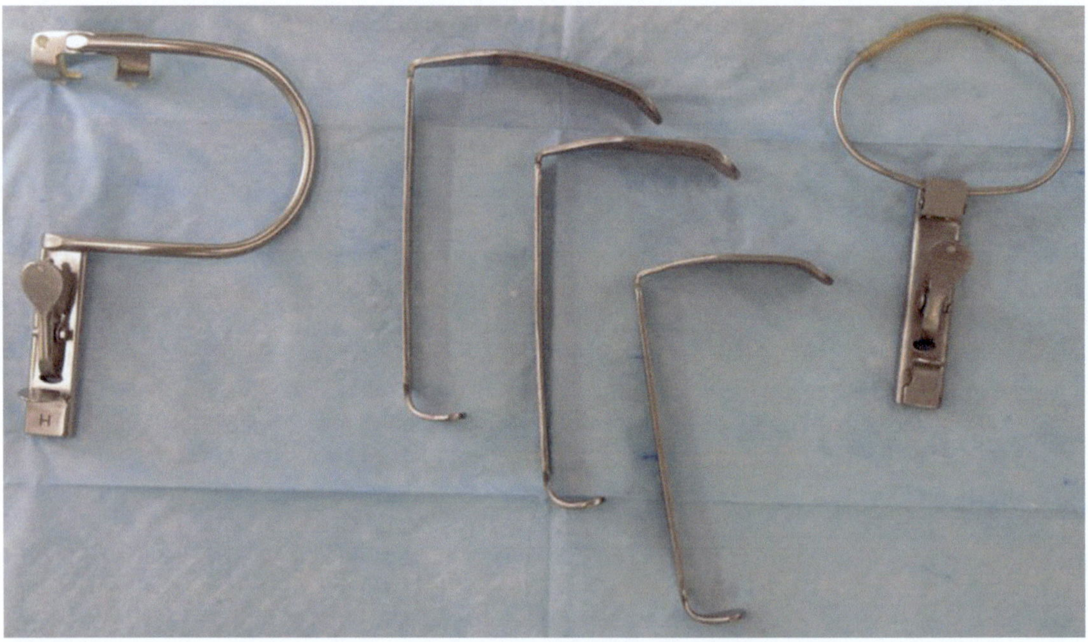

Fig. 6.1 Crowe-Davis (*left*) and McIvor (*right*) retractor systems with different-sized tongue blades

6.3 Dingman Retractor

In the 1960s, Dingman and Grabb [7] at the University of Michigan described a new, closed-frame retractor system to allow for improved visualization of the oral cavity and oropharynx. The Dingman gag includes not only the tongue retraction blade but also attachments to the lateral portion of the frame allowing for retraction of the cheeks. There are also springs on the inferior and superior portions of the frame to capture sutures that are placed through the palate or tongue for additional points and vectors of retraction (Fig. 6.2). This wide view and flexibility of retraction has made it a staple in surgery on the palate, primarily cleft surgery [8].

Again, given its wide availability and familiarity, the Dingman retractor has been adapted for use in TORS. Similar to the Crowe-Davis and McIvor, exposure of the oropharynx is excellent, although the closed frame restricts the motion of the robotic arms and camera. This limitation further increases as the surgeon moves to the base of tongue lesions and into the hypopharynx and larynx. There are few tongue retractor options with these systems, limiting the ability to obtain direct exposure of the base of tongue.

Given these restrictions, Hockstein et al. [9] describe a series of cadaveric dissections using the Dingman retractor, from laryngeal procedures such as vocal cord stripping and cordectomy to the base of tongue resections. In addition to the tongue and cheek retractors, retraction stitches through the oral tongue as well as the epiglottis are used and attached to the retractor to improve the field of view.

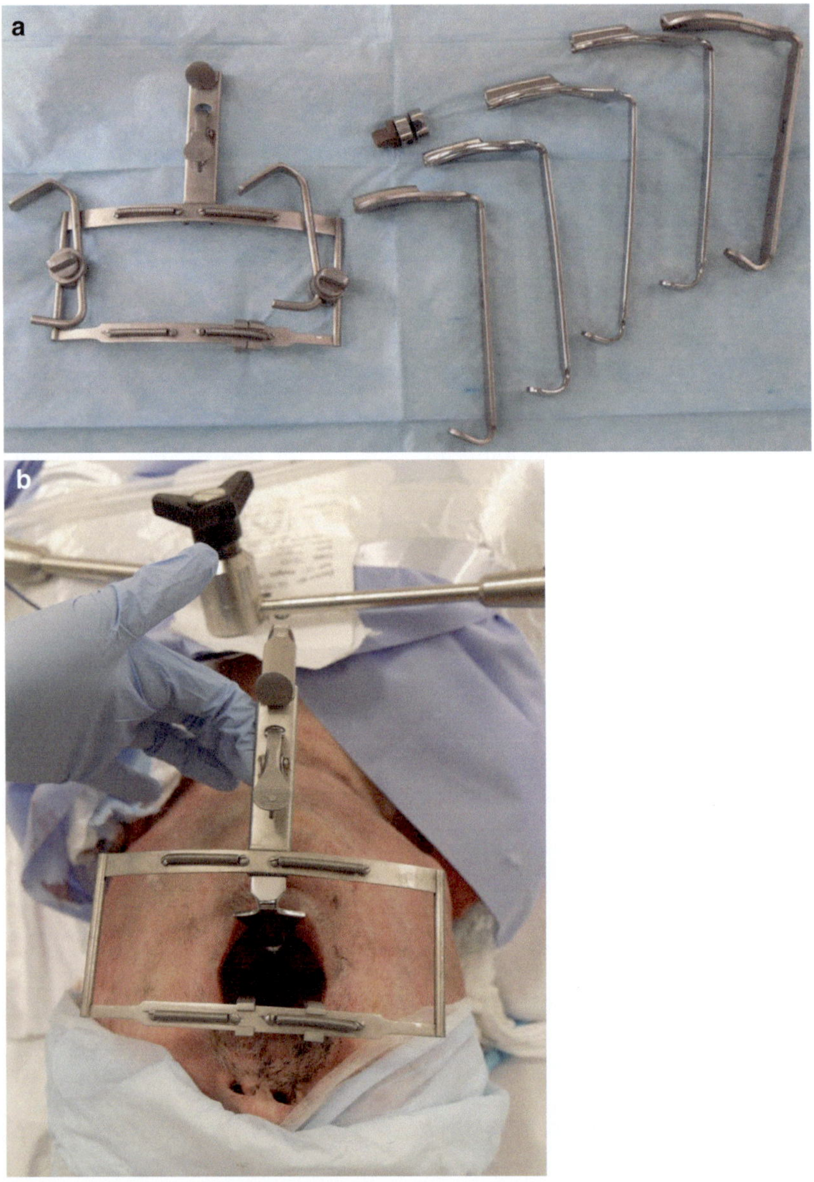

Fig. 6.2 (**a**) Dingman retractor system with different-sized tongue blades. (**b**) Dingman retractor in situ

6.4 Feyh-Kastenbauer Retractor

The Feyh-Kastenbauer (FK) retractor (Gyrus Medical Inc., Tuttlingen, Germany) is a versatile retraction system with unique applications in laryngeal, hypopharyngeal, and base of tongue procedures. The retractor features a closed rectangular frame, cheek retractors, tongue blades, laryngeal blades, and a vallecular blade [5]. The FK retraction system offers a variety of tongue blades with the ability to adjust both insertion depth and insertion angle. Some of these blades also offer the unique feature of "cutout" components designed for use in conjunction with the angle and depth adjustments to provide improved exposure of more distal operative sites (Fig. 6.3).

O'Malley and colleagues were one of the first groups to demonstrate the unique advantages offered by the FK retractor in TORS procedures of pharyngeal and base of tongue pathologies. In comparison to the Dingman and Crowe-Davis retractors, the FK is advantageous in base of tongue surgery as it provides a larger rectangular opening for the widest instrument working space with more space for robotic instrument movement. The two small articulating clamps of the FK allow for individualized articulation of each of the tongue and cheek retractor blades to be attached and manipulated for increased tissue exposure. The FK also includes integrated suction retractors that are not available in many other retraction systems. Modifications were made to the original FK retractor system by Weinstein and O'Malley, in order to optimize the retractor for use in conjunction with the da Vinci system, now named the FK-WO (Feyh-Kastenbauer Weinstein-O'Malley) [10]. These modifications included widening of the aperture at the frame to allow for more room for instruments and the camera, as well as new blades for exposure of the supraglottis (Fig. 6.3), making it useful in all transoral procedures.

In base of tongue cadaver studies, O'Malley and colleagues [5] determined that the FK had significant advantages with its lateral retractor attachments, a variety of tongue blades with and without cutouts, vallecular blade, cheek retractors, and three-dimensional adjustment capability that deemed it the most versatile retraction system at the time. Thus, it was chosen for use in the human base of tongue resections. The open laryngeal blade fit into the vallecula and provided visualization of the junction of the base of tongue and epiglottis, allowing for controlled inferior tissue incisions.

The FK retractor allows for TORS of the base of tongue, eliminating the requirement of mandibulotomy with a lip-split or transpharyngeal approaches that carry high risk of damage to delicate structures, with effects on mastication, swallowing, speech function, and cosmesis.

The FK retraction system is also the only retractor that has been reliably used for supraglottic partial laryngectomy and hypopharyngeal tumors as it is capable of exposing the larynx, a weakness of the Dingman and Crowe-Davis. In 2007, Weinstein and colleagues successfully utilized the FK retractor system for completion of supraglottic partial laryngectomies [11], and Park and colleagues describe the excision of supraglottic and glottic lesions in 2009 [12].

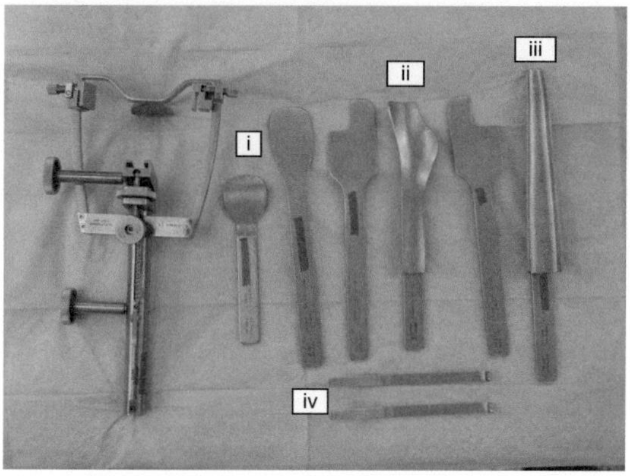

Fig. 6.3 FK-WO retractor system with blades available for exposure of different areas. (*i*) Tongue blades for exposure of oral cavity and oropharynx. (*ii*) Tongue blades for exposure of hypopharynx and base of tongue. (*iii*) Tongue blade for exposure of larynx. (*iv*) Cheek retractor attachments

6.5 Laryngeal Advanced Retractor System (LARS)

The laryngeal advanced retractor system is a newer design that was introduced to the field of TORS in 2011 by Remacle and colleagues [13]. The retractor features a rounded frame with blades that allow adjustment of both insertion depth and insertion angle, cheek retractors, tongue blades, and laryngeal blades [14]. The curved frame adapts to the shape of the patient's face and contains framework that extends in the horizontal plane to allow for ease of movement of the robot arms. There is also a ratchet system that is built into the frame to assist with vertical suspension of the device, a feature of standard laryngoscopes that is not available in other retractor systems (Fig. 6.4).

In addition to the FK retractor, the LARS is also capable of providing adequate exposure to the larynx and hypopharynx. It not only offers a repertoire of blades to choose from but has vertical attachment bars that allow for use of additional instruments if needed. The threaded adjustment system of this retractor provides the ability to slide the vertical blades upward and downward, as well as backward and forward. This single retractor can thus be used for procedures in the oral cavity, oropharynx, hypopharynx, larynx, and upper esophagus.

In the initial study in which the retractor was introduced, it was successfully used in five patients, two with oropharyngeal tumors, one with a supraglottic tumor, one with hypertrophy of the palatine tonsils, and one with a parapharyngeal space schwannoma. All procedures were completed with adequate exposure and without complications [13].

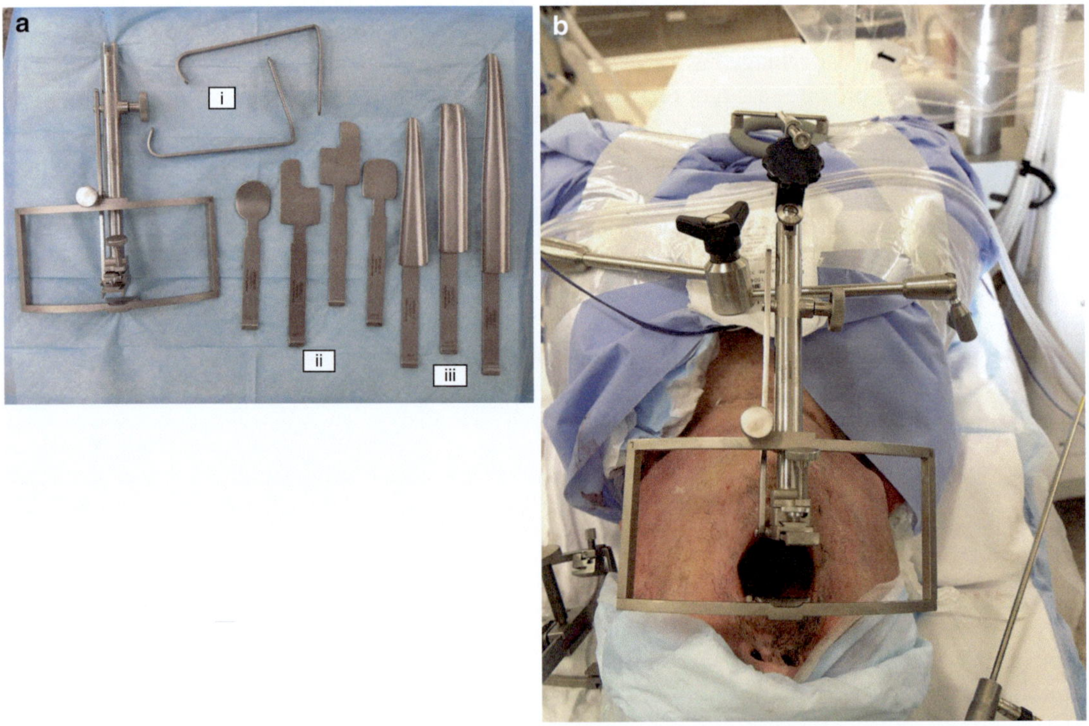

Fig. 6.4 (**a**) LARS retractor system with blades available for exposure of different areas. (*i*) Cheek retractor attachments. (*ii*) Tongue blades for exposure of oral cavity, base of tongue, and oropharynx. (*iii*) Tongue blades for exposure of the hypopharynx and larynx. (**b**) LARS retractor in situ

6.6 Medrobotics Flex Retractor System (FRS)

The first robotic system utilized and approved for TORS was the Intuitive Surgical da Vinci Si system. As this system was the only robot available for TORS, the evaluations of most retraction systems have predominantly used the da Vinci system. Recent advancements have led to the development of a smaller, flexible surgical robot designed with limited access sites such as the head and neck in mind, the FDA-approved Medrobotics Flex Robotic System (Raynham, Massachusetts, USA).

Along with the development of a new robotic system, a novel retractor system was designed for use with this robot, featuring interchangeable tongue retractors. The system integrates a large, rounded, closed frame with the various tongue retractors. This frame allows for attachment of cheek retractors similar to the Dingman retractor, with a frame size that increases the range of motion of the instruments (Fig. 6.5). In addition, the system includes a suction attachment to clear smoke created with electrocautery use, similar to that in the FK-WO.

This retractor system was designed in conjunction with the Flex robot; however, its usage is not limited to use with any specific robot. The authors have used the Medrobotics Flex Retractor System in cadaveric dissections with ease of use and placement, and excellent exposure was obtained while using the da Vinci Si system, performing oropharyngeal, base of tongue, hypopharyngeal, and supraglottic procedures (unpublished report/personal communication).

The unique design and primary advantage that the Flex retractor system allows are user-tunable adjustment of the angle and pitch of the tongue blade in the superior-inferior direction, the rotation of the blade axially, and depth of the blade. These adjustments, along with the variety of blades available, make the system useful in all transoral procedures, similar to the FK-WO. Hasskamp et al. [14] first describe the use of the Flex robot and retractor system in human patients. They found that the surgical exposure was excellent in all cases of oropharyngeal, base of tongue, and hypopharyngeal surgery. Laryngeal blades were still in development and thus not available for use from the company at the time of their testing.

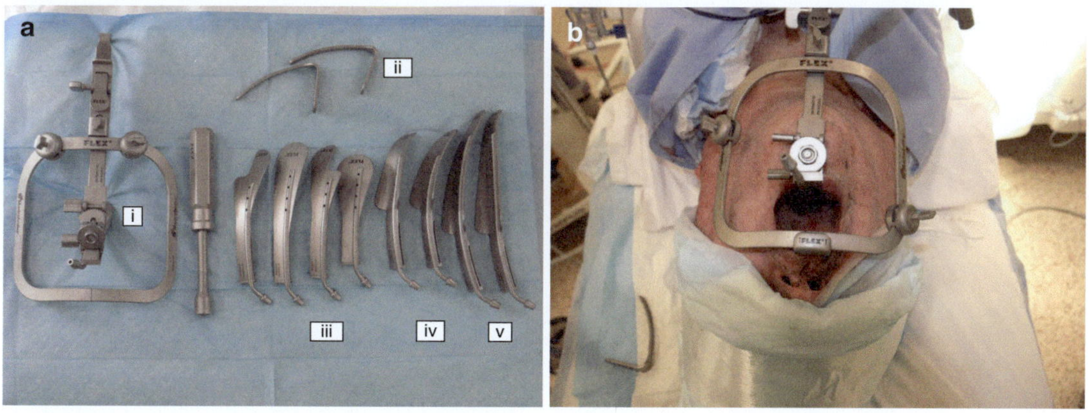

Fig. 6.5 (**a**) Flex retractor system with blades available for exposure of different areas. (*i*) Pitch and angle adjustment knobs. (*ii*) Cheek retractor attachments. (*iii*) Tongue blades for exposure of the oral cavity, base of tongue, and oropharynx. (*iv*) Tongue blades for exposure of the hypopharynx. (*v*) Tongue blades for exposure of the larynx. (**b**) Flex retractor in situ

6.7 Pediatric Applications of Retractor Systems

The application of robotic surgery in the pediatric population remains a challenging endeavor. The current size of robotic endoscope and instrument arms can be difficult to introduce into the pediatric oropharynx. In children, exposure can be particularly challenging, and specifically designed mouth retractors for infants and small children are currently not available. While the frame size is constant in available systems, some blades can be used for pediatric applications, particularly in procedures of the oropharynx. The Crowe-Davis, McIvor, and Dingman mouth gags offer tongue blades that are commonly used in the pediatric patient. While the Crowe-Davis and McIvor are commonly used in non-robotic tonsillectomies, the Dingman, FK, and McIvor retractors have been used in children undergoing lingual tonsillectomy [15].

Exposure of the larynx is much more challenging in the child as the laryngeal blades of the FK, LARS, and FRS are designed for the adult patient. However, exposure of the larynx for laryngeal cleft repair has been successful using the Crowe-Davis, FK, and Dingman mouth retractors [16, 17].

Conclusion

Transoral robotic surgery continues to expand and gain momentum. At this time, two robotic systems exist to facilitate TORS procedures. However, efficiently and safely using these systems does require adequate exposure of the surgical site. To this end, the head and neck surgeon must be familiar with the many retractor systems available to choose the ideal retractor.

A plethora of retractors have been developed to allow for adequate access without hindering visualization of lesions of the oropharynx, hypopharynx, and larynx (the reviewed retractors are summarized in Table 6.1). Notably, areas that require specific consideration are the base of tongue, where a retractor may cover the area of interest, and the larynx, where many retractors are not able to sufficiently elevate the tongue anteriorly and provide adequate exposure. As surgeons continue to expand the versatility of surgical robots, we suspect that the retractors used will continue to evolve and improve.

Table 6.1 Summary of the retractor systems currently available

Retractor	Studies	Features	Primary indications	Limitations
Crowe-Davis	Crowe [1], Davis [2], Weinstein and O'Malley [5]	Open lateral frame, easily accessible, familiar	Oral cavity, oropharynx	Limited base of tongue, hypopharynx, and larynx exposure
McIvor	McIvor [3]	Easily accessible, familiar, useful in edentulous patient	Oral cavity, oropharynx	Limited base of tongue, hypopharynx, and larynx exposure, closed frame
Dingman	Dingman and Grabb [7] Hockstein [9]	Wide frame, cheek retractors, tie down points, accessible	Oral cavity, oropharynx (especially palate)	Limited base of tongue, hypopharynx, and larynx exposure, closed frame
FK/FK-WO	Weinstein and O'Malley [5, 11], Park [12]	Wide frame, various blades designed for exposure of specific areas, integrated suction, modified for TORS (FK-WO)	Oropharynx, hypopharynx, larynx	Closed frame, expense?
LARS	Remacle [13]	Designed for laryngeal procedures, curved frame, various blades, vertically adjustable blades, instrument attachments	Larynx, oropharynx, hypopharynx	Closed frame, expense?
Medrobotics Flex (FRS)	Hasskamp [14]	Designed for TORS, curved frame various blades, blade adjustment in multiple planes, integrated suction	Oropharynx, hypopharynx, larynx	Closed frame, expense?

FK/FK-WO Feyh-Kastenbauer-Weinstein O'Malley, *LARS* laryngeal advanced retractor system, *TORS* transoral robotic surgery

References

1. Crowe SJ, Watkins SS, Rothholz AS. Relation of tonsillar and nasopharyngeal infections to general systemic disorders. Bull Johns Hopkins Hosp. 1917; 28:1–63.
2. Ameer F, Kumar S, Singh A. The story of mouth gags. J Cleft Lip Palate Craniofac Anom. 2014;1:70.
3. McIvor RJ. A new atraumatic mouth gag. Arch Otolaryngol. 1947;45:364.
4. Weinstein GS, O'Malley BW, Snyder W, Sherman E, Quon H. Transoral robotic surgery: radical tonsillectomy. Arch Otolaryngol Head Neck Surg. 2007;133: 1220–6.
5. O'Malley Jr BW, Weinstein GS, Snyder W, Hockstein NG. Transoral robotic surgery (TORS) for base of tongue neoplasms. Laryngoscope. 2006;116:1465–72.
6. Hockstein NG, Nolan JP, O'malley BW, Woo YJ. Robotic microlaryngeal surgery: a technical feasibility study using the daVinci surgical robot and an airway mannequin. Laryngoscope. 2005;115:780–5.
7. Dingman RO, Grabb WC. A new mouth gag. Plast Reconstr Surg Transplant Bull. 1962;29:208–9.
8. Rao LP, Peter S. Modification of the Dingman mouth gag for better visibility and access in the management of cleft palate. Cleft Palate Craniofac J Off Publ Am Cleft Palate Craniofac Assoc. 2015;52:250–3.
9. Hockstein NG, Nolan JP, O'Malley BW, Woo YJ. Robot-assisted pharyngeal and laryngeal microsurgery: results of robotic cadaver dissections. Laryngoscope. 2005;115:1003–8.
10. Weinstein GS, O'Malley BW. Transoral robotic surgery. (Plural, 2009) San Diego, CA, USA.
11. Weinstein GS, O'Malley BW, Desai SC, Quon H. Transoral robotic surgery: does the ends justify the means? Curr Opin Otolaryngol Head Neck Surg. 2009;17:126–31.
12. Park YM, et al. Transoral robotic surgery (TORS) in laryngeal and hypopharyngeal cancer. J Laparoendosc Adv Surg Tech A. 2009;19:361–8.
13. Remacle M, Matar N, Lawson G, Bachy V. Laryngeal advanced retractor system: a new retractor for transoral robotic surgery. Otolaryngol Head Neck Surg Off J Am Acad Otolaryngol Head Neck Surg. 2011;145:694–6.
14. Hasskamp P, Lang S, Holtmann L, Stuck BA, Mattheis S. First use of a new retractor in transoral robotic surgery (TORS). Eur Arch Otorhinolaryngol Off J Eur Fed Otorhinolaryngol Soc EUFOS Affil Ger Soc Otorhinolaryngol Head Neck Surg. 2015; doi:10.1007/s00405-015-3719-1.
15. Leonardis RL, Duvvuri U, Mehta D. Transoral robotic-assisted lingual tonsillectomy in the pediatric population. JAMA Otolaryngol Head Neck Surg. 2013;139:1032–6.
16. Rahbar R, Ferrari LR, Borer JG, Peters CA. Robotic surgery in the pediatric airway: application and safety. Arch Otolaryngol Head Neck Surg. 2007;133:46–50. discussion 50
17. Leonardis RL, Duvvuri U, Mehta D. Transoral robotic-assisted laryngeal cleft repair in the pediatric patient. Laryngoscope. 2014;124:2167–9.

Transoral Robotic Surgery for Tonsillar Cancer

7

Shivani Shah-Becker, Robert Saadi, and David Goldenberg

7.1 Introduction

Surgery for tonsillar cancer has previously been limited to early-stage and intra-tonsillar tumors due to inadequate visualization of the oropharynx via transoral approaches. Open approaches to the oropharynx are often quite morbid, requiring mandibulotomy or partial mandibulectomy and tracheotomy in order to achieve oncologic resection, followed by extensive reconstruction [1]. Until recently, trends have been to treat oropharyngeal carcinomas with primary radiation therapy. However, radiation therapy is also not without significant toxicity and side effects, including xerostomia, dental complications, and long-term dysphagia requiring a feeding tube [2]. Additionally, the use of radiation as a primary modality of treatment subsequently restricts its use in the case of recurrence or development of a second primary malignancy.

The introduction of robotic-assisted surgery in tonsillar cancer has allowed more advanced and extensive tumors to be treated with surgery. The transoral approach avoids the morbidity of an open procedure while still achieving complete oncologic resection, including margins. The magnified three-dimensional view along with the use of angled endoscopic cameras with 360° radius provides visualization beyond the tonsillar fossa to the great vessels laterally, the palate and nasopharynx superiorly, and the tongue base inferiorly, which could not be achieved using traditional transoral headlight or operative microscope alone.

7.2 History of Transoral Surgery for Tonsillar Cancer

A renewed interest in a surgical approach to oropharyngeal cancers has developed in the last decade, largely due to the increasing incidence of the HPV-associated squamous cell carcinoma affecting a younger demographic who are more susceptible to the delayed adverse effects of chemoradiation [3–5]. The transoral approach, a minimally invasive technique taking advantage of the access through the mouth, was first described in 1951 by the French surgeon Huet [6]. The poor visualization and reliance on rigid instruments made the approach unfavorable for resection deep within the oropharynx.

In 2003, Steiner utilized a carbon dioxide laser through a micromanipulater with a laryngoscope for visualization in the oropharynx [7]. In 2005, Holsinger et al. reported on the French experience, having achieved an 82% 5-year control rate with the use of transoral laser microsurgery

S. Shah-Becker, MD • R. Saadi, BS
D. Goldenberg, MD, FACS (✉)
Division of Otolaryngology-Head and Neck Surgery, Penn State Milton S. Hershey Medical Center, 500 University Drive, H091, Hershey, PA 17033, USA
e-mail: dgoldenberg@hmc.psu.edu

Z. Gil et al. (eds.), *Atlas of Head and Neck Robotic Surgery*, DOI 10.1007/978-3-319-49578-1_7

(TLM) in patients with early-stage tonsillar squamous cell carcinoma [8]. However, TLM has some shortcomings, particularly due to the line-of-site requirements of the CO_2 laser, as well as the challenges with manipulating the tumor to provide more deliberate dissection and complete visualization. Additionally, bleeding encountered during a TLM procedure can be difficult to manage with the laser and requires the surgeon to switch to electrocautery.

The introduction of the "robot" has reduced some of these challenges, and its use in carefully selected tongue base, tonsillar, and certain laryngeal and hypopharyngeal cases has shown great success. The robotic surgical system most widely used for transoral robotic surgery (TORS) procedures has been the *da Vinci Surgical System* developed by Intuitive Surgical (Sunnyvale, CA). With joysticks that control "wristed" surgical instruments in three-dimensional space, the da Vinci robot allows surgeons to cut, manipulate, and suture tissue via the minimally invasive approach.

In 2007, Weinstein et al. developed the TORS radical tonsillectomy based on the previous transoral technique with some basic modifications for the operating room setup and oral exposure. Their exclusion criteria were limited to unresectable neck nodes, mandibular invasion, involvement of >50% of the tongue base, involvement of >50% of the posterior pharyngeal wall, carotid artery involvement, or fixation to prevertebral fascia. Twenty-five of the 27 tumors were resected with negative margins, and there were no local or regional recurrences. Two patients required a tracheotomy, and only one experienced persistent difficulty swallowing [9]. Additional studies revealed the feasibility and safety of TORS, and preliminary outcome data showed optimal disease control with significantly better functional swallowing outcomes [10, 11]. In 2009, the US Food and Drug Administration (FDA) approved of the use of da Vinci robotics in head and neck benign disease and T1 and T2 malignancies.

Although visualization and anatomical access have been improved with this robotic system, the design of the long and rigid da Vinci end effector instruments does not provide for ideal, unhampered access to all anatomic sites within the upper aerodigestive tract [12]. A flexible robot was developed for minimally invasive surgery applications at Carnegie Mellon University. Originally designed for cardiac procedures, this robot is a device with 102 degrees of freedom and a snakelike advancement mechanism capable of steering a nonlinear, self-supported path. The flexible robot was further customized and transformed into the Medrobotics Flex System, developed specifically for use in surgical applications requiring nonlinear maneuverability such as transoral surgery. This flexible robot platform drives a chip-on-tip endoscope through nonlinear pathways and provides a platform for the delivery of flexible tools to perform a variety of surgical procedures. In 2015, the FDA approved the use of the Flex system for transoral resections of head and neck tumors (Fig. 7.1).

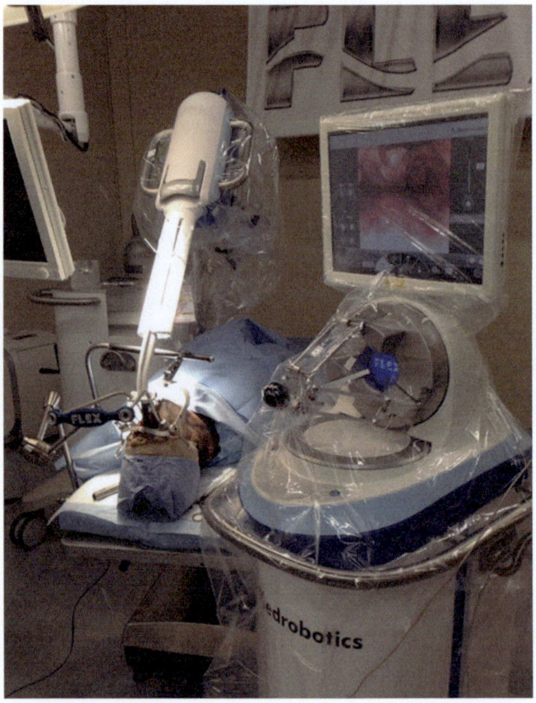

Fig. 7.1 Medrobotics Flex robot, approved for transoral robotic surgery in 2015

7.3 Indications

The current indications for robotic-assisted surgery for tonsillar cancer are tumors amenable to total resection with negative margins. The patients who are the best candidates typically have early-stage (T1 to T2) tumors and have the potential to avoid chemoradiation therapy. Those who have advanced-stage (T3 or T4) tumors will generally require chemoradiation therapy and may not always benefit as greatly from surgery. However, in the case of low-volume T3 disease, undergoing robotic surgery may still allow the patient to receive adjuvant radiation alone, without chemotherapy [9, 13, 14]. Therefore, advanced-stage disease is not a contraindication for TORS and is performed routinely at many institutions. Finally, robotic-assisted surgery may also be indicated in certain circumstances of salvage surgery for early T-stage tumors [15].

Contraindications of TORS for tonsillar cancer are separated into two major categories: tumor-related factors and patient-related factors. Factors that make the tumor unresectable include carotid artery involvement, fixation to the prevertebral fascia, and unresectable neck lymphadenopathy. T4a lesions with mandible invasion, hard palate invasion, >50% tongue base involvement, and >50% posterior pharyngeal wall involvement are also contraindicated [9, 13, 16]. Patient-related factors include anatomical issues such as trismus and kyphosis, retropharyngeal location of the internal carotid artery, and medical comorbidities precluding general anesthesia or inhibiting wound healing by secondary intention [9, 13, 16].

7.4 Operative Technique

When using the da Vinci robotic system, the setup for robotic-assisted radical tonsillectomy is similar to that in other transoral robotic head and neck surgery cases. The robot base is on the patient's left and the scrub nurse on the patient's right. A bedside assistant is seated at the head of the patient. Intubation can be achieved either transnasally or transorally using a RAE endotracheal tube. Exposure to the oropharynx is typically achieved using either a Crowe-Davis or Dingman mouth gag. The tongue blade accompanies the mouth gag to push the tongue inferiorly. Three robotic arms are inserted transorally [9] with the endoscope in the center and a spatula tip monopolar cautery and a Maryland dissector on the ipsilateral and contralateral arms, respectively, 30–45° from the center (Fig. 7.2). A 0 degree endoscope is typically utilized at the start of the case, but may be changed to a 30° scope later to better visualize the base of tongue. A retraction suture can be placed through the midline of the tongue for additional retraction. The bedside assistant should have suction in the oral cavity to remove smoke from the surgeon's view and an instrument for cheek retraction if necessary [9, 17–19].

When using the Flex robotic system, the robot is mounted to the surgical table rails and arranged to approach the oral cavity from the caudal direction (Fig. 7.3). The robot is then driven via the physician controller to enter the oral cavity and travel midline until the tonsillar region is reached (robot docking). Once the flexible robot had been docked in the desired position, the surgeon inserts flexible endoscopic instruments into the external accessory channels to perform the procedure. A 3.5 mm grasper is used for tissue retraction and manipulation, and a 3.5 mm cauterizing instrument and a laser guide are used for cutting. Flexible instrumentation can be inserted by the surgeon from the direction opposite the flexible robot, in this case from the cephalic direction [20].

Once adequate visualization of the tonsillar fossa is established using either robotic system, a dissector or other grasper is used to provide medial retraction of the tonsil. Monopolar cautery is used to make a mucosal incision in the anterior tonsillar pillar and soft palate (Figs. 7.4 and 7.5). The plane of dissection is developed deep to the superior constrictor muscle, leaving pharyngeal fat laterally. The spatula tip cautery or other instrument can be used for blunt dissection in this plane (Figs. 7.6 and 7.7). Pulsations from the carotid artery area easily visualized with the three-dimensional magnified view deep to the parapharyngeal fat. Dissection is carried to the styloglossus with the pterygoid muscles laterally.

Superiorly, the soft palate incision is carried down through both the palatoglossus and palatopharyngeus muscles to the prevertebral fascia. Here, again, the spatula cautery can be used to bluntly dissect the superior constrictor muscle off of the prevertebral fascia. Inferiorly, the use of the robot gives the surgeon complete visualization of the tongue base, allowing a cuff of tongue base muscle to be included as the inferior margin of the resection (Fig. 7.8). The styloglossus and stylopharyngeus muscles are encountered and carefully dissected circumferentially and typically transected [9, 17]. Branches of the external carotid, including lingual artery, are encountered 5–8 mm deep to the styloglossus muscle and should be carefully avoided or ligated with surgical clips.

The glossopharyngeal nerve can also be identified at the junction of the posterior tonsillar pillar and base of tongue. While distal branches and even the main trunk may require transection from an oncologic standpoint, the magnification and enhanced visualization of the robotic system can also give the surgeon the ability to trace the nerve and leave it intact [18].

Finally, the constrictor muscle is transected at the medial deep limit of the dissection and the posterior mucosal cut is completed, freeing up the specimen [9] (Figs. 7.9 and 7.10). Any bleeding which is encountered can be controlled with either monopolar cautery or vascular clips [17]. The bedside assistant may also be able to use bipolar forceps for hemostasis, or apply pressure to compress the lingual artery at the level of the hyoid to improve visualization [9].

The wound may be left open to heal by secondary intention or a skin graft can be placed to cover raw muscle edges. More extensive reconstruction is often unnecessary following TORS, as the intact buccopharyngeal fascia avoids exposure of any major vessels. If neck dissection is performed in a staged fashion, then fistulous connection to the neck is also avoided, precluding the need for local and/or free flap reconstruction [16].

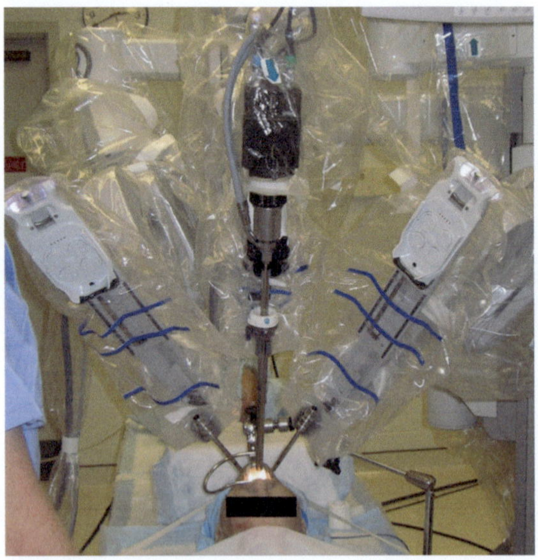

Fig. 7.2 Da Vinci robot setup with endoscope in the center and instruments on each side oriented at 45° from the center camera

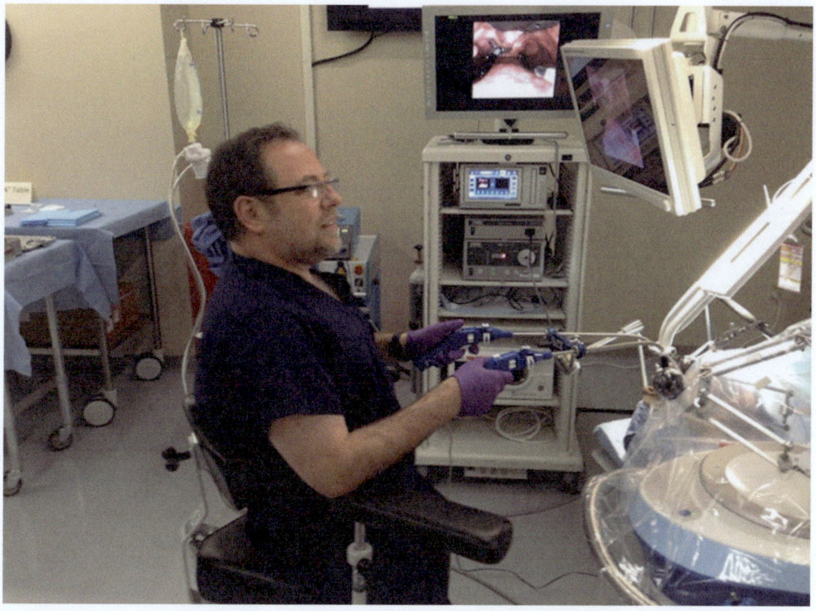

Fig. 7.3 Medrobotics Flex robot mounted to patient bed rails with surgeon at the patient's head controlling instruments

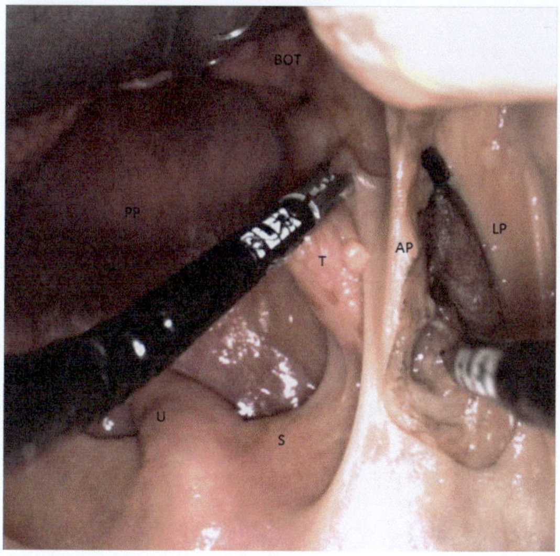

Fig. 7.4 Initial mucosal incision made in the anterior tonsillar pillar using monopolar cautery. *AP* anterior pillar, *U* uvula, *S* soft palate, *BOT* base of tongue, *T* tonsil, *PP* posterior pharyngeal wall, *LP* lateral pharyngeal wall

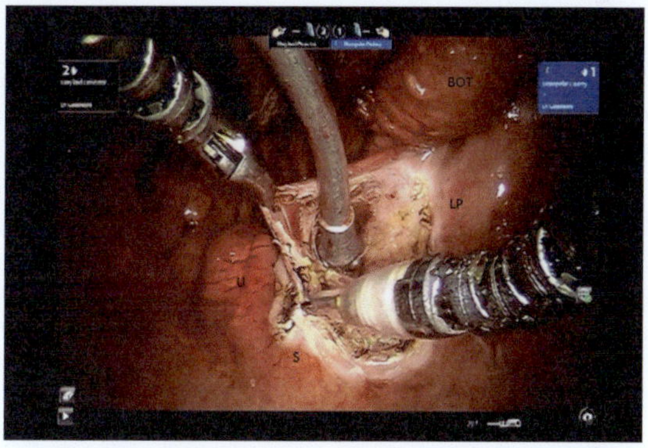

Fig. 7.5 Incision extended to soft palate using monopolar cautery, as seen through the Da Vinci console. *BOT* base of tongue, *U* uvula, *S* soft palate, *LP* lateral pharyngeal wall

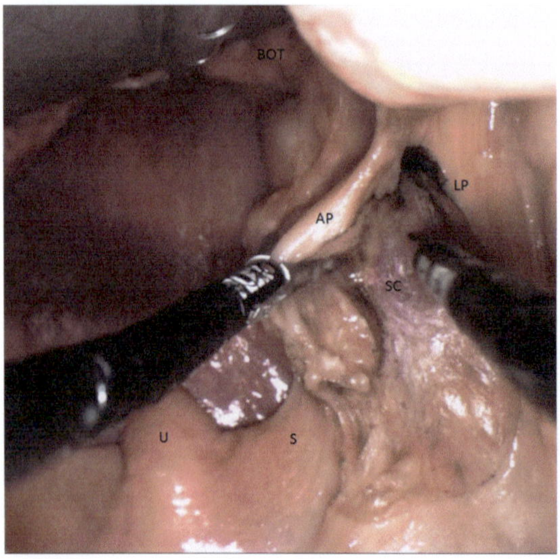

Fig. 7.6 A plane is bluntly developed deep to the superior constrictor muscle. *SC* superior constrictor muscle, *U* uvula, *S* soft palate, *AP* anterior pillar, *BOT* base of tongue, *LP* lateral pharyngeal wall

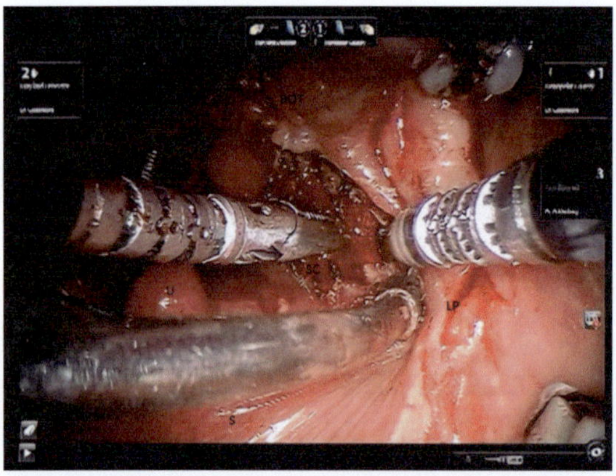

Fig. 7.7 Spatula tip cautery and suction continuing in blunt dissection in the established plane deep to the superior constrictor muscle. *SC* superior constrictor, *U* uvula, *S* soft palate, *BOT* base of tongue, *LP* lateral pharyngeal wall

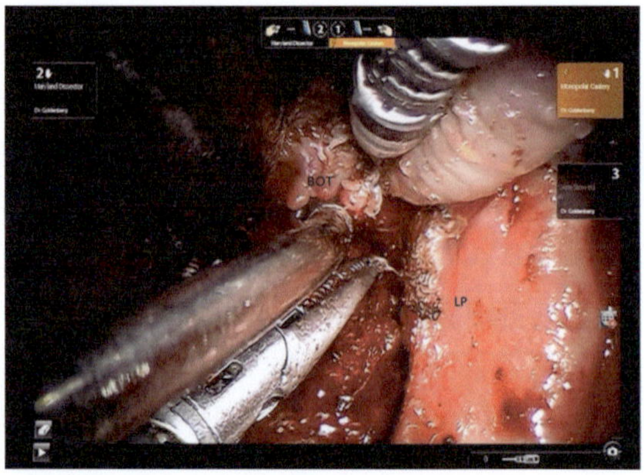

Fig. 7.8 A margin of tissue at the tongue base is taken inferiorly. *BOT* base of tongue, *LP* lateral pharyngeal all

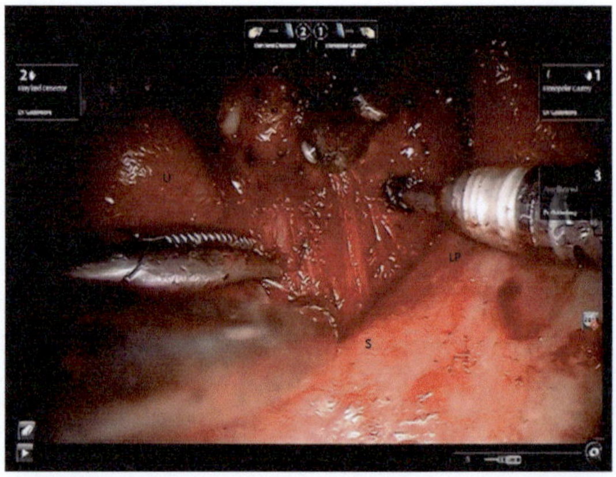

Fig. 7.9 Cephalad dissection is visualized as the specimen is retracted inferiorly. *U* uvula, *S* soft palate, *LP* lateral pharyngeal wall

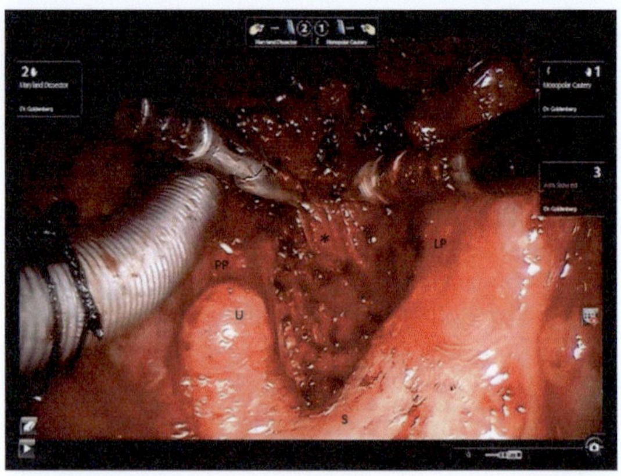

Fig. 7.10 Final cuts are made detaching the specimen from the posterior pharyngeal wall. *U* uvula, *S* soft palate, *PP* posterior pharyngeal wall, *LP* lateral pharyngeal wall, *asterisk* wound bed as posterior mucosal cut is completed

7.5 Complications

Reported complication rates following da Vinci TORS for tonsillar cancer are as high as 19% [9]. Bleeding is one of the most serious and potentially life-threatening acute complications. The incidence of bleeding following all transoral robotic surgery has been reported as 9.8%. The tonsil bed was found to be the second most common site of bleeding, following the base of tongue. T2 and T3 tumors trended toward higher bleeding rates than T1 tumors. Bleeding can be controlled by a variety of methods including silver nitrate cauterization, monopolar or bipolar cauterization, embolization, and transcervical arterial ligation. If the neck dissection is staged prior to resection of the primary tumor, the facial and lingual arteries can be ligated at their origin from the external carotid artery. Additionally, if performed concurrently with the primary tumor resection, the neck dissection should include ligation of the external carotid arterial branches, particularly the facial, lingual, and ascending pharyngeal branches. This theoretically can minimize post-TORS catastrophic bleeds. Airway protection is critical in post-TORS oropharyngeal hemorrhage and can prevent a catastrophic outcome [21].

The need for unplanned tracheotomy is another potentially life-threatening complication and has a reported incidence between 0% and 4% [9, 22]. Other reported minor complications from robotic oropharyngeal surgery include palatal insufficiency, nasopharyngeal stenosis, hypernasality, lingual nerve numbness, postoperative trismus, dysgeusia, and cervicalgia.

If en bloc concurrent resection of primary and cervical lymph nodes is performed, as opposed to staged neck dissection, the risk of creating a fistula to the neck is closer to 30%, and some reconstruction should be considered [23]. If a small connection is created (<1 cm), primary closure, tissue sealant, and cervical drain may be sufficient in management. If a larger defect is created, primary closure can be attempted, and local muscle coverage using the digastric, mylohyoid, and/or sternocleidomastoid muscle is indicated. Tissue sealant and cervical drains are still utilized, and NPO status is maintained for 48 h if leak is not suspected [23, 24].

7.6 Outcomes

7.6.1 Perioperative Outcomes

Average surgical time for TORS oropharyngeal resection is about 85 min [25]. Blood loss is typically low for an oncologic resection, averaging less than 90–100 ml. Patients have short hospital stays, ranging between 1 and 7 days, with most people staying in the hospital less than 4 days [25].

Anywhere from 0% to 31% of patients require tracheotomy at some point during their treatment, with patients with advanced-stage tumors requiring tracheotomy more frequently than those patients with early-stage tumors [26]. Due to the resultant aspiration and wound healing issues, patients undergoing salvage TORS for failed radiation therapy may benefit from elective tracheostomy at the time of surgery.

7.6.2 Oncologic Outcomes

Oncologic outcomes for early-staged patients are similar to patients undergoing primary chemoradiation therapy, but without any of the adverse effects of radiation or chemotherapy.

In early-stage oropharyngeal cancer treated with TORS alone, without adjuvant therapy, Weinstein et al. reported only a 3% rate of positive margins at resection and 97% local control at 18 months post-op. Regional control was achieved in 90% and distant control in 100%, with 100% survival at 18 months [25]. In a larger, multi-institutional study of oncologic outcomes of 410 patients, 2-year locoregional control in tonsillar cancers was 97.1%. The 2-year overall survival was 95.4% [27].

7.6.3 Functional Outcomes

Dysphagia is a frequently cited adverse effect of treatment for tonsillar cancer. Functional outcomes and swallowing are important to assess following any modality utilized for the treatment of these cancers, including TORS. Studies examining swallowing outcomes after TORS thus far are limited in follow-up to approximately 1–2 years [25, 26, 28].

For early-stage oropharyngeal cancers which were treated with TORS alone, greater than 90% of patients are able to take an oral diet on postoperative day 1 and 100% by the time of discharge from the hospital [26]. At 18 months after surgery, nearly all patients continue to take an oral diet without the use of a feeding tube [25]. With the addition of adjuvant therapy, more patients require feeding tube support in the short term, and only 70–85% are taking oral diet only [29].

For patients with advanced-stage tonsillar cancers, those patients treated with TORS followed by adjuvant therapy had significantly better swallowing outcomes and MDADI (MD Anderson Dysphagia Inventory) scores than those patients treated with primary chemoradiation at 6 and 12 months after surgery. This may be associated with the decreased dose of radiation given to patients during adjuvant therapy after TORS (54 Gy) compared to the average dose given during primary chemoradiation therapy (70 Gy) [28].

7.7 Limitations

TORS has predominantly been utilized and studied in early T1–T2 tonsillar cancers. Although there are reports of its use in more advanced tumors, one of the major benefits of utilizing robotic surgery is that it obviates the need for complex reconstruction. If the defect size would warrant free flap reconstruction, then the functional benefit from performing TORS may be more limited. Additionally, although there have been reports of TORS used in salvage surgery, patients are infrequently candidates for minimally invasive robotic surgery following chemoradiation therapy due to the extent of recurrence [16].

The management of intraoperative complications, such as hemorrhage, may be more challenging in minimally invasive robotic approaches compared to open approaches. More large-caliber vessels are likely to be encountered in the oropharynx than other sites in the head and neck for which TORS is utilized, and the management of these vessels has the potential to be more challenging. In the highly magnified view at the robotic console, even small quantities of blood can obscure the entire visual field. Despite this, surgeons experienced in TORS have been able to overcome this limitation using a number of standard monopolar and bipolar cautery tools, hemostasis clips, and the use of a capable bedside assistant [30].

Conclusion

Since the introduction of TORS into the head and neck surgeon's armamentarium, there has been widespread acceptance of its use at many institutions and a great deal of research documenting its effectiveness and outcomes. Indeed, since 2009, evidence from the National Cancer Data Base shows that surgical rates for oropharyngeal cancer have increased significantly after reaching a nadir prior to the FDA approval [31]. Among the many anatomical areas in the head and neck, TORS has been found to be extremely effective in the oropharynx, where it shows promise of becoming the treatment of choice and may allow for reduction or avoidance of adjuvant chemotherapy and radiation [32].

References

1. Galati LT, Myers EN, Johnson JT. Primary surgery as treatment for early squamous cell carcinoma of the tonsil. Head Neck. 2000;22(3):294–6.
2. May JT, Rao N, Sabater RD, Boutrid H, Caudell JJ, Merchant F, et al. Intensity-modulated radiation therapy as primary treatment for oropharyngeal squamous cell carcinoma. Head Neck. 2013;35(12):1796–800.
3. Clayburgh DR, Gross N. Surgical innovations. Otolaryngol Clin N Am. 2013;46(4):615–28.
4. Kelly K, Johnson-Obaseki S, Lumingu J, Corsten M. Oncologic, functional and surgical outcomes of primary transoral robotic surgery for early squamous cell cancer of the oropharynx: a systematic review. Oral Oncol. 2014;50(8):696–703.
5. Shah S, Goldenberg D. Robotic surgery for oropharyngeal cancer. Rambam Maimonides Med J. 2014;5(2):e0014.
6. HUET PC. Electrocoagulation in epitheliomas of the tonsils. Ann Otolaryngol. 1951;68(7):433–42.
7. Steiner W, Fierek O, Ambrosch P, Hommerich CP, Kron M. Transoral laser microsurgery for squa-

mous cell carcinoma of the base of the tongue. Arch Otolaryngol Head Neck Surg. 2003;129(1):36–43.
8. Holsinger FC, McWhorter AJ, Ménard M, Garcia D, Laccourreye O. Transoral lateral oropharyngectomy for squamous cell carcinoma of the tonsillar region: I. Technique, complications, and functional results. Arch Otolaryngol Head Neck Surg. 2005;131(7):583–91.
9. Weinstein GS, O'Malley BW, Snyder W, Sherman E, Quon H. Transoral robotic surgery: radical tonsillectomy. Arch Otolaryngol Head Neck Surg Am Med Assoc. 2007;133(12):1220–6.
10. Hockstein NG, O'Malley BW, Weinstein GS. Assessment of intraoperative safety in transoral robotic surgery. Laryngoscope. 2006;116(2):165–8.
11. Moore EJ, Olsen KD, Kasperbauer JL. Transoral robotic surgery for oropharyngeal squamous cell carcinoma: a prospective study of feasibility and functional outcomes. Laryngoscope. 2009;119(11):2156–64.
12. Parmar A, Grant DG, Loizou P. Robotic surgery in ear nose and throat. Eur Arch Otorhinolaryngol. 2010;267(4):625–33.
13. Brickman D, Gross ND. Robotic approaches to the pharynx: tonsil cancer. Otolaryngol Clin N Am. 2014;47(3):359–72.
14. Lee SY, Park YM, Byeon HK, Choi EC, Kim S-H. Comparison of oncologic and functional outcomes after transoral robotic lateral oropharyngectomy versus conventional surgery for T1 to T3 tonsillar cancer. Head Neck. 2014;36(8):1138–45.
15. Dean NR, Rosenthal EL, Carroll WR, Kostrzewa JP, Jones VL, Desmond RA, et al. Robotic-assisted surgery for primary or recurrent oropharyngeal carcinoma. Arch Otolaryngol Head Neck Surg. 2010;136(4):380–4.
16. Weinstein GS, O'Malley BW. Transoral Robotic Surgery (TORS). Plural Publishing; San Diego, California, USA, 2011. p. 253.
17. Granell J, Mendez-Benegassi I, Millas T, Garrido L, Gutierrez-Fonseca R. Transoral robotic surgery: step-by-step radical tonsillectomy. Case Rep Otolaryngol. 2014;2014:497528.
18. Lim CM, Mehta V, Chai R, Pinheiro C-ND, Rath T, Snyderman C, et al. Transoral anatomy of the tonsillar fossa and lateral pharyngeal wall: anatomic dissection with radiographic and clinical correlation. Laryngoscope. 2013;123(12):3021–5.
19. Goyal N, Yoo F, Setabutr D, Goldenberg D. Surgical anatomy of the supraglottic larynx using the da Vinci robot. Head Neck. 2014;36(8):1126–31.
20. Johnson PJ, Rivera Serrano CM, Castro M, Kuenzler R, Choset H, Tully S, et al. Demonstration of transoral surgery in cadaveric specimens with the medrobotics flex system. Laryngoscope. 2013;123(5):1168–72.
21. Mandal R, Duvvuri U, Ferris RL, Kaffenberger TM, Choby GW, Kim S. Analysis of post-transoral robotic-assisted surgery hemorrhage: frequency, outcomes, and prevention. Head Neck. 2015;Suppl 1:E776–82.
22. Richmon JD, Quon H, Gourin CG. The effect of transoral robotic surgery on short-term outcomes and cost of care after oropharyngeal cancer surgery. Laryngoscope. 2014;124(1):165–71.
23. Moore EJ, Olsen KD, Martin EJ. Concurrent neck dissection and transoral robotic surgery. Laryngoscope. 2011;121(3):541–4.
24. Nam I-C, Park J-O, Joo Y-H, Cho K-J, Kim M-S. Role of primary closure after transoral robotic surgery for tonsillar cancer. Auris Nasus Larynx. 2015;42(1):43–8.
25. Weinstein GS, Quon H, Newman HJ, Chalian JA, Malloy K, Lin A, et al. Transoral robotic surgery alone for oropharyngeal cancer: an analysis of local control. Arch Otolaryngol Head Neck Surg. 2012;138(7):628–34.
26. Hutcheson KA, Holsinger FC, Kupferman ME, Lewin JS. Functional outcomes after TORS for oropharyngeal cancer: a systematic review. Eur Arch Otorhinolaryngol. 2015;272(2):463–71.
27. de Almeida JR, Li R, Magnuson JS, Smith RV, Moore E, Lawson G, et al. Oncologic outcomes after transoral robotic surgery: a multi-institutional study. JAMA Otolaryngol Head Neck Surg. 2015;141(12):1043–51.
28. More YI, Tsue TT, Girod DA, Harbison J, Sykes KJ, Williams C, et al. Functional swallowing outcomes following transoral robotic surgery vs primary chemoradiotherapy in patients with advanced-stage oropharynx and supraglottis cancers. JAMA Otolaryngol Head Neck Surg. 2013;139(1):43–8.
29. Lörincz BB, Möckelmann N, Busch C-J, Knecht R. Functional outcomes, feasibility, and safety of resection of transoral robotic surgery: single-institution series of 35 consecutive cases of transoral robotic surgery for oropharyngeal squamous cell carcinoma. Head Neck. 2015;37(11):1618–24.
30. Hockstein NG, Weinstein GS, O'Malley Jr BW. Maintenance of hemostasis in transoral robotic surgery. ORL J Otorhinolaryngol Relat Spec. 2005;67(4):220–4.
31. Liederbach E, Lewis CM, Yao K, Brockstein BE, Wang C-H, Lutfi W, et al. A contemporary analysis of surgical trends in the treatment of squamous cell carcinoma of the oropharynx from 1998 to 2012: a report from the national cancer database. Ann Surg Oncol. 2015;22(13):4422–31.
32. Moore EJ, Olsen SM, Laborde RR, García JJ, Walsh FJ, Price DL, et al. Long-term functional and oncologic results of transoral robotic surgery for oropharyngeal squamous cell carcinoma. Mayo Clin Proc. 2012;87(3):219–25.

8 Transoral Robotic Surgery for Base of Tongue Cancer

J.K. Rasamny and Jason G. Newman

8.1 Introduction

Over the last few decades, there has been a marked increase in the incidence of squamous cell cancer (SCC) of the tongue base, coinciding with the increased prevalence of human papillomavirus (HPV) infection. Prior to advancements in the field of chemoradiation, these tumors were treated surgically either via transoral or open approaches. These approaches had several limitations. Transoral approaches were technically challenging due to limitations in visualization and the acquisition of hemostasis, frequently resulting in incomplete resections. Open approaches were looked upon unfavorably due to the relatively high morbidity associated with lip split and mandibulotomy required for access, in addition to the need for tracheotomy and gastrostomy tubes.

Following the results of the VA and ECOG trials in the 1990s, there was a large paradigm shift in the utilization of chemotherapy and radiation therapy for the treatment of squamous cell cancer of the upper aerodigestive tracts. While these trials were designed to demonstrate the efficacy of organ preservation therapy in the larynx, the results were quickly applied to other head and neck subsites. The tongue base and its associated malignancies, as much as any other subsite, served as an area ripe for the application of chemoradiation approaches due to the aforementioned obstacles associated with surgical resection. Consequently, chemoradiation was readily adopted and applied to treat patients with SCC of the tongue base.

Chemoradiation has resulted in equivalent oncologic control rates to those of open resection techniques [1]. With the success of chemoradiation techniques and the aforementioned challenges associated with older transoral and open techniques, surgery was mostly relegated to application in salvage scenarios. In spite of its increased utilization, chemoradiation has its drawbacks due to significant short- and long-term toxicities, most notably described in Machtay et al.'s review of the RTOG intensification trials, with severe late toxicity rates of 43 % [2]. HPV-induced SCC tends to occur in younger and healthier patients than their historical counterparts whose tumors were due to tobacco and alcohol exposure. Additionally, HPV-induced SCC has a more favorable prognosis. Both of these factors result in longer disease-free survival for patients after completing their treatment. As such, researchers have focused not only on oncologic control but also on functional outcomes and long-term sequela of cancer treatments. In this setting, researchers have turned back to the application of surgery in less invasive approaches to

J.K. Rasamny, MD
Department of Otolaryngology, Westchester Medical Center, Valhalla, NY, USA
email: JK.Rasamny@wmchealth.org

J.G. Newman, MD
Department of Otorhinolaryngology, Head and Neck Surgery Center for Cranial Base Surgery, University of Pennsylvania, Philadelphia, PA, USA

Z. Gil et al. (eds.), *Atlas of Head and Neck Robotic Surgery*, DOI 10.1007/978-3-319-49578-1_8

the treatment of tongue base cancers in hopes of maintaining excellent oncologic control and improving long-term functional outcomes.

Recently, there have been noted innovations in minimally invasive approaches to the tongue base, including transoral laser and robotic resections. Technological improvements, particularly in the field of transoral robotic surgery, have resulted in superior visualization due to innovations in the optics of the endoscopes, tremor filtration, motion scaling, and increasingly agile instrument movements [3]. When compared to prior open techniques, transoral approaches offer several benefits including decreased morbidity, decreased blood loss, shorter operative times, and decreased hospital stay [4]. The application of surgery when compared to chemoradiation demonstrates equivalent oncologic control with several studies reporting improved quality of life scores and long-term functional outcomes, particularly pertaining to decreased rates of PEG dependency [5, 6]. Consequently, there has been a trend in multiple centers nationally toward a new algorithm in the treatment of tongue base cancer where surgery is applied as the primary treatment modality [7].

8.2 Surgical Algorithm

The new algorithm of applying surgery up front in the treatment of tongue base cancers utilizes neck dissection as well as transoral resection of the primary lesion. Patients with tongue base cancers are first assessed with the in-office examination, including a flexible fiberoptic examination and palpation of the tongue base lesion to assess the extent of the tumor. Accurate understanding of the extent of the tumor requires cross-sectional imaging modalities including contrasted CT scan and MRI in addition to PET scans. The authors prefer to apply MRI to the assessment of all tongue base lesions given the superior soft tissue detail afforded, particularly as it relates to the lingual pedicle as well as the ability to assess the extent toward the midline of the tongue base. After office examination and the acquisition of axial imaging techniques, patients will frequently undergo a staging endoscopy under anesthesia, thereby permitting assessment of the extent of the primary, confirmation of the pathologic diagnosis, and ensuring adequate exposure can be obtained to perform a transoral resection. Following a staging examination, the patient can be scheduled for resection of both the primary tumor and the draining regional lymphatics. While neck dissection is beyond the scope of this chapter, surgeons have the options of either staged or concurrent neck dissection often combined with ligation of the external carotid arterial supply to the area of the primary. The authors prefer to perform a staged neck dissection one to weeks prior to the transoral resection to ligate the feeding arterial supply which in the case of tongue base lesions would include the facial and lingual arteries, as well as the superior laryngeal arterial branch from the superior thyroid artery which often supplies the vallecula.

In 2009, the FDA approved the use of the da Vinci robot for resections of T1 and T2 tongue base cancers. These cancers are ideal candidates for transoral robotic resections. There are oncologic, vascular, functional, and patient-specific contraindications that must be considered prior to resection. Oncologic contraindications include T4b disease, fixation to the retro- or parapharyngeal tissues, unresectable neck disease, and distant metastatic disease. Vascular contraindications within the tongue base include the need to spare the contralateral lingual vascular pedicle. In order to preserve swallowing function, tumors that extend beyond 50 % of the tongue base are considered poor surgical candidates due to the risk of future aspiration risks. Finally, patients may have their own specific contraindications such as trismus that precludes adequate exposure and medical comorbidities such as the need for anticoagulation which would result in unacceptable postoperative hemorrhage risks. If none of these conditions exist, then the patient is considered a candidate for resection.

8.3 Patient Setup

The patients should be intubated by an experienced anesthesiologist often with the use of a GlideScope or other fiberoptic approaches as injury to the tongue base during intubation may result in hemorrhage and an unsafe airway. A wire-reinforced endotracheal tube is required that should be secured contralaterally; our preference is to sew the tube to the contralateral melolabial crease to ensure it is not dislodged during the resection. The OR table is rotated 180° to allow for proper docking of the robot and its arms. Adequate eye protection is mandatory to reduce the risk of corneal injury. The patient should be completely paralyzed. Our preference is to give antibiotic prophylaxis with broad-spectrum antibiotics that cover anaerobes within the upper aerodigestive tract. Our protocol includes the use of Unasyn in penicillin-tolerant patients and clindamycin in penicillin-allergic patients.

The next step is proper exposure of the primary. A tongue stitch is applied anteriorly to retract the tongue anteriorly and aid in placement of the retractor. For tongue base cancers, we prefer the FK-WO retractor, while occasionally the Crowe-Davis retractor may be applied instead. Adequate exposure includes visualization of an acceptable cuff of tongue base anteriorly to ensure a clear margin as well the epiglottis to aid in the medial and inferior incisions through the vallecula. The retractor must be adequately stabilized by a side-arm device. After adequate visualization is obtained, the endotracheal tube is secured between the contralateral oral tongue and the retromolar trigone with a silk suture that we keep long and attached to a clamp so it is not forgotten about during extubation (Fig. 8.1).

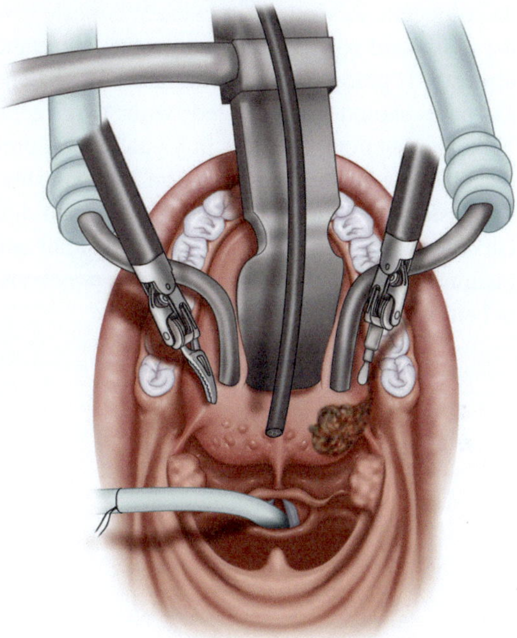

Fig. 8.1 Set up. View from head of bed with intubated patient in suspension with robotic arms in proper orientation, demonstrating suture securing endotracheal tube and tongue suture

8.4 Robot Setup

We typically use the 30° telescope for tongue base resections, as it more easily obtains a clear view of the anterior and deep margins during the resection. Without the 30° scope, surgeons may have the tendency to carry their anterior cut too superficial and risk transecting the specimen in the vallecula. A spatula tip cautery is placed on the ipsilateral robotic arm, while the Maryland dissector is placed on the contralateral arm. The assistant should be outfitted with two metal Yankauer suctions to assist in visualization during bleeding as well as retraction for exposure. The assistant will require both right and left curved manual clip appliers with both small and medium clips. Finally, a suction Bovie may assist in hemostasis.

8.5 Intraoperative Details

The following details our approach for resecting tongue base tumors; however we recognize that some natural variability exists due to individual surgeon preference. Our approach has always been to perform a standard resection in the same manner each time to make the resection easier to replicate for training the novice robotic surgeon. While other surgeons may approach the resection in a different order, the final defect should be identical.

First, an anterior cut is performed along the retractor taking care to carry the cut deep into tongue musculature. It is important to carefully note the extent of the preoperative imaging and utilize the excellent optics of robotic system to assess that tissue is clear of disease during dissection through deep tongue muscle (Fig. 8.2).

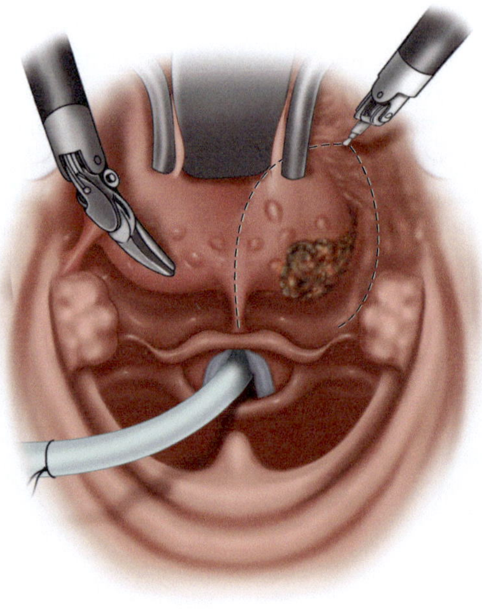

Fig. 8.2 Exposure. Exposed view of the tongue base after proper retractor placement

Next, the lateral cut is performed through the inferior aspect of the tonsil and constrictor with the exact location based upon the lateral extent of tumor. The incision is carried through to the styloglossus. Next, the styloglossus is divided by elevating the muscle with the spatula tip and grasping with Maryland prior to cutting on the Maryland with cautery. The lingual artery is identified deep and lateral, and several clips are applied; meticulous hemostasis is critical (Fig. 8.3).

Next, the medial cut is performed and carried through the midline of tongue base ensuring an adequate cuff of mucosa to obtain a clear margin. The incision is carried deep into the tongue base musculature and taken through to the inferior extent of the vallecula at the epiglottis. Finally, the posterior incision is made along posterior/inferior extent of the vallecular mucosa, often sacrificing mucosa along lingual surface of the epiglottis to obtain a clear inferior/posterior margin of mucosa. As mentioned earlier, exposure is key; as in an ideal scenario, the epiglottis will be visualized to ensure cut is carried through the vallecular mucosa in the proper location so that the malignancy is not transected prematurely (Fig. 8.4).

After the specimen has been completely extirpated, it is carefully oriented in vivo and carried to a side table where it is closely examined by the surgeon to assess for a grossly clear margin. If there is a close margin on exam, our approach is to apply methylene blue to the defect and excise an additional cuff of mucosa and deep tongue base muscle.

The specimen is then carried directly to pathology where the surgeon orients the specimen for the pathologist and observes the inking of the margins. The tumor is then incised vertically and horizontally to assess the deep margin. If necessary, the surgeon may have to repeat the inking of the defect and acquisition of additional deep tissue to obtain a clear margin.

Following the resection, attention is turned to hemostasis and reconstruction. Throughout the case, hemostasis is paramount. It is obtained with use of the robotic cautery and clips applied by the bedside assistant. Occasionally, suction Bovie electrocautery can be helpful as well. The defect is aggressively irrigated and Valsalva maneuvers are performed. Finally, our preference is to apply a hemostatic reagent to the defect; we have had success with Arista AH Hemostat®. In terms of reconstruction, the tongue base is left to granulate on its own, while a small pharyngoplasty may be performed as needed with horizontal mattress Vicryl sutures through the lateral aspect of the defect to reconstruct the resected tonsillar fossa laterally (Fig. 8.5).

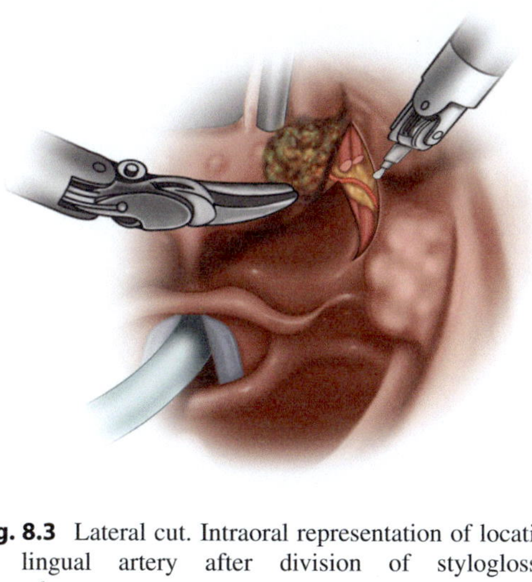

Fig. 8.3 Lateral cut. Intraoral representation of location of lingual artery after division of styloglossus musculature

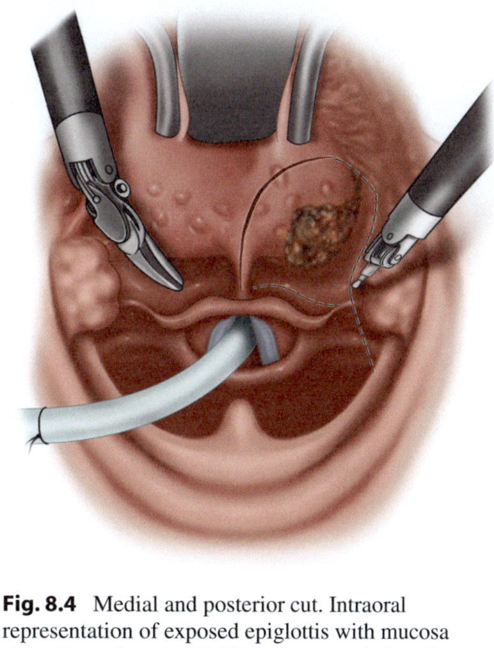

Fig. 8.4 Medial and posterior cut. Intraoral representation of exposed epiglottis with mucosa along lingual aspect divided after completing the medial incision

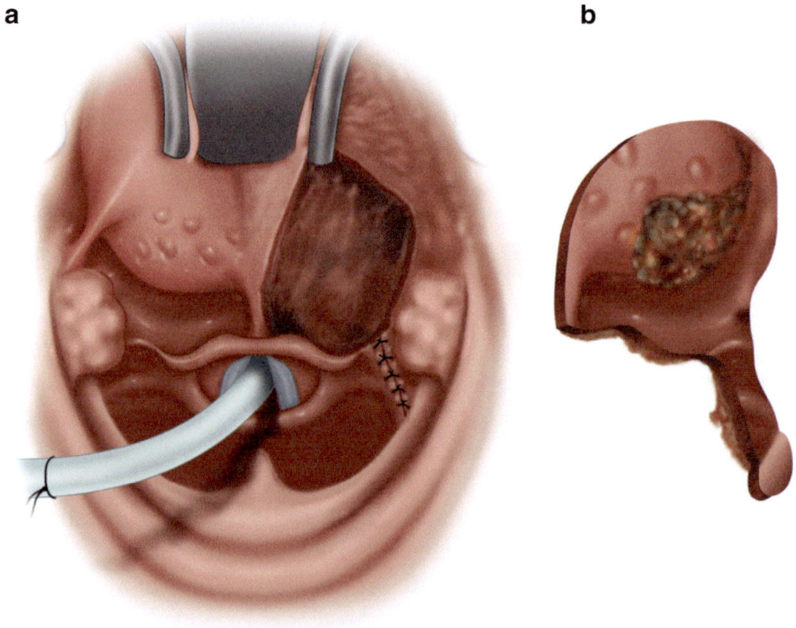

Fig. 8.5 Resection bed and reconstruction. (**a**) Surgical defect with exposed epiglottis and tongue base margins as well as pharyngoplasty completed along inferior tonsillar pole. (**b**) Excised specimen with labels

8.6 Perioperative Considerations

8.6.1 Airway Concerns

Tongue base resections distort anatomy making intubation in the postoperative period quite difficult and dangerous, particularly if accompanied by postoperative hemorrhage. As such, our early protocol was to keep all tongue base resections intubated for 48–72 h postoperatively. Currently, patients are being extubated more liberally after this procedure, but judicious management is the rule. In cases for which we anticipate the patient remaining intubated, we remove the robotic arms as well as the retractors and perform a direct laryngoscopy to place the patient into suspension. With the patient suspended, we place a dual-port endotracheal tube over a 0° endoscope prior to removal of the original reinforced endotracheal tube. Once the appropriate location is verified, the original tube is removed. The advantage of the new endotracheal tube is the second lumen represents a suction port to allow for clearance of the pharyngeal secretions above the cuff of the balloon by attaching the suction port to wall suction in the postoperative period. This obviates the need for nursing or respiratory care to perform deep suctioning at the bedside in a patient with a healing tongue base defect. Finally, a nasogastric tube is placed for enteral access in the recovery period. The tube is secured with transeptal sutures to decrease the likelihood of displacement, as replacement at bedside in the freshly operated field is challenging and could lead to bleeding. Other centers routinely extubate patients postoperatively, and if there is concern for progressive airway edema, a tracheostomy should be strongly considered.

8.7 Postoperative Care

The patient is then transported to the ICU. Our protocol in the vast majority of tongue base resections is to keep the patient intubated for 48–72 h postoperatively. The patient is started on PCA analgesics and enteral feeding is slowly advanced. If the drainage from the suction port is minimal, then the patients are extubated and observed for a short period in the ICU. After transfer to floor status, they are evaluated by our speech and swallow team, typically on POD 3. If they pass their evaluation, then oral feedings are initiated. The NGT stays in place until the patient is adequately able to maintain their hydration and pain control with PO intake. The typical tongue base resection patient is discharged on POD 4–5. If the choice is made to extubate in the OR, patients are closely monitored and allowed to initiate small amounts of oral intake in the postoperative period. The nasogastric tube is removed when adequate fluid intake is achieved.

References

1. Parsons JT, Mendenhall WM, Stringer SP, et al. Squamous cell carcinoma of the oropharynx. Cancer. 2002;94(11):2967–80.
2. Machtay M, Moughan J, Trotti A, et al. Factors associated with severe late toxicity after concurrent chemoradiation for locally advanced head and neck cancer: an RTOG analysis. J Clin Oncol. 2008;26:3582–9.
3. Weinstein GS, O'Malley Jr BW, Snyder W, Sherman E, Quon H. Transoral robotic surgery: radical tonsillectomy. Arch Otolaryngol Head Neck Surg. 2007;133(12):1220–6.
4. Dean NR, Rosenthal EL, Carroll WR, et al. Robotic-assisted surgery for primary or recurrent oropharyngeal carcinoma. Arch Otolaryngol Head Neck Surg. 2010;136(4):380–4.
5. Leonhardt FD, Quon H, Abrahão M, O'Malley BW, Weinstein GS. Transoral robotic surgery for oropharyngeal carcinoma and its impact on patient-reported quality of life and function. Head Neck. 2012;34(2):146–54. doi:10.1002/hed.21688.
6. Dziegielewski PT, Teknos TN, Durmus K, et al. Transoral robotic surgery for oropharyngeal cancer: long-term quality of life and functional outcomes. JAMA Otolaryngol Head Neck Surg. 2013;139(11): 1099–108.
7. de Almeida JR, Li R, Magnuson J, et al. Oncologic outcomes after transoral robotic surgery: a multi-institutional study. JAMA Otolaryngol Head Neck Surg. 2015;141(12):1043–51.

Laryngeal Robotic Surgery

9

James R. Bekeny and Enver Ozer

9.1 Background

Laryngeal cancer has seen a variety of treatment modalities through history. Originally in a surgical disease managed by total laryngectomy, larynx-preserving treatments evolved with the development of partial laryngectomy techniques (both open and endoscopic). These partial techniques allow for the maintenance of a unified aerodigestive tract through which a patient is able to phonate, breath, and swallow. Since the publication of the Department of Veterans Affairs Laryngeal Cancer Study Group results, showing patients with advanced laryngeal cancer who received chemoradiation therapy had equivalent survival to patients treated surgically, and 64% of patients were able to preserve their laryngeal function for some period of time after surgery [1]. Therefore, partial laryngeal surgery and total laryngectomy became less commonplace as chemoradiation became the favored treatment modality for early-stage disease. Initial laryngectomy does tend toward improved survival in patients with T4 disease, and generally these patients have poor function to begin with and are good candidates for laryngectomy [2]. As patients who have received chemoradiation are followed longer, late complications of chemoradiation therapy have been found to be extremely debilitating, causing long-term problems with swallowing, breathing, and vocal function. The addition of chemotherapy to radiation improves survival between 8% and 15% [3], but also increases the severity of the functional side effects [4]. These effects significantly impact patient quality of life, and a significant portion of patients ultimately requires total laryngectomy for nonfunctional larynx [5]. Therefore, there is an increasing interest in minimally invasive partial laryngeal surgery to treat limited disease and prevent the need for functionally devastating adjuvant treatment.

As for minimally invasive, natural orifice surgery, there are two major treatment modalities for the larynx: transoral laser microsurgery (TLM) and transoral robotic surgery (TORS). TLM has a fairly long history, with descriptions of use for laryngeal cancers as early as 2002 [6]. TLM has been shown to be successful and equivalent to open partial laryngeal surgery in terms of survival and cure of primary cancer with excellent

J.R. Bekeny
Head and Neck Surgical Oncology & Microvascular Reconstruction, Florida Hospital Celebration, 410 Celebration Place, Suite #305, Celebration, FL, USA
e-mail: bekeny.james@gmail.com

E. Ozer, MD (✉)
Department of Otolaryngology- Head and Neck Surgery, Wexner Medical Center at the Ohio State University, Starling Loving Hall – Room B221, 320 West 10th Avenue, Columbus, OH 43210, USA
e-mail: Enver.ozer@osumc.edu

Z. Gil et al. (eds.), *Atlas of Head and Neck Robotic Surgery*, DOI 10.1007/978-3-319-49578-1_9

functional outcomes [7–14]. In TLM, a microscope, laser, and microdissection instruments are used to remove tumor through a rigid endoscope. Generally the tumor is removed in sections, and the margins are evaluated intraoperatively to insure clearance of the tumor. TORS for laryngeal surgery on the other hand has a more limited history. Initial work in 2005 in a canine model showed the ability to perform glottic and supraglottic procedures with the assistance of the da Vinci robot [15, 16]. The first case series of supraglottic laryngectomy in three humans was published in 2007 by Weinstein et al. [17]. TORS differs from laser microsurgery in several regards. First, a binocular endoscope provides a high-definition three-dimensional image of the surgical field. Second, the wristed action of the instruments allows for increased dexterity. Furthermore, the robot can reduce tremor allowing for increased precision. These attributes often allow the tumor to be completely resected under direct visualization. There has been no direct study of survival or functional outcomes comparing TLM and TORS. However, these endoscopic methods have improved swallowing outcomes as compared to chemoradiation therapy [11, 18–22]. With transoral robotic resection of the supraglottic larynx, the need for tracheostomy, as standard in open partial laryngeal surgery, is avoided. This chapter will focus on the current status and future of robotic laryngeal surgery.

9.2 Anatomical Considerations

The larynx is the gatekeeper to the airway and has three important functions. First, the larynx must divert solid and liquid boluses from the airway and into the hypopharynx. Second, it must open to allow air passage during respiration. Finally, it must allow contact of mucosal edges to generate acoustic vibration during phonation. The ultimate goal of partial laryngeal surgery is to maintain a unified aerodigestive tract and preserve these three functions. Therefore, patients should have an intact glottis with normally functioning vocal cords to be a candidate for TORS supraglottic laryngectomy and expect a reasonable functional outcome. The glottic level is the only barrier to aspiration after supraglottic laryngectomy and thus must be preserved.

As with all transoral surgery, the surgeon must be familiar with inside-out anatomy when performing robotic laryngeal surgery. In this chapter, we focus on the supraglottic larynx where robotic surgery has proven most useful to date. The supraglottic larynx is comprised of the laryngeal surface of the epiglottis, the aryepiglottic folds, the arytenoids, the false vocal cords, and the laryngeal ventricle. The region is bound by the vallecula, preepiglottic space, and hyoid bone anteriorly, the pharynx and hypopharynx posteriorly, and the true vocal cords inferiorly. The anatomical subunit removed in

TORS supraglottic laryngectomy includes the epiglottis, the preepiglottic space and paraglottic space contents, the aryepiglottic folds, the false vocal cords, and the ventricular mucosa. Extended approaches can be utilized where a small amount of tongue base, limited portions of the medial piriform sinus wall, and small amounts of arytenoid mucosa can be resected to gain adequate margins.

Endoscopic inspection of the supraglottis reveals the pharyngoepiglottic fold, through which runs the superior laryngeal artery and the internal branch of the superior laryngeal nerve as seen in Fig. 9.1. This neurovascular bundle provides the majority of the blood flow and sensory input to the supraglottic larynx. Surgical control of the artery and its branches with either hemoclips or electrocautery is essential to prevent postoperative bleeding complications. In our experience, branches of the artery medial to the hyoid bone can be controlled with targeted electrocautery alone. Any branches of the superior laryngeal nerve should be preserved if possible to allow for sensation to the superior glottis to help with prevention of aspiration. However, it often must be transected to allow for appropriate oncologic resection [23].

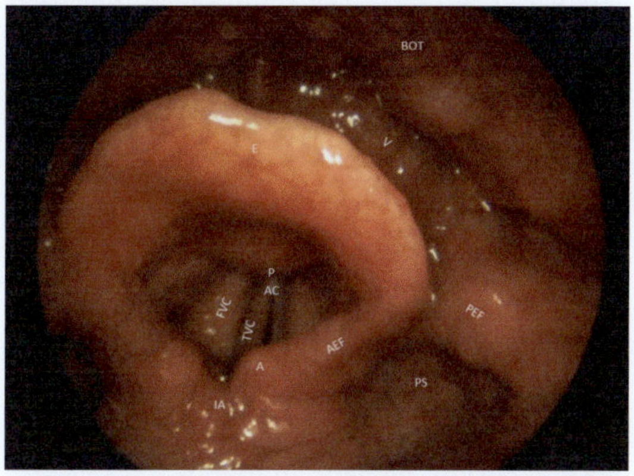

Fig. 9.1 Endoscopic view of the normal larynx, labeled with surface anatomy. base of tongue (BOT); Vallecula (V); Petiole (P); false vocal cord (FVC); true vocal cord (TVC); arytenoid (A); aryepiglottic fold (AEF); epiglottis (E); Anterior commussure (AC); interarytenoid (IA); Pyriform sinus (PS); Pyriform epiglottis fold (PEF)

9.3 Preoperative Planning

Through experience with open partial laryngectomy and TLM procedures, guidelines for patient selection for transoral supraglottic laryngectomy have been developed. The authors have organized this into inclusion and exclusion criteria as shown in Table 9.1 and Table 9.2 [24]. TORS supraglottic laryngectomy is not necessarily contraindicated in patients with a history of prior radiation therapy; however, exposure may be challenging secondary to trismus and neck scarring, and tissue planes may not be well preserved.

Exposure of the supraglottis is perhaps the most challenging portion of a transoral robotic supraglottic laryngectomy. There are several major commercial retractors for obtaining adequate exposure, namely, the Feyh-Kastenbauer retractor, the Fentex Medical LARS retractor, and the Medrobotics Flex retractor. The LARS and Flex retractors were designed specifically for robotic use, whereas the Feyh-Kastenbauer retractor predates transoral robotic surgery and was modified by O'Malley and Weinstein for use in TORS. Both are adequate and retractor selection is ultimately a matter of personal preference. It is a luxury to have both available to optimize exposure in individual patients. Placing the operating bed in a slight Trendelenburg position may be useful in accommodating the robotic arms.

Often when exposure is difficult, the instinct is to open the retractor as wide as possible. However, experience indicates that increasing the mouth opening at the level of the teeth is not helpful in better exposing the supraglottic larynx and is in fact counterproductive. As the mouth opens wider, the tongue blade actually begins to rotate toward the posterior pharyngeal wall blocking access for the endoscope and robotic arms. The key to exposure is opening the mouth just enough to allow entry of the instruments while lifting the tongue base forward. As compared to oropharyngeal exposure, the angle of the workspace is more parallel to the axis of the posterior pharyngeal wall as shown in Fig. 9.2.

Table 9.1 Indications for TORS-SGL

T1 or T2 supraglottic carcinoma
Selected T3 supraglottic carcinoma
Preepiglottic space invasion
Ability to preserve 50% of the tongue base with an oncological resection
Mobile vocal cords
Minimal piriform sinus involvement
Ability to achieve adequate transoral exposure of the tumor and its margins

Table 9.2 Contraindications for TORS-SGL

Vocal cord fixation
Bilateral arytenoid cartilage involvement
Thyroid or cricoid cartilage involvement
Anterior or posterior commissure involvement
Poor pulmonary reserve (FEV1/FVC <50%)

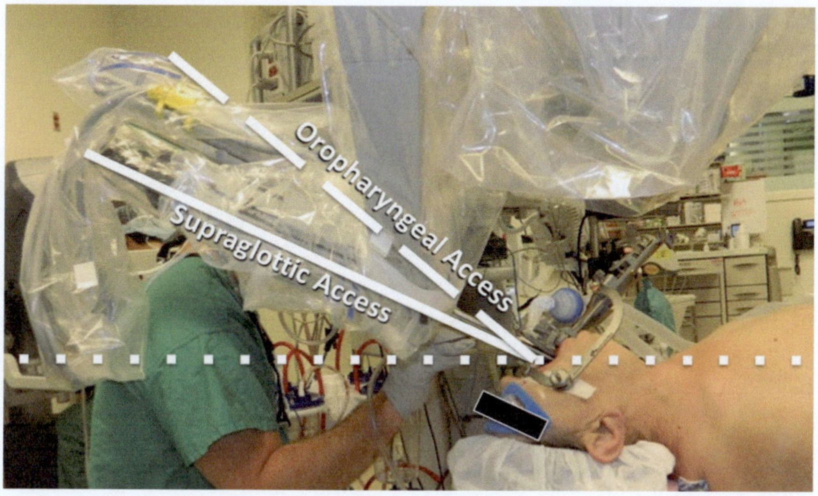

Fig. 9.2 Positioning of the robotic arms for TORS supraglottic laryngectomy differs as compared to oropharyngeal surgery. The angle of approach is less steep as demonstrated in this diagram. The dotted line represents the long access of the patient's body. The dashed line represents the steep trajectory utilized for oropharyngeal TORS with a 0° endoscope. The solid line demonstrates the more gradual angulation of the robotic arms used to access the supraglottis and visualize this area with the 30° endoscope

9.4 Procedural Considerations for TORS Supraglottic Laryngectomy

Transnasal intubation is preferred for supraglottic laryngectomy, as this allows the tube to lie along the posterior pharyngeal wall. A reinforced or laser safe tube may be considered to decrease risk of violating the tube with the electrocautery. The fraction of inspired oxygen should be kept at or below 30% to prevent airway fires while electrocautery is being utilized. Intraoperative airway dose steroids (i.e., 10 mg dexamethasone IV) are given to help reduce edema.

An articulating Bovie, a Maryland dissector, and an anteriorly facing 30-degree endoscope are the most commonly utilized instruments for this procedure. An assistant at the head of the bed, as seen in Fig. 9.2, utilizes two Yankauer suctions to evacuate smoke, secretions, and blood, while also providing additional tissue retraction as needed.

The preferred retractor is placed carefully into the oral cavity, using caution to prevent damage to the teeth and lips. Once the retractor is in place, the 30-degree endoscope can be used to check the exposure before docking the robot.

Once exposure is adequate, the robot is docked and the arms are positioned. The Bovie and the Maryland dissector may need to be switched at some point through the case to prevent crossing of the robotic arms and to provide adequate tissue retraction.

Some authors have advocated splitting the supraglottic laryngectomy specimen and begin the procedure by dividing the epiglottis down the midline. With adequate exposure, the authors advocate for an en bloc resection.

9.5 Step-by-Step TORS Supraglottic Laryngectomy

A case example is given here to demonstrate the steps of a TORS supraglottic laryngectomy. Figure 9.3 demonstrates the preoperative in office endoscopy showing a supraglottic tumor on the laryngeal surface of the epiglottis. Figure 9.4 shows the step-by-step procedure with corresponding commentary below.

Image 1 Robotic exposure of the supraglottic larynx is shown here. The tongue blade is placed in the vallecula holding the tongue base forward. The ulcerative lesion can be seen on the laryngeal surface of the epiglottis. A reinforced endotracheal tube is utilized to prevent damage to the tube and decrease risk of airway fire

Image 2 Prior to making mucosal incisions, the tumor is inspected under 3D HD visualization to verify candidacy for TORS supraglottic laryngectomy. Demonstrated here the right arytenoid complex and true vocal cord are visualized to ensure they are free of tumor. Other key areas to examine include the anterior commissure, the vallecula, and the contralateral arytenoid and true vocal cord

Image 3 The right-sided mucosal incision is made in the vallecula and toward the tongue base, cutting toward the tongue blade. As this area is traversed, the branches of the superior laryngeal neurovascular bundle may be encountered. Generally the bleeding can be controlled with electrocautery when these vessels are transected medial to the hyoid bone. Any large vessels should be controlled with hemoclips applied transorally

Image 4 A similar mucosal incision is made in the contralateral lateral vallecular region and onto the tongue base. This incision is deepened down and carried forward including a small cuff of tongue base anterior to the vallecula

Image 5 Dissection is carried on in an anterior direction, almost cutting upward and beyond the tip of the tongue blade as shown here. The internal surface of the hyoid bone should be identified. The hyoid can be identified by palpation of the tissue with the robot. This results in mass movement of the entire hyoid bone, making a bilateral mass movement that is distinct from the movement seen when palpating soft tissue alone. Transcervical palpation can also aid in identification of the hyoid bone. Note that the tongue blade can push the hyoid bone anteriorly, and the hyoid will not be encountered with dissection, as it will be on the other side of the retractor. Adjusting the retractor to release the hyoid bone may be necessary

Image 6 Here the two vallecular cuts have been joined in the midline. Dissection has been carried down to reveal the superior border of the thyroid cartilage. Again, palpation is useful in identifying this landmark. At this point, the pre-epiglottic contents are removed off of the internal aspect of the thyroid cartilage. Dissection is carried only partially inferiorly in this region to prevent disruption of the anterior commissure

Image 7 With the anterior attachments released, dissection focuses on the posterior aspect attachments. In this example, the lesion was essentially midline; however, it is generally best to start on the side with the least amount of disease. As the procedure continues, the exposure of the contralateral side will improve allowing for better determination of adequate margins

Image 8 Here the aryepiglottic fold is being transected just anterior to the arytenoid complex. Small portions of the superior arytenoid and the arytenoid mucosa can be resected to gain adequate margins. At times, extension of these cuts onto the medial wall of the piriform sinus and removing some of this mucosa may be necessary

Image 9 The paraglottic space contents and false cords are released from their posterior attachments near the arytenoid, and the ventricle is identified. Here the posterior aspect of the laryngeal ventricle is being entered. Anterior to the Bovie tip, a small hole in the false cord can be seen showing the ventricular space and the true vocal cord lying below

Image 10 The dissection is then carried forward toward the anterior commissure, releasing all of the paraglottic space contents on the right. The anterior commissure is checked carefully again to ensure the disease is completely cleared

Image 11 The petiole region is divided and the contralateral vocal cord is now visible. Anterior attachments are divided at the level of the laryngeal ventricle. Placing the tip of the electrocautery in the ventricle and cutting upward through the false cord, while ensuring no contact with the true vocal cord below, can be a useful maneuver to release this area

Image 12 Now the posterior cuts are made on the contralateral arytenoid region. Here a mucosal incision from the posterior ventricle along the anterior surface of the arytenoid is made leaving the arytenoid and its mucosa intact

Image 13 The remaining lateral attachments of the paraglottic space contents, false cords, and ventricular mucosa are released

Image 14 The specimen is nearly free at this point and the uninjured vocal cord can be seen deep to the ventricle

Image 15 The assistant grasps the tip of the epiglottis to remove the supraglottis en bloc. The orientation of the lesion is noted prior to removal from the pharynx. The specimen should be immediately oriented with sutures or surgical clips once it is removed

Image 16 The final defect shows the bilateral true vocal cords and preserved arytenoids with absent false cords and the surrounding paraglottic tissues. The anterior commissure is preserved without injury

Following removal of the specimen, margins may be taken from the specimen itself or from the surgical bed. Taking adequate tissue and preventing char are critical in margin analysis. Often standard cupped forceps can be utilized to take samples from the margins and prevent further cautery artifact. The surgical site is then irrigated copiously and complete hemostasis is achieved.

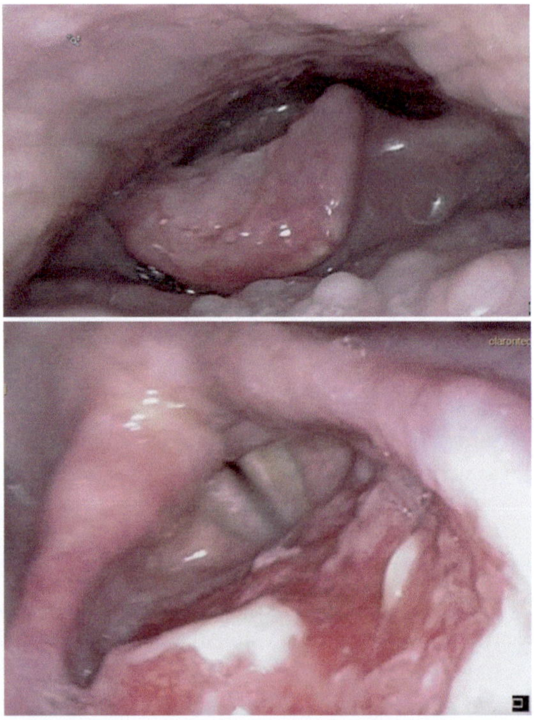

Fig. 9.3 Preoperative endoscopy demonstrating an ulcerative lesion on the laryngeal surface of the epiglottis. Preoperative evaluation consists of careful inspection of the lesion to determine candidacy for supraglottic laryngectomy. The arytenoids, aryepiglottic folds, vallecula, tongue base, piriform sinuses, anterior commissure, and true vocal cords. Here there is ulceration extending to the tip of the epiglottis from the laryngeal surface; however, the lingual surface, vallecula, and tongue base are clear. The disease is contained within the limits of the aryepiglottic folds and extends toward the anterior commissure, but on closer inspection (not shown here), there was adequate margin between the lesion and the commissure

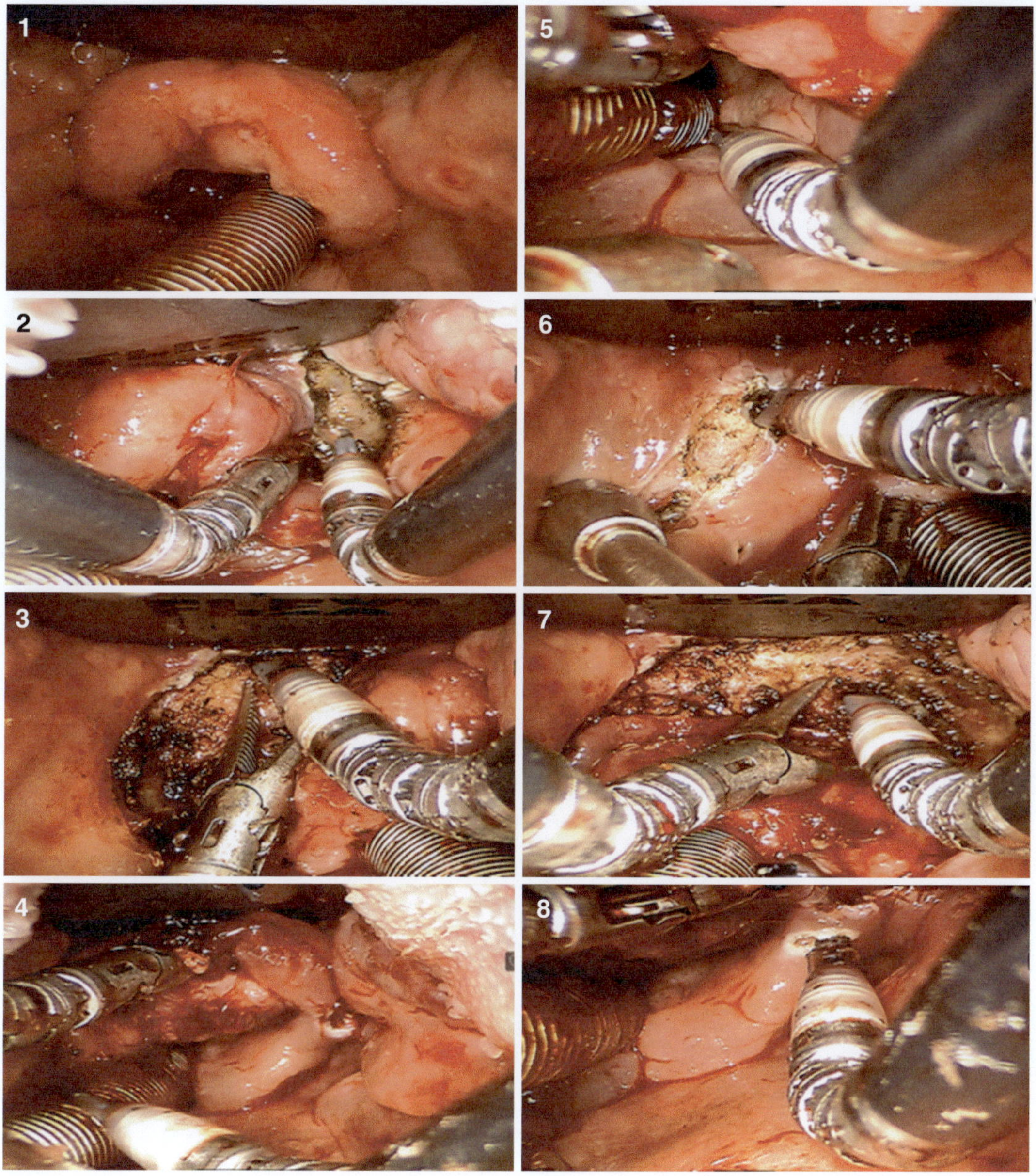

Fig. 9.4 Step-by-step TORS supraglottic laryngectomy intraoperative photos. See text for descriptions of each step depicted

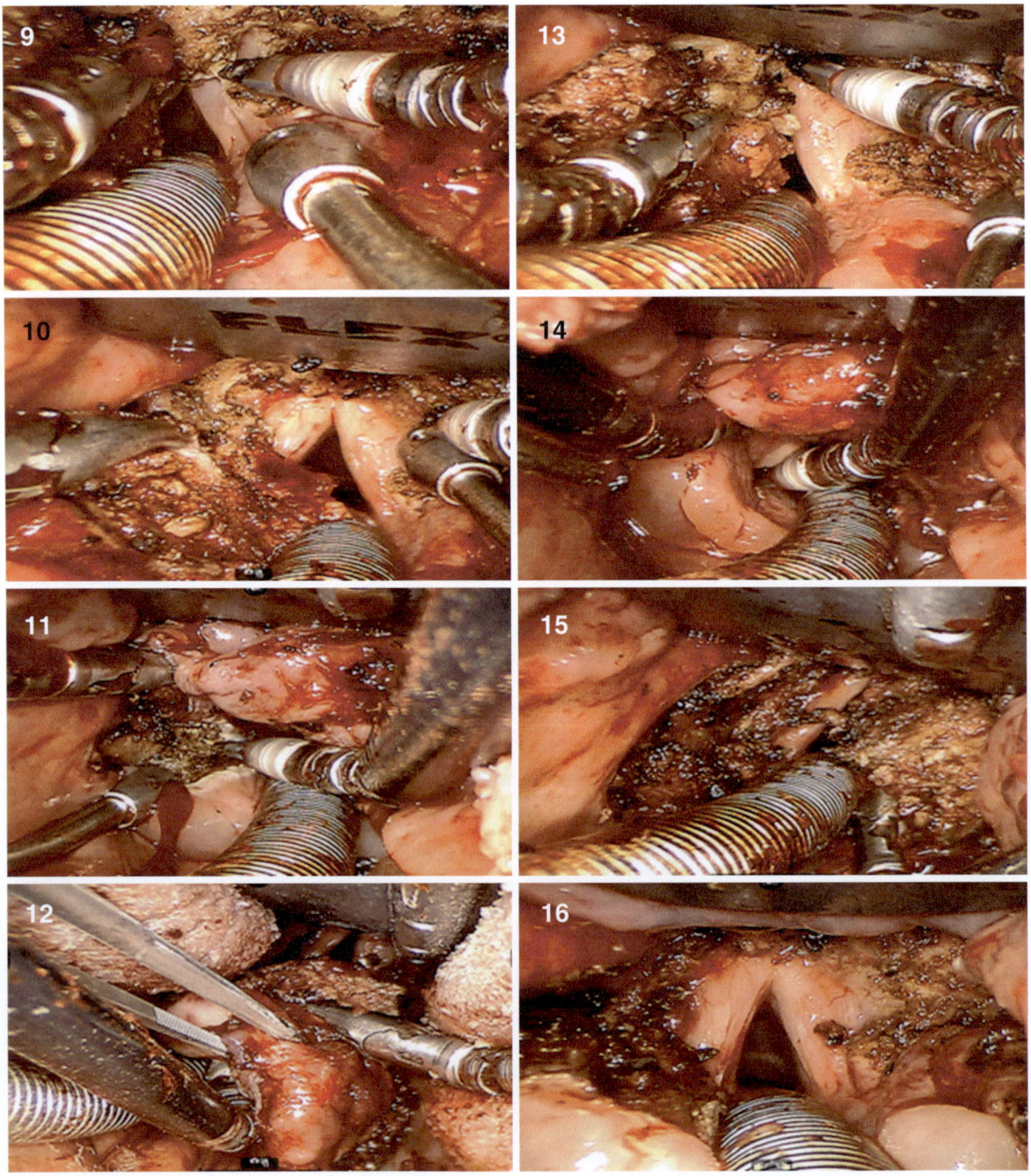

Fig. 9.4 (continued)

9.6 Postoperative Considerations

Patients are generally able to be extubated in the operating room; however, delayed intubation may be considered if the surgeon has concern for airway obstruction postoperatively. Following recovery from anesthesia, patients are transferred to a monitored unit. Emergency airway equipment should be readily available. Dexamethasone can be given at an interval of every 6–8 h to assist with airway edema during the first 24–48 h. Three days of antibiotics and 6 weeks of proton pump inhibitors are prescribed during the postoperative phase. The speech and swallow therapy team sees the patient on postoperative day one, and a bedside swallow evaluation is conducted, and the diet is advanced as tolerated. The majority of these patients are able to resume adequate nutrition transorally and a nasogastric tube is not required.

Patients are discharged from the hospital once they achieve adequate nutrition either orally or via nasogastric tube, vital signs are stable, and pain is controlled. Average hospital stay at the author's institution is 4 days [18, 24].

9.7 Complications of TORS Supraglottic Laryngectomy

Complications arising from TORS supraglottic laryngectomy are no different than other TORS subsites. Airway compromise and bleeding are two major immediate postoperative concerns, and they should be managed as in other subsites. Acute airway compromise warrants reintubation. Bleeding patients should be intubated or have a tracheostomy performed to protect the airway. Bleeding should be controlled in the operative setting using electrocautery and hemoclips as indicated. Endovascular or open control of cervical blood vessels may also be indicated if transoral control cannot be obtained. Late complications include dysphagia, dysphonia, and laryngeal stricture. Dysphagia and dysphonia are managed conservatively with the use of speech and swallow therapy. Laryngeal stricture may require revision surgery with lysis of adhesions. During the initial procedure, care should be taken to prevent violation of opposing mucosal surfaces to prevent adhesive scarring. The anterior and posterior commissures are most prone to this type of scarring.

9.8 Outcomes of TORS Supraglottic Laryngectomy

Robotic supraglottic laryngectomy is now a standard TORS procedure, although compared to oropharyngeal TORS, there is substantially less data. Ozer et al. published a case series of 13 patients who underwent TORS supraglottic laryngectomy demonstrating safety and good functional outcomes. All 13 patients were able to be resected to negative margins and 11 were able to tolerate an oral diet within 24 h [18]. Survival data in this population is limited, with Olsen first reporting a 2-year disease-specific survival of 88% in 9 patients [25] and Mendelsohn et al. reporting 2-year survival data in 18 patients (local regional control 83%, disease-specific survival 100%, overall survival 89%) [19]. Park et al. showed a 2 year disease-free survival rate of 91%. These patients were matched to a cohort of patients who underwent open supraglottic laryngectomy, and the TORS group demonstrated earlier oral feeding, decreased time to decannulation, and decreased hospital stay [26]. Factors predictive of difficulty with swallowing include being male, patients with T3 tumors, postoperative vocal fold hypomobility, or undergoing simultaneous neck dissection [19]. These results suggest that TORS supraglottic laryngectomy is a valuable tool for managing patients with supraglottic tumors and warrants continued study.

9.9 Frontiers in Laryngeal TORS

Several other robotic laryngeal procedures other than supraglottic laryngectomy have been described in the literature. These include cordectomy and the removal of an assortment of benign laryngeal lesions [27, 28, 29]. Perhaps the most intriguing newly described procedure is the robotic-assisted total laryngectomy. Smith et al. published a multi-institutional series of seven patients who underwent attempted transoral robotic laryngectomy [30, 31]. Five of the procedures were completed successfully, while two required conversion to a standard open approach. The authors suggest that this procedure might be particularly valuable in surgical salvage patients and in patients with nonfunctional larynx after radiation therapy. The limited dissection is thought to potentially lead to fewer wound healing complications. Further study is required before this technique will become widely endorsed. A description of the procedure can be found in the original articles [18, 19].

Conclusion

TORS laryngeal surgery is a useful tool for patients with laryngeal disease. Supraglottic laryngectomy has become a standard procedure for patients with limited supraglottic disease. To date, the results indicate equivalent local control and survival to other standard approaches. Outcomes also suggest acceptable morbidity of the TORS approach. The future role of robotic laryngeal surgery may include robot-assisted total laryngectomy. As technology improves and new robotic systems are developed, the ability to perform intricate tasks within the larynx will likely expand our abilities to better treat glottic and subglottic lesions.

References

1. Induction chemotherapy plus radiation compared with surgery plus radiation in patients with advanced laryngeal cancer. N Engl J Med. 1991;324(24):1685–90. doi:10.1056/NEJM199106133242402.
2. Gourin CG, Conger BT, Chris Sheils W, Bilodeau PA, Coleman TA, Porubsky ES. The effect of treatment on survival in patients with advanced laryngeal carcinoma. Laryngoscope. 2009;119(7):1312–7. doi:10.1002/lary.20477.
3. Pignon JP, le Maître A, Bourhis J, and MACH-NC Collaborative Group. Meta-analyses of chemotherapy in head and neck cancer (MACH-NC): an update. Int J Radiat Oncol Biol Phys. 2007;69(2 Suppl):S112–14. doi:10.1016/j.ijrobp.2007.04.088.
4. Machtay M, Moughan J, Trotti A, Garden AS, Weber RS, Cooper JS, Forastiere A, Ang KK. Factors associated with severe late toxicity after concurrent chemoradiation for locally advanced head and neck cancer: an RTOG analysis. J Clin Oncol. 2008;26(21):3582–9. doi:10.1200/JCO.2007.14.8841.
5. Theunissen EAR, Timmermans AJ, Zuur CL, Hamming-Vrieze O, de Boer JP, Hilgers FJM, van den Brekel MWM. Total laryngectomy for a dysfunctional larynx after (Chemo)radiotherapy. Arch Otolaryngol Head Neck Surg. 2012;138(6):548. doi:10.1001/archoto.2012.862.
6. Gallo A, de Vincentiis M, Manciocco V, Simonelli M, Fiorella ML, Shah JP. CO2 laser cordectomy for early-stage glottic carcinoma: a long-term follow-up of 156 cases. Laryngoscope. 2002;112(2):370–4. doi:10.1097/00005537-200202000-00030.
7. Lee HS, Chun B-G, Kim SW, Kim ST, Oh JH, Hong JC, Lee KD. Transoral laser microsurgery for early glottic cancer as one-stage single-modality therapy: transoral laser microsurgery. Laryngoscope. 2013;123(11):2670–4. doi:10.1002/lary.24080.
8. Arshad H, Jayaprakash V, Gupta V, Cohan DM, Ambujakshan D, Rigual NR, Singh AK, Hicks WL. Survival differences between organ preservation surgery and definitive radiotherapy in early supraglottic squamous cell carcinoma. Otolaryngol Head Neck Surg. 2014;150(2):237–44. doi:10.1177/0194599813512783.
9. Peretti G, Piazza C, Cocco D, De Benedetto L, Del Bon F, De Zinis LOR, Nicolai P. Transoral CO2 laser treatment for Tis-T3 glottic cancer: The University of Brescia experience on 595 patients. Head Neck. 2009;32(8):977–83. doi:10.1002/hed.21278.
10. Peretti G, Piazza C, Cattaneo A, De Benedetto L, Martin E, Nicolai P. Comparison of functional outcomes after endoscopic versus open-neck supraglottic laryngectomies. Ann Otol Rhinol Laryngol. 2006;115(11):827–32. doi:10.1177/000348940611501106.
11. Peretti G, Piazza C, Del Bon F, Mora R, Grazioli P, Barbieri D, Mangili S, Nicolai P. Function preservation using transoral laser surgery for T2–T3 glottic cancer: oncologic, vocal, and swallowing outcomes. Eur Arch Otorhinolaryngol. 2013;270(8):2275–81. doi:10.1007/s00405-013-2461-9.
12. Mantsopoulos K, Psychogios G, Koch M, Zenk J, Waldfahrer F, Iro H. Comparison of different surgical approaches in T2 glottic cancer. Head Neck. 2012;34(1):73–7. doi:10.1002/hed.21687.
13. Canis M, Martin A, Ihler F, Wolff HA, Kron M, Matthias C, Steiner W. Results of transoral laser microsurgery for supraglottic carcinoma in 277 patients. Eur Arch Otorhinolaryngol. 2013;270(8):2315–26. doi:10.1007/s00405-012-2327-6.
14. Bussu F, Almadori G, De Corso E, Rizzo D, Rigante M, Parrilla C, Valentini V, Paludetti G. Endoscopic horizontal partial laryngectomy by CO_2 laser in the management of supraglottic squamous cell carcinoma. Head Neck. 2009;31(9):1196–206. doi:10.1002/hed.21085.

15. O'Malley BW, Weinstein GS, Hockstein NG. Transoral robotic surgery (TORS): glottic microsurgery in a canine model. J Voice. 2006;20(2):263–8. doi:10.1016/j.jvoice.2005.10.004.
16. Weinstein GS, O'Malley BW, Hockstein NG. Transoral robotic surgery: supraglottic laryngectomy in a canine model. Laryngoscope. 2005;115(7):1315–9. doi:10.1097/01.MLG.0000170848.76045.47.
17. Weinstein GS, O'Malley BW, Snyder W, Hockstein NG. Transoral robotic surgery: supraglottic partial laryngectomy. Ann Otol Rhinol Laryngol. 2007;116(1):19–23. doi:10.1177/000348940711600104.
18. Ozer E, Alvarez B, Kakarala K, Durmus K, Teknos TN, Carrau RL. Clinical outcomes of transoral robotic supraglottic laryngectomy. Head Neck. 2013;35(8):1158–61. doi:10.1002/hed.23101.
19. Mendelsohn AH, Remacle M, Van Der Vorst S, Bachy V, Lawson G. Outcomes following transoral robotic surgery: supraglottic laryngectomy: TORS supraglottic laryngectomy. Laryngoscope. 2013;123(1):208–14. doi:10.1002/lary.23621.
20. Hurtuk AM, Marcinow A, Agrawal A, Old M, Teknos TN, Ozer E. Quality-of-life outcomes in transoral robotic surgery. Otolaryngol Head Neck Surg. 2012;146(1):68–73. doi:10.1177/0194599811421298.
21. More YI, Tsue TT, Girod DA, Harbison J, Sykes KJ, Williams C, Shnayder Y. Functional swallowing outcomes following transoral robotic surgery vs primary chemoradiotherapy in patients with advanced-stage oropharynx and supraglottis cancers. JAMA Otolaryngol Head Neck Surg. 2013;139(1):43. doi:10.1001/jamaoto.2013.1074.
22. Hinni ML, Salassa JR, Grant DG, Pearson BW, Hayden RE, Martin A, Christiansen H, Haughey BH, Nussenbaum B, Steiner W. Transoral laser microsurgery for advanced laryngeal cancer. Arch Otolaryngol–Head Neck Surg. 2007;133(12):1198. doi:10.1001/archotol.133.12.1198.
23. Gun R, Ozer E. Surgical anatomy of oropharynx and supraglottic larynx for transoral robotic surgery: transoral surgical anatomy for TORS. J Surg Oncol. 2015;112(7):690–6. doi:10.1002/jso.24020.
24. Dziegielewski PT, Ozer E. Transoral robotic surgery: supraglottic laryngectomy. Oper Tech Otolaryngol Head Neck Surg Robot. 2013;24(2):86–91. doi:10.1016/j.otot.2013.04.003.
25. Olsen SM, Moore EJ, Koch CA, Price DL, Kasperbauer JL, Olsen KD. Transoral robotic surgery for supraglottic squamous cell carcinoma. Am J Otolaryngol. 2012;33(4):379–84. doi:10.1016/j.amjoto.2011.10.007.
26. Park YM, Kim WS, Byeon HK, Lee SY, Kim S-H. Surgical techniques and treatment outcomes of transoral robotic supraglottic partial laryngectomy. Laryngoscope. 2013;123(3):670–7. doi:10.1002/lary.23767.
27. Kayhan FT, Kaya KH, Sayin I. Transoral robotic cordectomy for early glottic carcinoma. Ann Otol Rhinol Laryngol. August 2012;121(8):497–502.
28. Kayhan FT, Kaya KH, Ylmazbayhan ED. Transoral robotic approach for Schwannoma of the larynx. J Craniofac Surg. 2011;22(3):1000–2. doi:10.1097/SCS.0b013e3182101580.
29. Ciabatti PG, Burali G, D'Ascanio L. Transoral robotic surgery for large mixed laryngocoele. J Laryngol Otol. 2013;127(04):435–7. doi:10.1017/S0022215113000236.
30. Smith RV, Schiff BA, Sarta C, Hans S, Brasnu D. Transoral robotic total laryngectomy. Laryngoscope. 2013;123(3):678–82. doi:10.1002/lary.23842.
31. Dowthwaite S, Nichols AC, Yoo J, Smith RV, Dhaliwal S, Basmaji J, Franklin JH, Fung K. Transoral robotic total laryngectomy: report of 3 cases: Head Neck. 2013;35(11):E338–42. doi:10.1002/hed.23226.

Robotic Thyroidectomy

10

Naomi Rabinovics, Raphael Feinmesser, Patrick Aidan, and Gideon Bachar

10.1 Introduction

It was in the nineteenth century when Kocher developed and refined the classical cervical thyroidectomy; however, it has remained almost unchanged since [1]. The cervical approach has been proven as highly reliable and relatively fast but unfortunately leaves an obvious scar in the anterior cervical region. In recent years, advances in surgical instrumentation have introduced the minimally invasive thyroid surgery. The endoscopic thyroid surgery, popularized by Miccoli from Italy (the minimally invasive video-assisted thyroidectomy (MIVAT)), resulted in less morbidity and smaller surgical scars [2]. However, the endoscopic cervical approach is relatively challenging due to the use of straight and rigid instruments with no articulations. Moreover, the neck is a very confined space to use CO2 insufflation, with risk of PaCO2 elevation, subcutaneous emphysema, and air embolism [3].

The non-cervical, remote-access approaches were developed primarily due to cosmetic concerns and unfavorable scarring, particularly in certain ethnic groups, and the aversion to neck scars in the Asian culture [4]. The transaxillary endoscopic thyroidectomy was first introduced by Ikeda et al. in 2000 [5].

With the introduction of the da Vinci robot (Intuitive Surgical, Sunnyvale, CA, USA), surgeons have implemented its advantages to thyroid surgery. In late 2007, Chung and his team from Seoul started implementing the robotic-assisted transaxillary thyroid surgery (RATS) and introduced it in 2009 [6, 7]. This approach was described later, in 2011 in the USA, by Kuppersmith and Holsinger, where body habitus is considerably different than that of the Asian population [8]. Originally, the RATS was performed with two incisions (axillary and anterior chest wall), but later a modification using only a single axillary incision was described [5]. Since 2008, thousands of RATS procedures have been performed worldwide, almost half of those in South Korea [9]. Among the other robot-assisted thyroidectomy (RT) approaches, the transaxillary became the most popular.

Since the RATS was introduced, it has gained much interest worldwide with several teams publishing their initial successful experience [10]. However, since the conventional approach has long been proven to be safe and effective, some surgeons are hesitant regarding the clinical use of robotic thyroid surgery [11]. Robotic thyroidectomy remains controversial, especially in North America, where the FDA has revoked the approval on robotic thyroidectomy in 2011 [10].

N. Rabinovics, MD (✉) • R. Feinmesser, MD
G. Bachar, MD
Department of Otolaryngology Head and Neck Surgery, Rabin Medical Center, Sackler Faculty of Medicine, Tel Aviv University, Tel Aviv-Yafo, Israel
e-mail: naomirab@gmail.com; gidybahar@gmail.com

P. Aidan, MD
Department of ENT Head and Neck Surgery, The American Hospital, Paris, France

Z. Gil et al. (eds.), *Atlas of Head and Neck Robotic Surgery*, DOI 10.1007/978-3-319-49578-1_10

Several criteria for candidates to RATS were described, but there are no standard selection criteria [12]. Recommended absolute contraindications are previous neck surgery or radiation, retrosternal thyroid extension, and advanced thyroid disease (invasion of the trachea, esophagus, distant metastases). Relative contraindications include patient comorbidities, advanced age, obesity, very large goiters, well-differentiated carcinomas with a diameter larger than 2 cm, lateral neck metastases, and known ipsilateral shoulder dysfunction [5, 13, 14].

During the same period the RATS was introduced, multiple other remote-access robot-assisted thyroidectomy approaches were described. This chapter will discuss the more widely described RATS approach.

10.2 Transaxillary Approach: Surgical Technique

The RATS can be divided into three surgical stages

10.2.1 Working Space

The surgery is performed under general anesthesia. The use of an endotracheal tube with laryngeal nerve monitoring is recommended.

The dissection area is outlined by anatomical landmarks. The axillary incision is defined in its inferior border by a horizontal line, from the sternal notch, and the superior border—by an oblique line—at a 60° angle from the thyroid notch. The incision itself is performed in the anterior axillary line (Fig. 10.1).

The axillary incision may be marked, while the patient is sitting, with the arms relaxed in a neutral position, to verify it is well camouflaged.

Following anesthesia, the patient is placed in a supine position with the neck mildly extended. The patient's arm is placed in an extended position over the forehead, with the elbow flexed at 90° (Fig. 10.1). The arm should be carefully rotated and padded. Eye protection should be applied to avoid any injuries from the robotic arms during surgery.

Following the axillary incision (5–6 cm), a subcutaneous dissection is performed and carried superficial to the pectoralis major muscle, to the direction of the clavicle. At the sternoclavicular joint, the sternal and clavicular heads of the sternocleidomastoid muscle are identified. The dissection then continues between these two heads, at which point the strap muscles are identified and deeper to it, the thyroid gland. Care should be taken during this step to avoid injury to the internal and external jugular veins. At this point, a retractor is inserted to elevate the skin flap, thereby creating a tunnel from the axilla to the thyroid gland (Fig. 10.2).

10.2.2 Docking of the Robot

The da Vinci cart is positioned in the contralateral side, while the robotic arms extend over the patient. The three arms and the camera are inserted through the axillary incision and along the working space

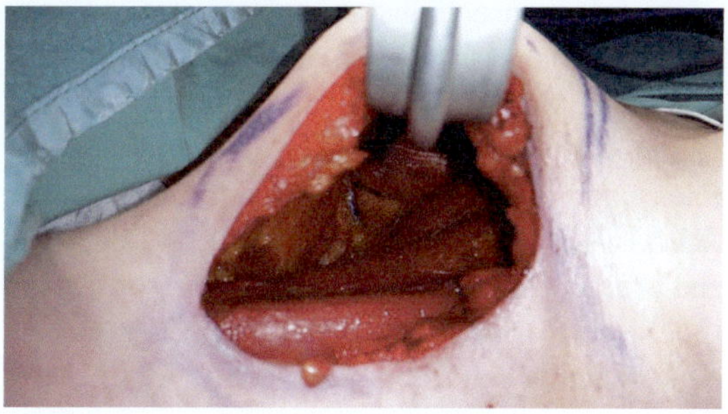

Fig. 10.2 View of working space after retractor insertion

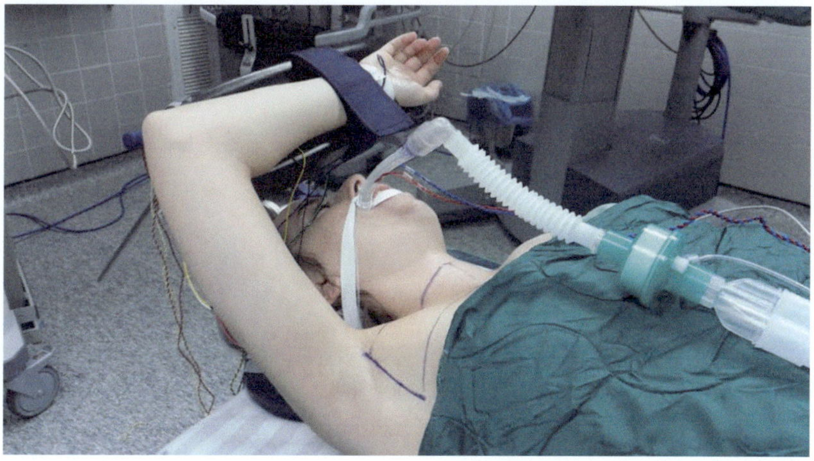

Fig. 10.1 Ipsilateral hand position: extended over the forehead, elbow flexed at 90°

(ProGrasp forceps, harmonic shears, and Maryland dissector). The correct alignment of the robotic arms within the tunnel is crucial to avoid collision of the robotic arms inside the working space, during the console time. The recommended alignment of the robotic arms is with the forceps used for retraction at the top of the working space, the Harmonic scalpel (Harmonic ACE® curved shears) on the inferior cephalad side, the dissector on the inferior caudal, and the camera in the middle inferior of the surgical field. The assistant may further retract the strap muscles using the suction catheter.

10.2.3 Robotic Thyroidectomy (Console Time, Figs. 10.3–10.10)

The thyroidectomy is performed in the classical order: first, dissecting the superior pole off the cricothyroid muscle, using the harmonic shears, and safely transecting the superior thyroid vessels close to the gland as to avoid external branch of SLN injury; second, the thyroid lobe is retracted medially in order to expose the parathyroid glands and the recurrent laryngeal nerve (RLN). After ligating the inferior thyroid vessels and identifying the trachea, further mobilization is achieved, and further medial dissection is carried out while carefully preserving the RLN. The lobe is carefully dissected from Berry's ligament and extracted through the axillary incision. Saline irrigations may assist in preventing thermal injury to the RLN from the harmonic shears. A clip demonstrating the robotic hemithyroidectomy is attached.

A total thyroidectomy is performed via the same axillary incision used for the ipsilateral lobe. The decision regarding which lobe to dissect first should not differ from the cervical approach where the surgeon would usually favor resecting the larger lobe or nodule side first. The axillary incision should be performed ipsilateral to that lobe, and the resection should be carried out in the same fashion detailed above, before attempting to resect the contralateral lobe. After the extraction of the ipsilateral lobe, the assistant should retract the trachea downward, while the superior pole of the contralateral lobe is retracted upward using the ProGrasp forceps. The deep aspect of the lobe is then dissected away from the trachea using the harmonic shears. It should be noted that the contralateral RLN is not easily visible as is the ipsilateral one so care must be taken to avoid injury.

Some surgeons advocate removing the thyroid with an endo-bag as to avoid any tissue spillage. Lastly, a drain is placed in the thyroid bed [12, 15].

10.2.4 Advantages of RATS

The most considerable advantage of RATS over conventional cervical thyroidectomy is that it avoids any cervical incision. This cosmetic aspect makes RATS appealing especially to young female patients, which is the majority of the patient population, and those with a tendency toward keloid or hypertrophic scar formation. An example of an axillary scar can be seen in Fig. 10.3.

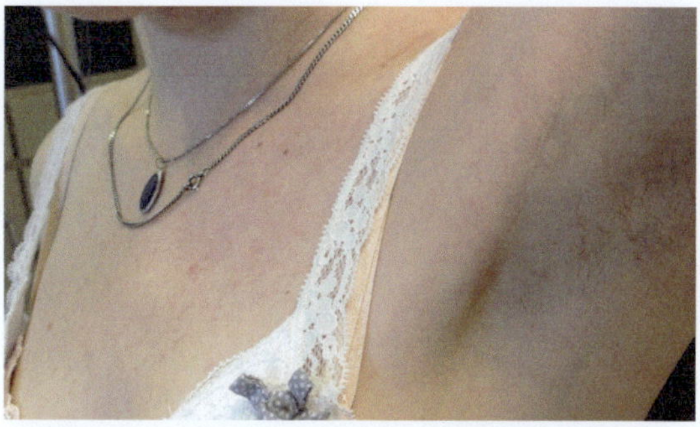

Fig. 10.3 Postoperative axillary scar (Contributed by Dr. Patrick Aidan, The American Hospital in Paris, France)

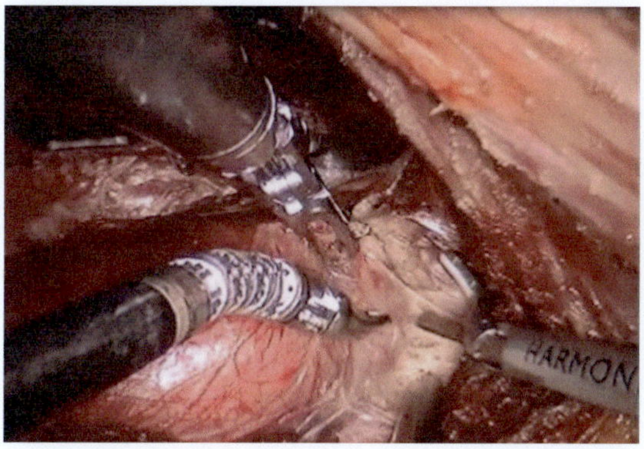

Fig. 10.4 Dissection of the superior pole of the thyroid lobe with the harmonic scalpel. General view (landmarks): left thyroid lobe, trachea, internal jogular vein (blue hue at the bottom), Omohyoid muscle retracted at the right and bottom of photo, Cricothyroid muscle at the top right

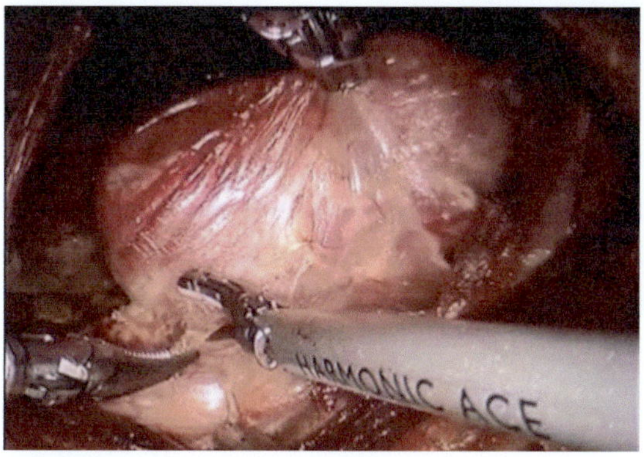

Fig. 10.5 Dissection of the inferior pole of the thyroid lobe with the harmonic scalpel while lobe is retracted upwards by the prograsp

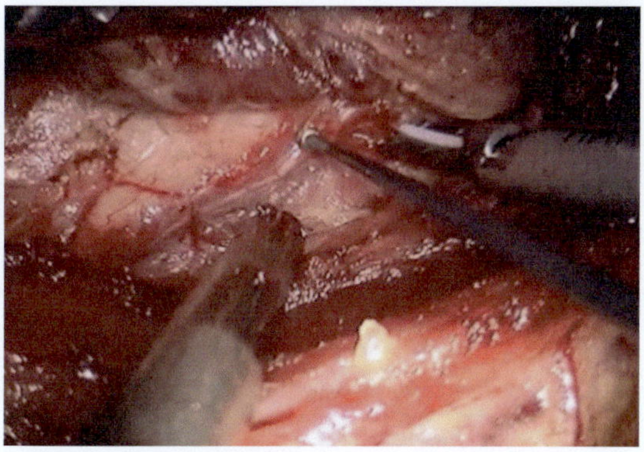

Fig. 10.6 RLN is visible and stimulated by the nerve stimulator for verification

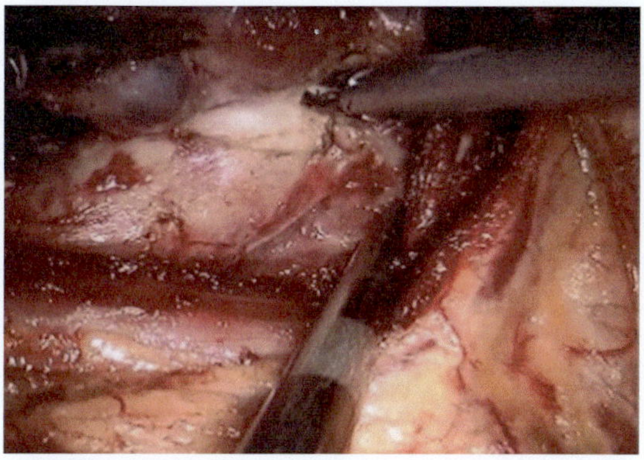

Fig. 10.7 Once the RLN has been identified, carefull dissection of the thyroid lobe off the trachea is performed using the harmonic scalpel

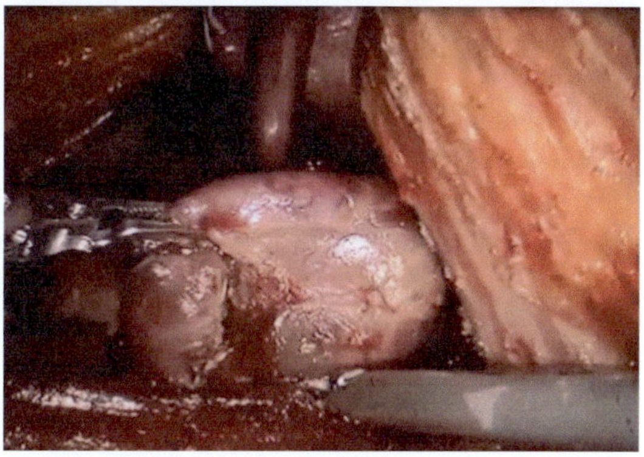

Fig. 10.8 Separating the isthmus

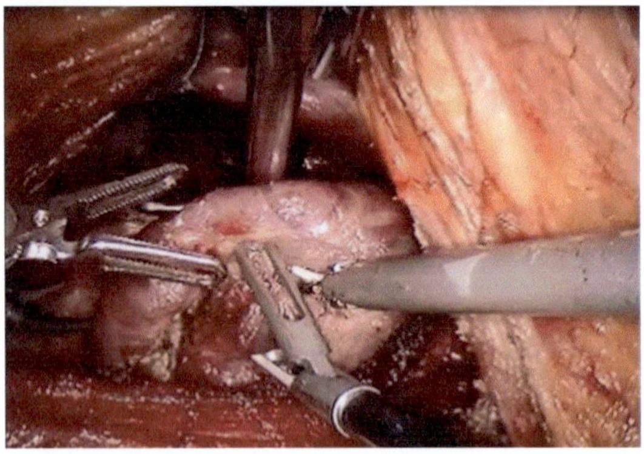

Fig. 10.9 The disconnected lobe is removed through the axilla

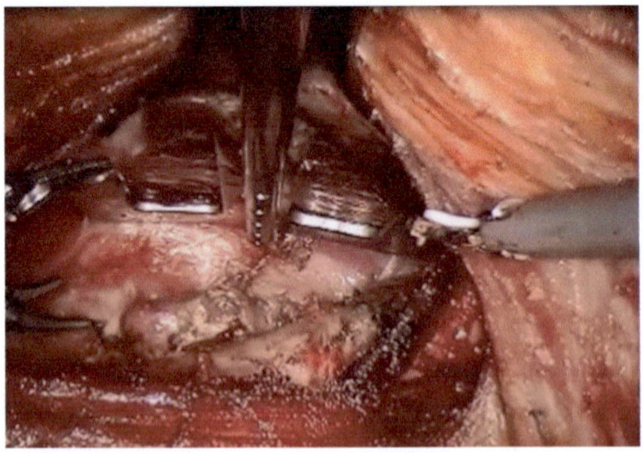

Fig. 10.10 View s/p hemithyroidectomy: trachea and isthmus of contralateral lobe

The RATS has some major technical advantages. First, the robotic camera provides three-dimensional high-resolution visualization, which enables an easier identification of the RLN and parathyroid glands compared to the cervical approach; second, the robotic arms eliminate the natural surgeon tremor; and, third, it provides a wider range of motion through the robot's EndoWrist and the articulations of the arms. In addition, the improved visualization and surgical ergonomics have been reported to reduce musculoskeletal discomfort to the surgeon compared with open or endoscopic surgery [7].

Lastly, with regard to patients' quality of life, RATS was found to yield better patient outcomes, including reduced pain and increased cosmetic satisfaction, as well as lower rates of paresthesia over the neck, postoperative voice change, and swallowing discomfort [16, 17].

10.2.5 Disadvantages of RATS

This relative new approach to the thyroid gland, in terms of the surrounding anatomy and the loss of tactile sensation, may expose the patient to potential new complications such as tracheal, esophageal, or brachial plexus injury. Very few studies accounted for such complications, with minimal attention to the conversion rate to open thyroidectomy. Due to the ipsilateral arm position, there is a risk of brachial plexus neuropathy. This risk can be reduced by placing the arm in a flexed overhead 90° position, thereby reducing the chance of stretching the nerves. Care must be taken to avoid local pressure from the robotic arm. Intraoperative neurophysiological monitoring of the ulnar, radial, and median nerves may further reduce the possibility of brachial plexus injury, by identification of any impending damage to these nerves and enabling the patient to be repositioned as needed [18]. Intraoperative monitoring has shown to decrease rates of hypoesthesia and pain and improve shoulder movement, as well as higher quality of life, in the early postoperative period [19]. Despite the benefits of intraoperative monitoring, it is not obligatory in RATS.

Another disadvantage of RATS is the longer operative time mainly due to the extra time needed for the creation of the working space and the robot docking. In different studies, it is assessed as 1.5–3 times compared to the cervical approach. However, several studies have examined the learning curves of the RT and have shown that increased experience led to decreased total operative time [1]. RATS involves a relatively challenging learning curve, compared to the conventional approach. However, it has been demonstrated that RT required 35–40 procedures, much lower compared to the endoscopic approach [7]. Park et al. examined the learning curves of surgeons with little or no experience, performing transaxillary RT on 125 patients. They showed excellent results compared to those in a larger series of more experienced surgeons and, specifically, that the operation times gradually decreased, reaching a plateau after 20 procedures [20]. Another disadvantage of RATS is the limitation in the body habitus and BMI. With RATS, the working space dissection is relatively more challenging in obese patients (BMI >30). However, it has been demonstrated, and per the authors' experience, that in skilled hands, the body habitus limitation is irrelevant [21, 22].

In terms of economic considerations, RT is a more expensive procedure compared to open thyroidectomy, primarily due to the cost of the equipment (da Vinci robot itself and periodic maintenance of the robotic arms), staff training, and longer operative time. However, RT actually eliminates the need for an additional surgical assistant, and, combined with the potentially shorter hospital stay and the expected decrease in the maintenance cost of the robot, this may lower the costs of the procedure.

10.3 RATS Experience

RATS is being practiced mainly in South Korea and Asia and, to a smaller extent, in Europe and North America. With the rising popularity of RT, several meta-analyses were conducted in order to examine both the surgical and oncological safety of RT compared to conventional and endoscopic approaches.

In 2015, Kandil et al. summarized 18 studies, including 4878 patients, and concluded that RT was associated with longer total operative time (mean difference 43 min) and had similar risks of total postoperative complications and similar oncological results [23].

Another meta-analysis published in 2014 by Jackson et al. [1] summarized a total of nine studies with 2881 patients, 1122 of whom underwent RT. They conclude that RT is as effective as endoscopic and open thyroidectomy, with equivalent postoperative results, shorter hospitalization, and higher patient satisfaction. Several other meta-analyses with overall 1000–3000 patients demonstrated similar results, in addition to lower blood loss and lower level of swallowing impairment [16, 24–26].

Lee et al. have also published their experience with 2014 patients who underwent RATS, with a low complication rate of 1% for major complications (e.g., permanent RLN or brachial injury, conversion to open thyroidectomy) and 19% for minor ones (transient hypocalcemia, seroma, etc.). Interestingly, this group also found that in terms of the surgeon's musculoskeletal ergonomic parameters, RATS resulted in less neck and back discomfort than did the endoscopic or open thyroidectomy [7].

One of the relative contraindications of RATS is Graves' disease, due to the usually large-volume thyroid glands and hypervascularity. However, some surgeons have already reported their successful experience with Graves' patients showing similar complication rates, blood loss, and hospital stay [27, 28]. The largest European experience from Paris, France, with over 350 robotic thyroidectomies and neck dissections, is also very promising with low complication rates. Interestingly, almost 60% of their RT involved large-volume thyroid glands (over 20 mL) [29]. It should be noted that all patients received potassium iodide preoperatively.

In skillful hands, RATS can be feasible and safe for patients with large-volume thyroid glands such as Graves' and MNG patients.

10.4 RATS in Papillary Thyroid Carcinoma

The incidence of thyroid cancer is gradually increasing worldwide, and in accordance with that, the proportion of papillary thyroid microcarcinomas. Since early-stage PTC has an excellent prognosis with minimal mortality and low recurrence rates, the patients' quality of life issues, including cosmetic concerns, play a major role [9, 19].

In 2011, Lee et al. published their experience with RT on 1043 patients with low-risk well-differentiated thyroid carcinoma. They showed that the RATS was feasible and offered outcomes similar to conventional and endoscopic thyroidectomies [30]. Another study published recently explored the efficacy of RATS in North American population with thyroid cancer, compared to the conventional approach—they found similar operative times and blood loss, with negative margins for malignancy and similar thyroglobulin levels [3].

Ban et al. have described the surgical complications in their experience of 3000 patients who underwent RT for thyroid cancer. Hypocalcemia was the most common complication, 1% permanent; permanent RLN injury, 0.27%; tracheal injury, 0.2%; carotid artery injury, 0.03%; skin flap injury, 0.1%; and brachial plexopathy, 0.13%. The mortality rate was 0% [31]. Male gender, overweight BMI, a large thyroid gland, and coexistent thyroiditis are factors that were found to adversely affect the surgical outcome of RT in DTC cases, namely, longer operative times [9].

The resection of the contralateral thyroid lobe in total thyroidectomy is surgically challenging via a single axillary incision. Therefore some surgeons doubted the surgical completeness of the procedure. A recently published meta-analysis compared the surgical completeness and oncological outcome between RT and conventional open thyroidectomy (OT) in low-risk DTC. Ten studies were analyzed, including 752 patients who had RT and 1453 patients who had OT. RT was associated with fewer central lymph nodes retrieval and less-complete resection (based on Tg levels), compared to OT, probably due to residual tissue in the contralateral side. Nevertheless, no locoregional recurrence was found in the RT group; therefore, the authors concluded that using RT was unlikely to compromise the outcomes of low-risk DTC [10]. Other studies and meta-analyses investigated the completeness of the thyroidectomy, comparing it to conventional thyroidectomy using stimulated thyroglobulin levels, RAI uptake, and postoperative sonography. These studies ultimately demonstrated that the surgical completeness of RT is comparable to conventional thyroidectomy, if performed by experienced surgeons [32–36].

Some criticism arose regarding the oncological assessment of RT in thyroid cancer due to the relatively short follow-up period in most studies, compared to the long-term risk of recurrence in these tumors. In addition, some argued against bias as the RT procedures were performed mainly for microcarcinomas and other early-stage thyroid cancers. To address these issues, the South Korean team recently compared longer-term oncologic outcomes (over 5 years after surgery), in patients who underwent robotic (245 patients) or conventional total thyroidectomy (494 patients) and central neck dissection for PTC. To avoid selection bias, the groups were matched for age, gender, tumor size, extrathyroidal invasion, multiplicity, bilaterality, and TNM stage. They found similar serum thyroglobulin (Tg) and anti-thyroglobulin antibody (TgAb) levels. Nine patients experienced locoregional recurrence, six in the conventional group and three in the robotic group, with all recurrences in regional LNs. Disease-free survival was similar [37].

A newly reported use of the RATS for modified radical neck dissection (MRND) suggests that the precise movements and magnified 3D vision enable a meticulous and safe dissection with recovery of similar numbers of lymph nodes as an open procedure with similar recovery of neck and shoulder disability [35, 38].

10.5 Other Robotic Thyroidectomy Approaches

Alternate robotic remote-access thyroidectomy approaches were also described in recent years. These included the bilateral axillo-breast approach (BABA), currently performed mainly in Korea with successful outcome [39]; transoral and infraclavicular approaches, with very limited experience in humans [40, 41]; and the facelift approaches.

The robotic facelift, or retroauricular thyroidectomy, was first introduced by Terris in 2011. It was developed to overcome the concerns and complications of robotic axillary thyroidectomy, namely, brachial plexus injury and anterior chest wall discomfort, and to adjust the procedure to the western population. It presents a growing body of evidence supporting its feasibility and safety [42, 43].

Conclusions

RATS has gained much popularity in recent years, mainly in Asia and Europe. It is considered an oncologically and surgically safe alternative to cervical thyroidectomy, with increased patient satisfaction. RATS should be performed in high-volume centers, by skilled surgeons, and presented to suitable patients, especially those with aesthetic concerns; with increasing experience and improvement in the robotic technology, the indications for RATs will continue to expand.

References

1. Jackson NR, Yao L, Tufano RP, et al. Safety of robotic thyroidectomy approaches: meta-analysis and systematic review. Head Neck. 2014;36:137–43.
2. Miccoli P, Bellantone R, Mourad M, et al. Minimally invasive video-assisted thyroidectomy: multiinstitutional experience. World J Surg. 2002;26:972–5.
3. Noureldine SI, Jackson NR, Tufano RP, et al. A comparative North American experience of robotic thyroidectomy in a thyroid cancer population. Langenbeck's Arch Surg. 2013;398:1069–74.
4. Terris DJ. Surgical approaches to the thyroid gland: which is the best for you and your patient? JAMA Otolaryngol Head Neck Surg. 2013;139:515–7.
5. Ikeda Y, Takami H, Sasaki Y, et al. Clinical benefits in endoscopic thyroidectomy by the axillary approach. J Am Coll Surg. 2003;196:189–95.
6. Kang SW, Jeong JJ, Yun JS, Sung TY, Lee SC, Lee YS, Nam KH, Chang HS, Chung WY, Park CS. Robot-assisted endoscopic surgery for thyroid cancer: experience with the first 100 patients. Surg Endosc. 2009;23(11):2399–406.
7. Lee J, Kang SW, Jung JJ, et al. Multicenter study of robotic thyroidectomy: short-term postoperative outcomes and surgeon ergonomic considerations. Ann Surg Oncol. 2011;18:2538–47.
8. Kuppersmith RB, Holsinger FC. Robotic thyroid surgery: an initial experience with North American patients. Laryngoscope. 2011;121:521–6.
9. Son H, Park S, Lee CR, et al. Factors contributing to surgical outcomes of transaxillary robotic thyroidectomy for papillary thyroid carcinoma. Surg Endosc. 2014;28:3134–42.
10. Lang BH, Wong CK, Tsang JS, et al. A systematic review and meta-analysis evaluating completeness and outcomes of robotic thyroidectomy. Laryngoscope. 2015;125:509–18.
11. Chung WY. Pros of robotic transaxillary thyroid surgery: its impact on cancer control and surgical quality. Thyroid. 2012;22:986–7.
12. Lin HS, Folbe AJ, Carron MA, et al. Single-incision transaxillary robotic thyroidectomy: challenges and limitations in a North American population. Otolaryngol Head Neck Surg. 2012;147:1041–6.
13. Perrier ND, Randolph GW, Inabnet WB, et al. Robotic thyroidectomy: a framework for new technology assessment and safe implementation. Thyroid. 2010; 20:1327–32.
14. Lee YM, Yi O, Sung TY, et al. Surgical outcomes of robotic thyroid surgery using a double incision gasless transaxillary approach: analysis of 400 cases treated by the same surgeon. Head Neck. 2014;36: 1413–9.
15. Holsinger FC, Chung WY. Robotic thyroidectomy. Otolaryngol Clin N Am. 2014;47:373–8.
16. Sun GH, Peress L, Pynnonen MA. Systematic review and meta-analysis of robotic vs conventional thyroidectomy approaches for thyroid disease. Otolaryngol Head Neck Surg. 2014;150:520–32.

17. Song CM, Yun BR, Ji YB, Sung ES, Kim KR, Tae K. Long-term voice outcomes after robotic thyroidectomy. World J Surg. 2016;40(1):110–6.
18. Davis SF, Abdel Khalek M, Giles J, Fox C, Lirette L, Kandil E. Detection and prevention of impending brachial plexus injury secondary to arm positioning using ulnar nerve somatosensory evoked potentials during transaxillary approach for thyroid lobectomy. Am J Electroneurodiagnostic Technol. 2011;51(4): 274–9.
19. Alkan U, Zarchi O, Rabinovics N, Nachalon Y, Feinmesser R, Bachar G. The cause of brachial plexopathy in robot-assisted transaxillary thyroidectomy-A neurophysiological investigation. Laryngoscope. 2016;126(9):2187–93.
20. Park JH, Lee J, Hakim NA, et al. Robotic thyroidectomy learning curve for beginning surgeons with little or no experience of endoscopic surgery. Head Neck. 2015;37(12):1705–11.
21. Kandil E, Abdelghani S, Noureldine SI, et al. Transaxillary gasless robotic thyroidectomy: a single surgeon's experience in North America. Arch Otolaryngol Head Neck Surg. 2012;138:113–7.
22. Kandil EH, Noureldine SI, Yao L, et al. Robotic transaxillary thyroidectomy: an examination of the first one hundred cases. J Am Coll Surg. 2012;214:558–564; discussion 564–6.
23. Kandil E, Hammad AY, Walvekar RR, Hu T, Masoodi H, Mohamed SE, Deniwar A, Stack BC Jr. Robotic thyroidectomy versus nonrobotic approaches: a meta-analysis examining surgical outcomes. Surg Innov. 2016;23(3):317–25.
24. Lang BH, Wong CK, Tsang JS, Wong KP, Wan KY. A systematic review and meta-analysis comparing surgically-related complications between robotic-assisted thyroidectomy and conventional open thyroidectomy. Ann Surg Oncol. 2014;21(3):850–61.
25. Son SK, Kim JH, Bae JS, Lee SH. Surgical safety and oncologic effectiveness in robotic versus conventional open thyroidectomy in thyroid cancer: a systematic review and meta-analysis. Ann Surg Oncol. 2015;22(9):3022–32.
26. Shen H, Shan C, Qiu M. Systematic review and meta-analysis of transaxillary robotic thyroidectomy versus open thyroidectomy. Surg Laparosc Endosc Percutan Tech. 2014;24(3):199–206.
27. Kwon H, Koo do H, Choi JY, et al. Bilateral axillo-breast approach robotic thyroidectomy for Graves' disease: an initial experience in a single institute. World J Surg. 2013;37:1576–81. 30
28. Noureldine SI, Yao L, Wavekar RR, et al. Thyroidectomy for Graves' disease: a feasibility study of the robotic transaxillary approach. ORL J Otorhinolaryngol Relat Spec. 2013;75:350–6.
29. Rabinovics N, Aidan P. Robotic transaxillary thyroid surgery. Gland Surg. 2015;4(5):397–402.
30. Lee J, Yun JH, Nam KH, et al. Perioperative clinical outcomes after robotic thyroidectomy for thyroid carcinoma: a multicenter study. Surg Endosc. 2011;25:906–12.
31. Ban EJ, Yoo JY, Kim WW, et al. Surgical complications after robotic thyroidectomy for thyroid carcinoma: a single center experience with 3,000 patients. Surg Endosc. 2014;28:2555–63.
32. Lee S, Lee CR, Lee SC, et al. Surgical completeness of robotic thyroidectomy: a prospective comparison with conventional open thyroidectomy in papillary thyroid carcinoma patients. Surg Endosc. 2014;28: 1068–75.
33. Tae K, Song CM, Ji YB, et al. Comparison of surgical completeness between robotic total thyroidectomy versus open thyroidectomy. Laryngoscope. 2014;124: 1042–7.
34. Yi O, Yoon JH, Lee YM, et al. Technical and oncologic safety of robotic thyroid surgery. Ann Surg Oncol. 2013;20:1927–33.
35. Lee J, Kwon IS, Bae EH, et al. Comparative analysis of oncological outcomes and quality of life after robotic versus conventional open thyroidectomy with modified radical neck dissection in patients with papillary thyroid carcinoma and lateral neck node metastases. J Clin Endocrinol Metab. 2013;98:2701–8.
36. Wang YC, Liu K, Ong JJ, Zhu JQ. Robotic thyroidectomy versus conventional open thyroidectomy for differentiated thyroid cancer: meta-analysis. J Laryngol Otol. 2015;129(6):558–67.
37. Lee SG, Lee J, Kim MJ, Choi JB, Kim TH, Ban EJ, Lee CR, Kang SW, Jeong JJ, Nam KH, Jo YS, Chung WY. Long term oncologic outcome of robotic versus open total thyroidectomy in PTC: a case-matched retrospective study. Surg Endosc. 2016;30(8):3474–9.
38. Kang SW, Chung WY. Transaxillary single-incision robotic neck dissection for metastatic thyroid cancer. Gland Surg. 2015;4(5):388–96.
39. Lee KE, Kim E, Koo do H, Choi JY, Kim KH, Youn YK. Robotic thyroidectomy by bilateral axillo-breast approach: review of 1,026 cases and surgical completeness. Surg Endosc. 2013;27(8):2955–62.
40. Clark JH, Kim HY, Richmon JD. Transoral robotic thyroid surgery. Gland Surg. 2015;4(5):429–34.
41. Lallemant B, Chambon G, Rupp D, Reynaud C, Alovisetti C, Kacha S, Lallemant JG, Trevillot V. Robotic thyroid surgery: our experience with the infraclavicular approach. Head Neck. 2012;34(9): 1247–50.
42. Bomeli SR, Duke WS, Terris DJ. Robotic facelift thyroid surgery. Gland Surg. 2015;4(5):403–9.
43. Byeon HK, Kim DH, Chang JW, Ban MJ, Park JH, Kim WS, Choi EC, Koh YW. Comprehensive application of robotic retroauricular thyroidectomy: the evolution of robotic thyroidectomy. Laryngoscope. 2016;126(8):1952–7.

11 Single-Port Transaxillary Robotic Parathyroidectomy

George Garas, Ara Darzi, Asit Arora, and Neil Tolley

Surgical steps

1. *Preoperative considerations*
2. *Informed consent*
3. *Patient positioning*
4. *Surgical equipment*
5. *Transaxillary access to the neck*
6. *Preparation of the robotic field*
7. *Robotic surgery*
8. *Postoperative care and follow-up*
9. *Surgical complications*
10. *Mentoring and proctorship*

11.1 Preoperative Considerations

As with all surgical operations, patient selection is paramount. Prior to offering the approach to a patient, a multidisciplinary evaluation with an endocrinologist and radiologist is mandatory. This is to confirm the presence of primary hyperparathyroidism (pHPT), localize the adenoma, and exclude conditions such as vitamin D deficiency or familial hypocalciuric hypercalcemia (FHH) which do not require surgical intervention [1].

Single-port transaxillary robotic parathyroidectomy (RP) constitutes an advanced remote-access targeted parathyroidectomy approach. When considering the indications, the approach is an option when a single adenoma has been clearly identified and there is concordance between different imaging modalities. To minimize the risk of failure and need for revision surgery, we advocate triple modality concordance using ultrasonography, sestamibi scintigraphy, and single-photon emission computed tomography (SPECT-CT).

Adenoma size is not a limitation nor is adenoma location. With the exception of giant parathyroid adenomas that are exquisitely rare, parathyroid adenomas are usually relatively small [2]. Ectopic parathyroid adenomas located in the mediastinum and retropharyngeal space have also been successfully removed using the robotic technique. However, access to these locations is not the same (thoracoscopic and transoral routes, respectively) and beyond the scope of this chapter [3–7].

Other important considerations prior to offering RP include body habitus, comorbidities, and patient psyche. A list of contraindications to RP is presented in Table 11.1.

G. Garas, BSc, MBBS, MRCS, DOHNS (✉)
A. Darzi, MD, KBE, FRCS • A. Arora, PhD, DIC, FRCS, DOHNS • N. Tolley, MD, FRCS, DLO
Department of Surgery and Cancer, Imperial College London, St. Mary's Hospital, London W2 1NY, UK
e-mail: g.garas@imperial.ac.uk

Z. Gil et al. (eds.), *Atlas of Head and Neck Robotic Surgery*, DOI 10.1007/978-3-319-49578-1_11

The ideal RP patient would be slim with a preoperatively localized parathyroid adenoma. Individuals with a predisposition to hypertrophic scarring and keloid formation are ideal candidates as the avoidance of a neck scar is particularly desirable [8].

Table 11.1 Contraindications to single-port transaxillary robotic parathyroidectomy

Obesity (BMI >30 kgm^{-2})
Large ipsilateral goiter
Previous surgery to the neck
Previous radiotherapy to the neck
Important co-comorbidity (ASA>2)
Suspicion of parathyroid carcinoma
Ipsilateral acromioclavicular osteoarthritis

11.2 Informed Consent

Informed consent is undertaken by the attending surgeon. RP may be offered as an alternative to the conventional cervical approach, and both options should be discussed with the patient.

The risks associated with RP are the same as for conventional parathyroidectomy with regard to the recurrent laryngeal nerve (RLN), infection, hematoma, seroma, persistent hyperparathyroidism, and need for revision surgery. The literature does not support an increased infection rate with RP compared to cervical parathyroidectomy [9].

Additional points that should be explained to the patient include the fact that there will still be a scar though this will be concealed in the axilla. Moreover, it is very likely that they will experience dysesthesia on the chest over the area that the subcutaneous flap has been raised. This almost always resolves though may take several months. Pain is not a particular problem with RP [9, 10]. The patient should also be made aware of the risk of brachial plexus neurapraxia. This is rare and becomes almost a "theoretical" risk when the ipsilateral arm is placed in the "extended salute" position (see Sect. 3, "Patient Positioning").

With regard to the latter risks (axillary scar, dysesthesia on chest, and potential for brachial plexus neurapraxia) and the prolonged operative time, it should be made clear to the patient that these are specific to RP and not associated with conventional parathyroidectomy so that they can subsequently make an informed decision. The inpatient stay and time off work are similar to the conventional open technique [9, 11].

11.3 Patient Positioning

It is important to position the patient's ipsilateral arm when they are awake in order to ensure comfort and thus minimize the risk of traction on the brachial plexus (and associated neurapraxia) [12]. The ipsilateral arm must be free of identification bracelets, lines, blood pressure cuffs, or EKG leads. Arm positioning involves the back of the patient's hand touching the central portion of the forehead, in an "extended salute" position (Fig. 11.1). This has been shown to minimize the risk of brachial plexus neurapraxia [13].

A 5–6 cm axillary incision is also marked at this point as in our experience this is the optimal way to plan where to place the incision to prevent subsequent migration. The incision may need to be extended superiorly in a curvilinear fashion so that it sits in a natural skin crease. This reduces tension and a tendency toward hypertrophic and pigmented scarring. Laterality (side of surgery) is indicated by a skin marker (arrow).

Following this, the anesthesiologist intubates the patient and ventilates them via a transoral endotracheal tube with electrodes (NIM EMG Endotracheal Tube, Medtronic, Inc., Jacksonville, FL). The correct positioning of the NIM EMG endotracheal tube with the electrodes at the level of the glottis is confirmed by direct laryngoscopy. Visualization of the electromyographic waveform on the nerve integrity monitor (NIM) following insertion of the stimulator and earth leads serves as additional confirmation. An extended tip of the NIM must be available due to the long distance between the axillary incision and neck. At induction, the patient is routinely administered intravenously 1.2 g co-amoxiclav and 4 mg dexamethasone.

Contrary to conventional parathyroid surgery, a shoulder roll is not placed under the shoulders as this leads to neck extension moving the parathyroid adenoma away from the robotic instruments. Instead, a pillow is placed under the patient's head and shoulders to provide adequate and comfortable support in a subtle "sniffing the morning air" position. The head of the table is then dropped to about 20° to widen the angle between the arm and chest.

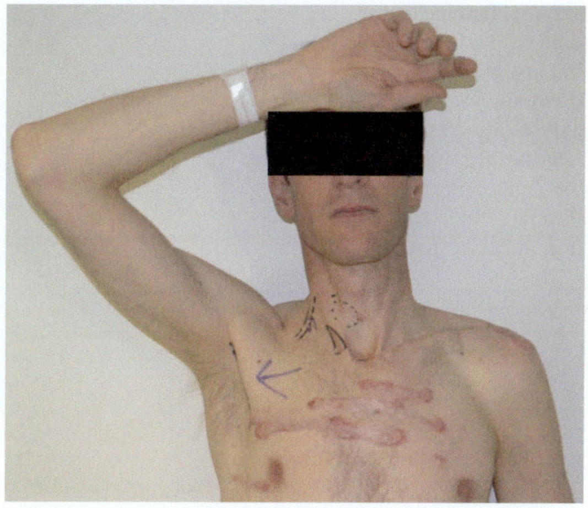

Fig. 11.1 The "extended salute" position for single-port transaxillary robotic parathyroidectomy. By adjusting the position of the ipsilateral arm with the patient awake to assess for comfort, the risk of traction injury to the brachial plexus is minimized. Doing so and marking the incision immediately prior to surgery constitute vital components of preoperative planning. The laterality is pre-marked with an *arrow* as is the external jugular vein, sternal head of sternocleidomastoid muscle, parathyroid adenoma location, and the 5–6 cm axillary incision. This is rechecked once the patient is positioned on the operating table as in our experience this is the optimal way to plan where to place the incision to prevent subsequent migration. Note extensive scaring on the chest from chickenpox (anteriorly) and right lateral minithoracotomy hypertrophic scar from previous bullectomy to treat pneumothorax. This is a patient who had valid reasons for wanting to avoid a visible neck scar and seeking a transaxillary approach for his parathyroidectomy

11.4 Surgical Equipment

The surgical equipment consists of the non-robotic trays (used for the single-port transaxillary access) and the robotic instruments. These are illustrated in Figs. 11.2, 11.3, 11.4, 11.5, 11.6, and 11.7.

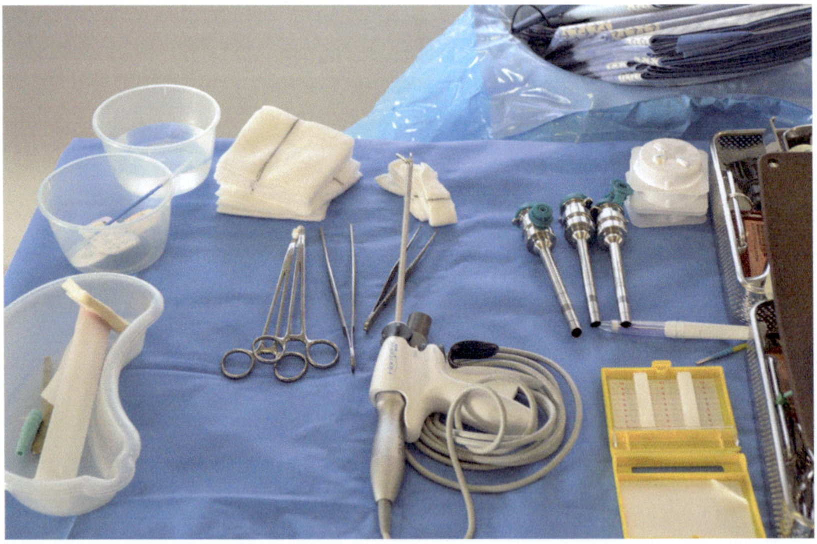

Fig. 11.2 Non-robotic instruments used for establishing the single-port transaxillary access. These include a Bovie (monopolar electrocautery) with a long extension and insulated tip, Harmonic scalpel (Ethicon Endo-Surgery, Inc., Johnson & Johnson, Cincinnati, OH), pledgets (Teleflex® Inc., NC), and Langenbeck retractors

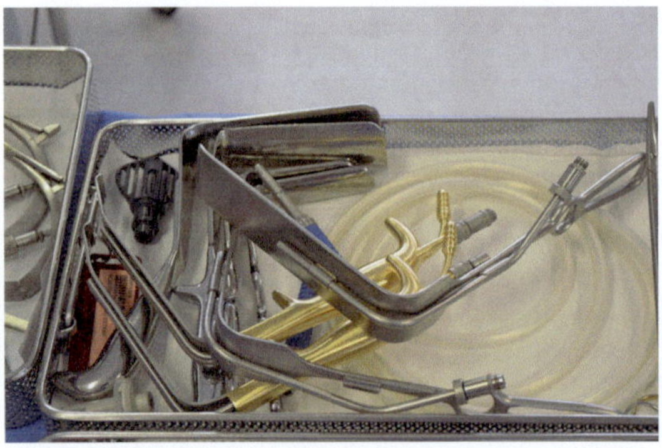

Fig. 11.3 Self-illuminating retractor used for raising the subcutaneous flap for single-port transaxillary access to the neck

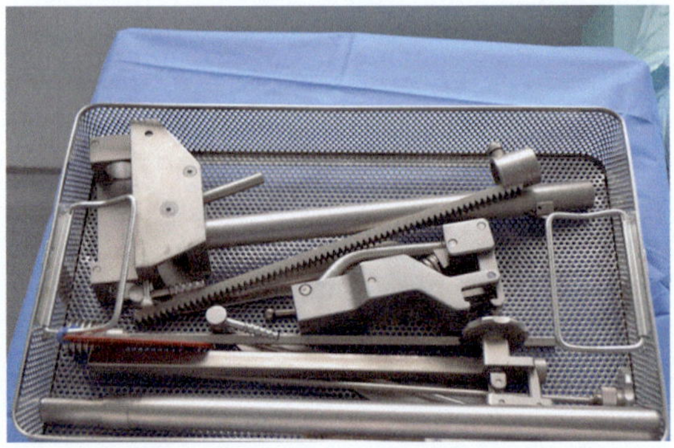

Fig. 11.4 The Modena surgical modular retractor (CEATEC® Medizintechnik) is introduced once the flap has been raised and prior to docking the da Vinci robot (Intuitive Surgical, Sunnyvale, CA). It incorporates a suction tube to its blade to prevent fogging of the robotic dual-channel endoscope intraoperatively

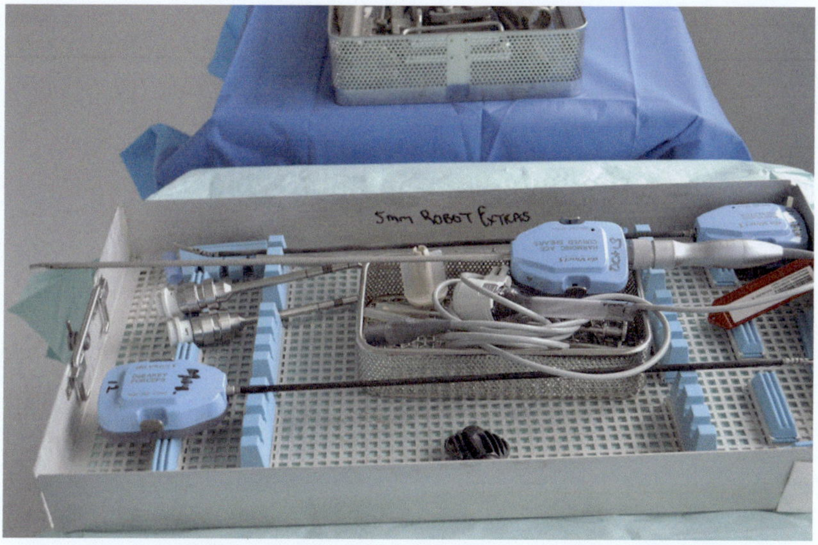

Fig. 11.5 The three robotic arms used: Harmonic ACE curved shears, DeBakey forceps, and Maryland dissector used in single-port transaxillary robotic parathyroidectomy. The fourth assistant arm holds the 8 mm ProGrasp which serves mainly for retraction of the ipsilateral thyroid lobe (see Fig. 11.17). Following insertion into their trochars, all robotic arms and camera are inserted through the axillary incision

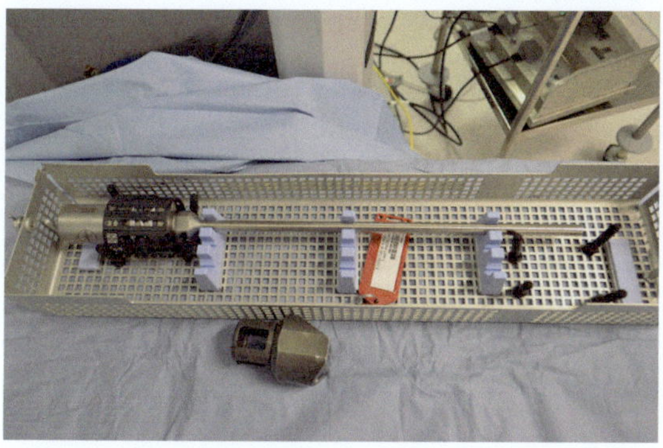

Fig. 11.6 A 30° down, 12 mm dual-channel endoscope is used. The endoscope and all robotic arms are inserted through the axillary incision

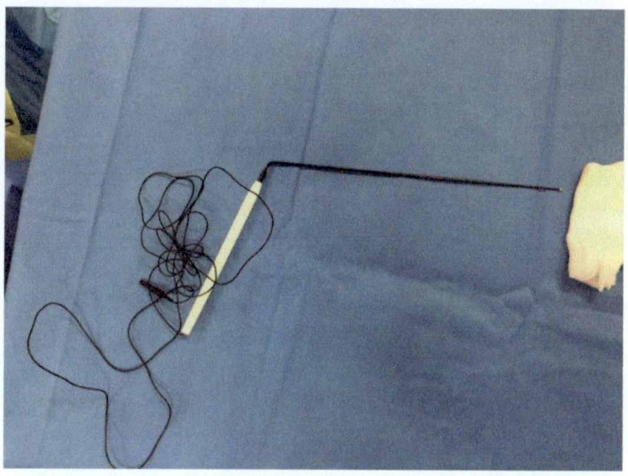

Fig. 11.7 The extended tip of the nerve integrity monitor required during robotic dissection for stimulation of the recurrent laryngeal nerve due to the long distance between the axillary incision and neck

11.5 Transaxillary Access to the Neck

This follows patient positioning (Fig. 11.8), sterilization, and draping. It provides access to the operative field and precedes the robotic part of the operation. A step-by-step narrative is provided in Figs. 11.9, 11.10, 11.11, 11.12, 11.13, 11.14, and 11.15.

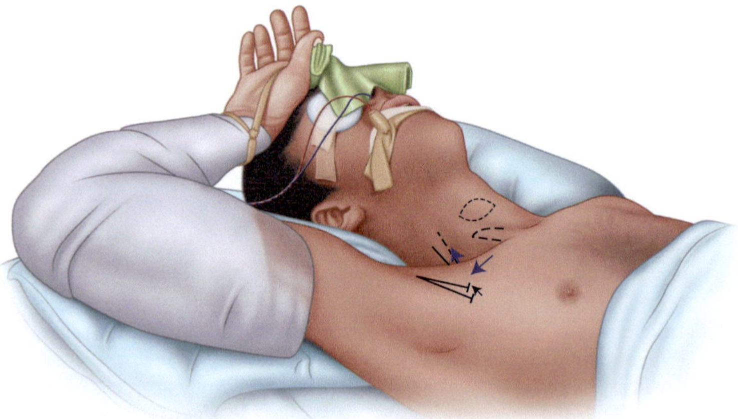

Fig. 11.8 The "extended salute" position for right single-port transaxillary robotic parathyroidectomy (laterality pre-marked with *arrow*). This position shortens the distance between the incision site and parathyroid adenoma by elevating and externally rotating the clavicle while protecting the brachial plexus from traction. This is a modification to Chung's method for transaxillary robotic thyroidectomy where the arm is fully extended over the head [14]. We advise against the fully extended arm position as this puts the brachial plexus at risk through traction. We have had no such problems since modifying Chung's method of arm positioning. Adjusting the position of the ipsilateral arm with the patient awake to assess for comfort and marking the incision immediately prior to surgery constitute vital components of preoperative planning. The 5–6 cm axillary incision has been pre-marked and rechecked once the patient is positioned on the operating table as in our experience this is the optimal way to plan where to place the incision to prevent subsequent migration. Note the NIM EMG endotracheal tube, eye protection, and special arm rest to support the arm which is abducted and flexed with the forearm being pronated so that the back of the hand rests on the central portion of the forehead. A Velcro coin is attached to the hand and forehead to maintain the position

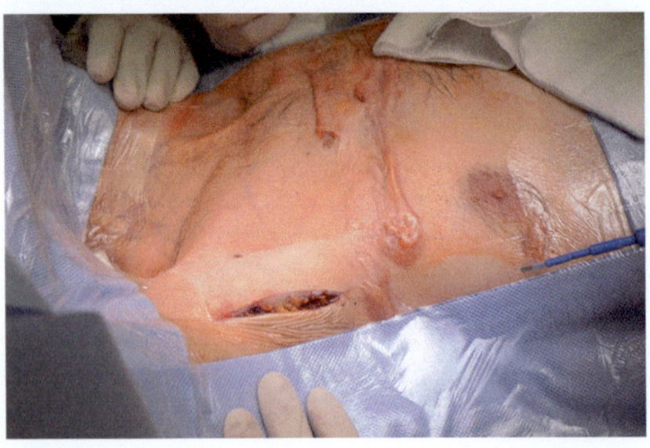

Fig. 11.9 The axillary incision. Note the sterile field includes the neck, anterior thorax, and ipsilateral axilla. EKG leads are placed on the back so as not to interfere with the sterile field

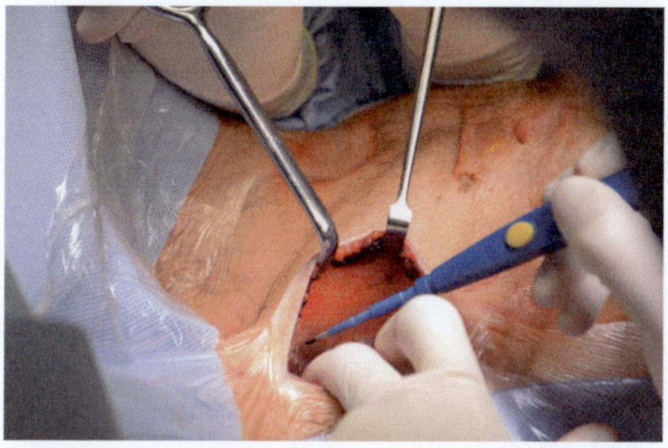

Fig. 11.10 Following the axillary incision, a subcutaneous flap is raised superficial to the clavipectoral fascia. The superior and inferior points of the axillary incision are extended to the thyroid cartilage and sternal notch, respectively. The resulting shape of the flap is that of a trapezoid. In taller patients, if the distance from the axilla to the sternal notch exceeds the limit of the instruments, the robot can be docked in earlier to perform the last (most distal) part of the subcutaneous flap raising. The technique for entering the neck is identical to the one described below but is performed robotically. This modification expands the range of patients to whom single-port transaxillary robotic parathyroidectomy can be offered [15]

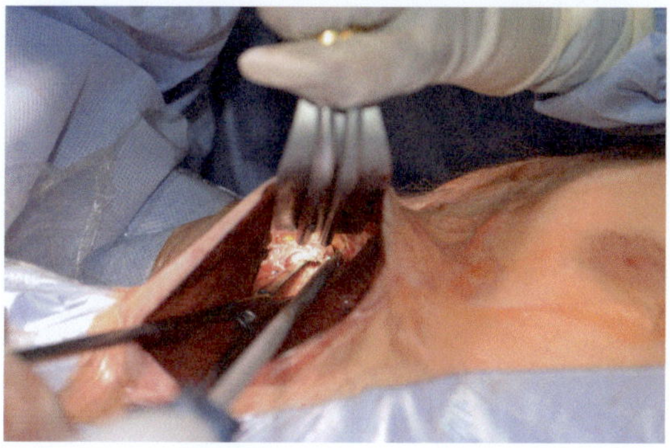

Fig. 11.11 Once the subcutaneous flap is raised, dissection is continued above the pectoralis major and over the clavicle until the sternal and clavicular heads of the sternocleidomastoid muscle are reached

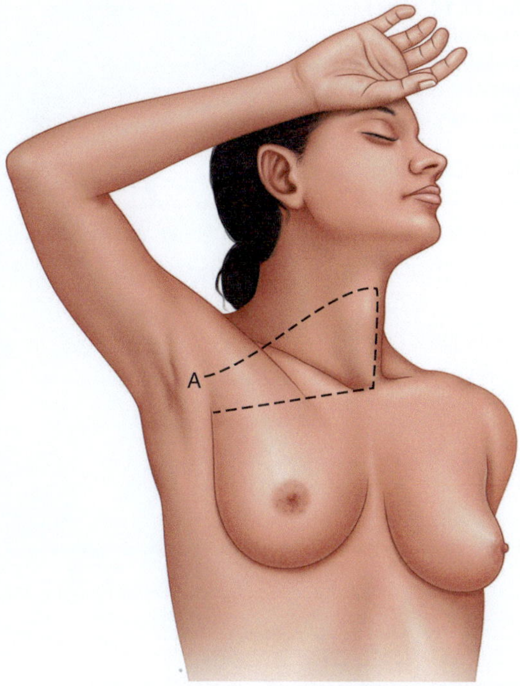

Fig. 11.12 Schematic representation of the incision and anatomical boundaries of the subcutaneous flap needed for right single-port transaxillary robotic parathyroidectomy. The superior and inferior points of the axillary incision are extended to the thyroid cartilage and sternal notch, respectively, resulting in a trapezoid-shaped flap as shown

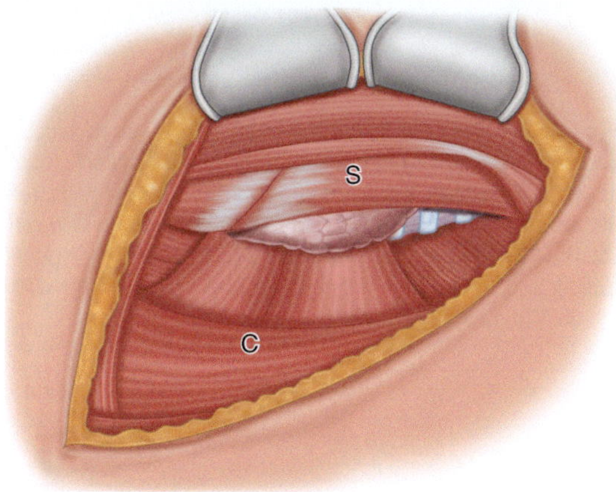

Fig. 11.13 Close-up view of the sternal (S) and clavicular (C) heads of the sternocleidomastoid muscle and the natural dehiscence between the two. The surgical planes are then developed as in a standard parathyroidectomy exposing the ipsilateral internal jugular vein, common carotid artery, and omohyoid and sternohyoid muscles (see Fig. 11.20)

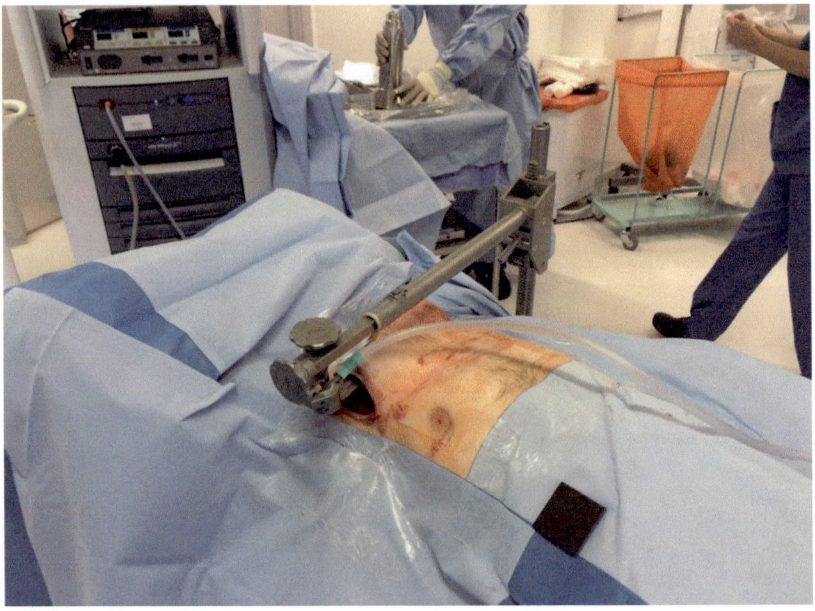

Fig. 11.14 The Modena retractor in situ. Once placed, it is important to connect its port to a suction tube so as to prevent fogging of the robotic dual-channel endoscope once it is inserted

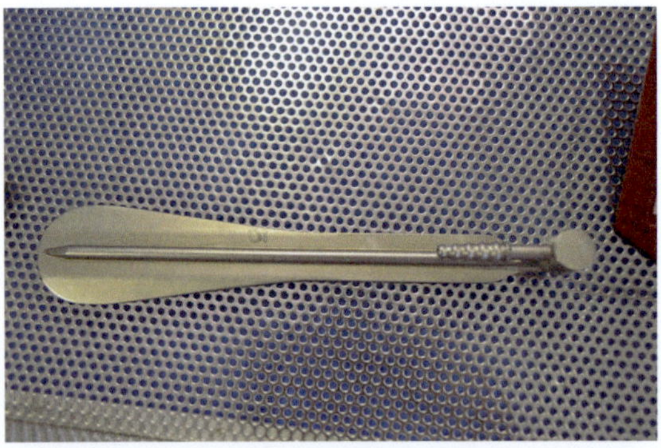

Fig. 11.15 The Modena retractor blade. This is placed under the flap and strap muscles to retract them and create sufficient working space for the robotic arms to be introduced and for them to be able to move freely without clashing. No gas insufflation is required. Once this is positioned and adequate visualization and space confirmed, the da Vinci robot is docked

11.6 Preparation of the Robotic Field

The setup of the operating room (OR) for right single-port transaxillary robotic parathyroidectomy is schematically shown in Fig. 11.16 and the introduction and orientation of the robotic arms and 3D endoscope through the axillary incision explained in Fig. 11.17.

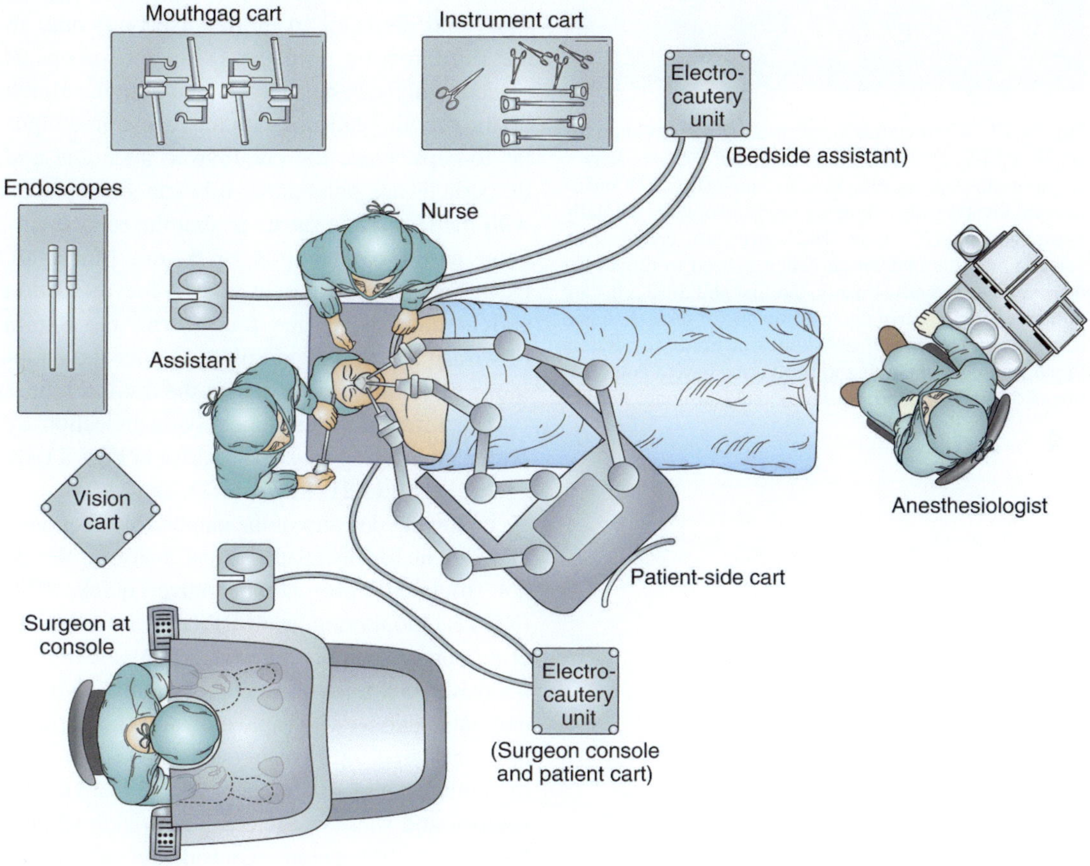

Fig. 11.16 Operating room configuration for right single-port transaxillary robotic parathyroidectomy. Note the cart is docked at right angles to the operating table on the contralateral side to the adenoma

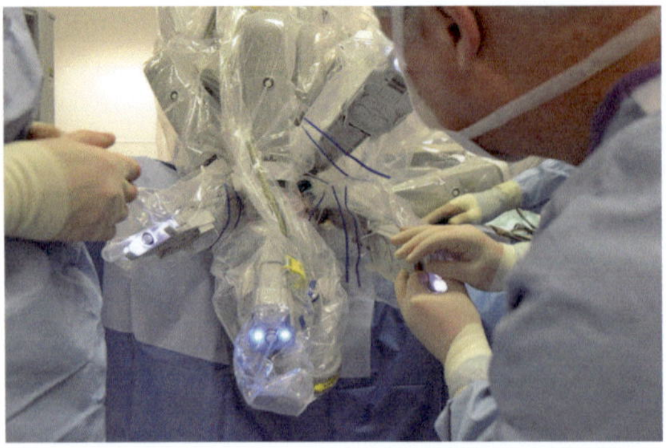

Fig. 11.17 All three robotic arms are placed through the single axillary incision. The 30° down 12 mm stereoscopic endoscope is placed at an angle of 220° and is inserted low laterally extending high and upward medially toward the thyroid gland. The fourth arm can then be placed under the endoscope which is used to retract the thyroid lobe medially. Finally, the first and third arms are positioned which carry the instruments for dissection and hemostasis. The fourth assistant arm holds the 8 mm ProGrasp, while the first and third arms have a combination of 5 mm Maryland, DeBakey, and Harmonic shears

11.7 Robotic Surgery

Following docking of the da Vinci surgical robot, the instruments are placed through their corresponding ports in the respective robotic arms. Initially, provided the robotic surgeon is right-handed, the fenestrated bipolar forceps is placed in the right (first) robotic arm and the 5 mm Maryland dissector in the left (second) one. In the third robotic arm, the DeBakey forceps is placed which can be interchanged with the clutch on the robotic platform with the fenestrated bipolar forceps. Once the parathyroid adenoma and its pedicle are delineated, this can be replaced with the Harmonic shears so that the robotic surgeon has a combination of 5 mm Maryland, DeBakey, and Harmonic shears for dissection and hemostasis. In the fourth arm, the 8 mm ProGrasp is inserted and placed under the endoscope to contralaterally retract the thyroid lobe.

The different stages of the robotic dissection are presented in a step-by-step narrative in Figs. 11.18, 11.19, 11.20, 11.21, 11.22, 11.23, and 11.24.

Following delivery of the parathyroid adenoma, this is sent for histopathological analysis. We do not routinely use intraoperative quick PTH (iQPTH) monitoring as all RP cases in our endocrine surgery tertiary referral center undergo an intensive multidisciplinary preoperative workup and only patients with triple modality concordance are considered for this approach. This is precisely to minimize the risk of persistent hyperparathyroidism and subsequent need for revision surgery (see Sect. 1, "Preoperative Considerations"). We do however use iQPTH routinely if no triple modality concordance exists or there is any other doubt about adenoma location or the presence of parathyroid hyperplasia, though, as already discussed, such patients would not constitute candidates for robotic surgery. In the presence of preoperative triple modality concordance, iQPTH monitoring can be safely omitted when performing focused parathyroidectomy for most cases of pHPT [17, 18].

As with all parathyroid surgery, hemostasis should be meticulous. The anesthesiologist is asked to bring the blood pressure up to normal and a reversed Trendelenburg position and Valsalva maneuver applied. Any remaining bleeding points are addressed at this stage to ensure hemostasis. As in conventional parathyroid surgery, no drain is applied. We have not found this to be a problem.

Following hemostasis, the da Vinci robot is withdrawn and 2-layer closure completed with 4-0 subcuticular Vicryl Rapide sutures (Ethicon Products, Inc., Johnson & Johnson, Cincinnati, OH) followed by application of Dermabond (Ethicon Products, Inc., Johnson & Johnson, Cincinnati, OH) tissue glue on the wound (Fig. 11.25). An anterior chest wall compression dressing is applied overnight (Fig. 11.26).

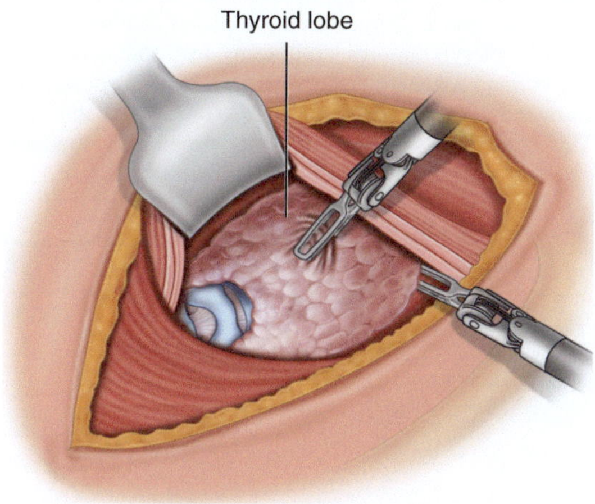

Fig. 11.18 Entering the natural dehiscence between the sternal and clavicular heads of the sternocleidomastoid muscle. As the flap and strap muscles are retracted by the Modena retractor, the first structure to encounter is the ipsilateral thyroid lobe

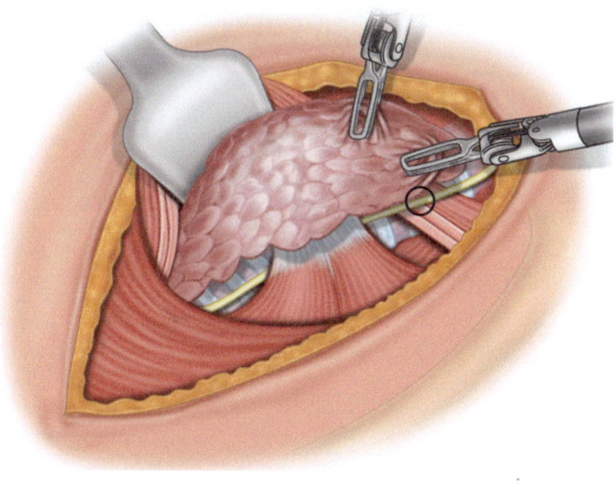

Fig. 11.19 The thyroid lobe is retracted medially and the recurrent laryngeal nerve (*circled*) identified in the tracheoesophageal groove

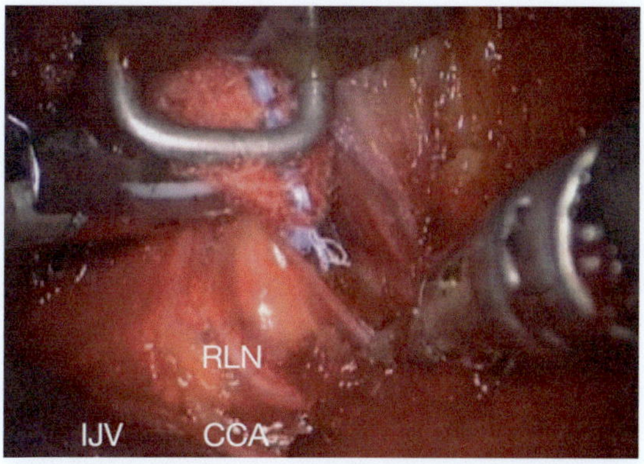

Fig. 11.20 The great vessels of the neck, the common carotid artery (CCA), and the internal jugular vein (IJV) are also identified while keeping into view the recurrent laryngeal nerve (RLN)

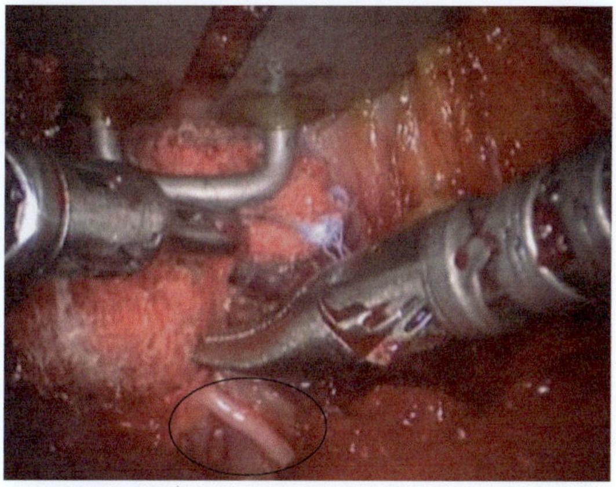

Fig. 11.21 Following identification of all relevant neurovascular structures, the recurrent laryngeal nerve (*circled*) is carefully dissected, stimulated, and subsequently gently displaced laterally out of the operative field and protected with a pledget

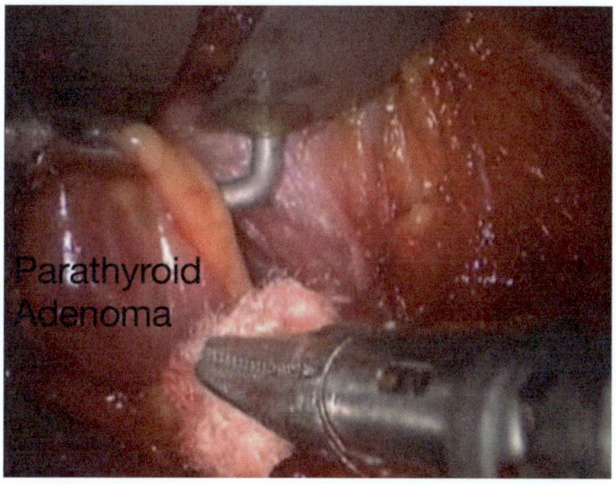

Fig. 11.22 Next, the parathyroid adenoma is identified posterior to the thyroid and bluntly dissected with a pledget

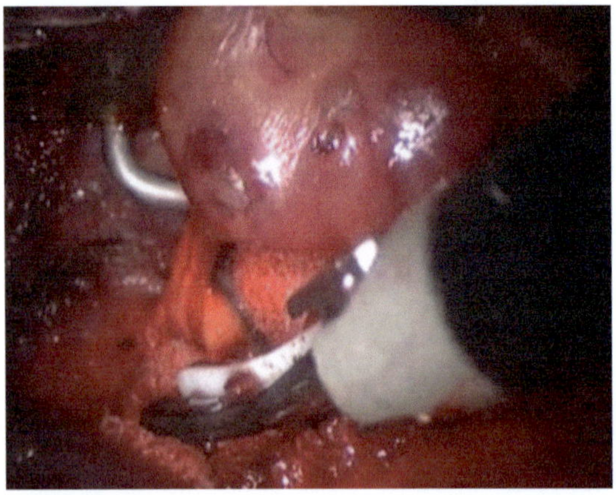

Fig. 11.23 Following blunt dissection of the parathyroid adenoma, its vascular pedicle is delineated. At this point, the Harmonic shears is introduced

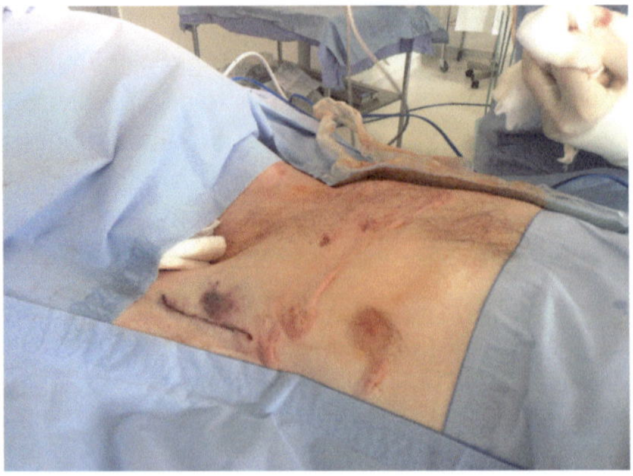

Fig. 11.25 Following hemostasis, the da Vinci robot is withdrawn and 2-layer closure completed with 4-0 subcuticular Vicryl sutures followed by application of Dermabond tissue glue on the wound. Note the ecchymosis over the distal flap just superior to the axillary incision. This commonly appears due to the prolonged retraction and resolves after about 2 week following surgery

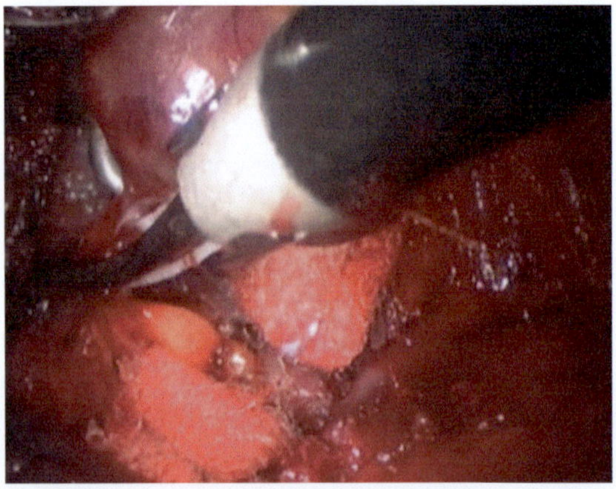

Fig. 11.24 The Harmonic shears is used to ligate and divide the vascular pedicle. Prior to doing so, it is vital to reconfirm the position of the recurrent laryngeal nerve, protect it again with a pledget, and keep the Harmonic shears at a clear distance from it, as illustrated, to prevent nerve damage from lateral thermal spread [16]. Subsequently, the parathyroid adenoma can be delivered through the axillary incision by the assistant surgeon

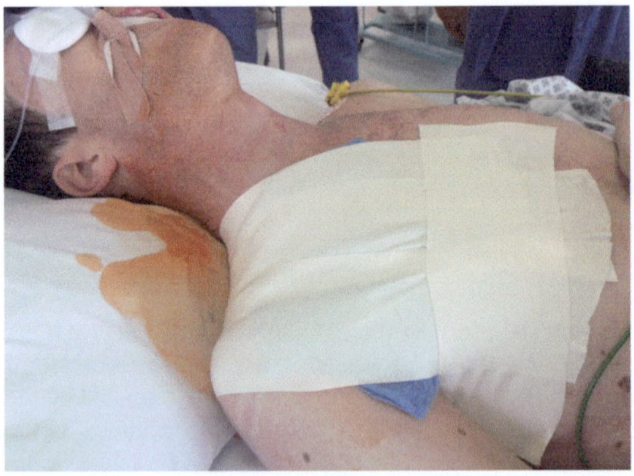

Fig. 11.26 Following wound closure, the ipsilateral arm is brought back to the neutral position, and an anterior chest wall compression dressing is applied overnight

11.8 Postoperative Care and Follow-Up

Patients are discharged the following morning once corrected calcium and PTH levels have been checked and confirmed to be normal (<24 h hospital stay). They are advised to wear a sports bra or vest for 2 weeks to provide light compression to the anterior chest wall. Antibiotics (co-amoxiclav 625 mg three times a day) are routinely given for 7 days and analgesia (acetaminophen 1 g four times a day for 7 days) as required. Regular follow-up at 2 weeks, 3, 6, 12, 18, and 24 months allows prospective long-term evaluation.

11.9 Surgical Complications

As discussed, the risks associated with RP are the same as for conventional parathyroidectomy with regard to the recurrent laryngeal nerve (RLN), infection, hematoma, seroma, persistent hyperparathyroidism, and need for revision surgery. Thus, preventing and managing those complications involves the same measures as in conventional parathyroid surgery. The only exception relates to the prevention of hematoma and seroma where following wound closure, an anterior chest wall compression dressing is applied overnight. The next morning, this is removed, and the patient is advised to wear a sports bra or vest for 2 weeks to provide light compression to the anterior chest wall.

This section will address those complications that relate specifically to RP. These are dysesthesia on the chest over the area of the subcutaneous flap and brachial plexus neurapraxia.

Regarding dysesthesia over the chest wall, it is important to mention this to the patient before surgery so that they expect it. As a matter of fact, this is not a complication but a natural occurrence following subcutaneous flap elevation. All patients will experience this to a certain extent. It is equally important to explain to the patient that it almost always resolves though can take several months to do so. Pain is not a particular problem with RP [9, 10].

The other risk is brachial plexus neurapraxia. Patients need to be also made aware of this, but at the same time, they need to be explained so that this is exquisitely rare, provided the correct preventative measures have been employed. These are described below.

The key to preventing brachial plexus neurapraxia is by placing the arm in the "correct" position and maintaining this for the duration of the operation. The reason for this is that the mechanism underlining this complication involves hyperextension of the brachial plexus. By "correct" we mean a position where the ipsilateral arm is comfortable for the patient while ensuring optimal transaxillary access to the neck. The only way to achieve this is by positioning the patient's arm when they are awake in order to assess for comfort (and thus prevent hyperextension of the brachial plexus) [12]. The position we advise for the arm is the "extended salute" position described in detail in Fig. 11.1. This position shortens the distance between the incision site and parathyroid adenoma by elevating and externally rotating the clavicle whilst protecting the brachial plexus from traction. A Velcro coin is attached to the hand and forehead to maintain the position during surgery.

As part of the routine postoperative check in the recovery room, it is vital not only to ask the patient for any abnormal sensation or weakness along their arm but also formally assess the neurovascular status of their upper limb. If any neurological deficit or shoulder stiffness is identified that has not resolved by the next morning, it is paramount to involve a physiotherapist at an early stage, i.e., prior to discharge to teach the patient what exercises to do daily and follow them up on an outpatient basis until full resolution occurs.

11.10 Mentoring and Proctorship

The most important influence on outcomes in parathyroid surgery is the experience and volume of the surgeon [19]. Thus, mentoring and proctorship are vital to optimize surgical results and minimize complications [20].

RP should only be undertaken by appropriately trained surgeons with sufficient experience in parathyroid surgery employed in high-volume institutions that possess the necessary equipment and access to technical support [11]. Finally, there needs to be a dedicated robotic nursing team too with the appropriate training and experience so as to enhance the performance of the robotic team.

References

1. Tolley N, Arora A, Palazzo F, Garas G, Dhawan R, Cox J, Darzi A. Robotic-assisted parathyroidectomy: a feasibility study. Otolaryngol Head Neck Surg. 2011;144(6):859–66.
2. Garas G, Poulasouchidou M, Dimoulas A, Hytiroglou P, Kita M, Zacharakis E. Radiological considerations and surgical planning in the treatment of giant parathyroid adenomas. Ann R Coll Surg Engl. 2015;97(4):e64–6.
3. Bearelly S, Prendes BL, Wang SJ, Glastonbury C, Orloff LA. Transoral robotic-assisted surgical excision of a retropharyngeal parathyroid adenoma: a case report. Head Neck. 2015;37(11):E150–2.
4. Bodner J, Profanter C, Prommegger R, Greiner A, Margreiter R, Schmid T. Mediastinal parathyroidectomy with the da Vinci robot: presentation of a new technique. J Thorac Cardiovasc Surg. 2004; 127(6):1831–2.
5. Chan AP, Wan IY, Wong RH, Hsin MK, Underwood MJ. Robot-assisted excision of ectopic mediastinal parathyroid adenoma. Asian Cardiovasc Thorac Ann. 2010;18(1):65–7.
6. Ismail M, Maza S, Swierzy M, Tsilimparis N, Rogalla P, Sandrock D, Ruckert RI, Muller JM, Ruckert JC. Resection of ectopic mediastinal parathyroid glands with the da Vinci robotic system. Br J Surg. 2010;97(3):337–43.
7. Van Dessel E, Hendriks JM, Lauwers P, Ysebaert D, Ruyssers Jr N, Van Schil PE. Mediastinal parathyroidectomy with the da Vinci robot. Innovations (Phila). 2011;6(4):262–4.
8. Arora A, Swords C, Garas G, Chaidas K, Prichard A, Budge J, Davies DC, Tolley N. The perception of scar cosmesis following thyroid and parathyroid surgery: a prospective cohort study. Int J Surg. 2016;25:38–43.
9. Tolley N, Garas G, Palazzo F, Prichard A, Chaidas K, Cox J, Darzi A, Arora A. Long-term prospective evaluation comparing robotic parathyroidectomy with minimally invasive open parathyroidectomy for primary hyperparathyroidism. Head Neck. 2014;38 Suppl 1:E300–6.
10. Garas G, Holsinger FC, Grant DG, Athanasiou T, Arora A, Tolley N. Is robotic parathyroidectomy a feasible and safe alternative to targeted open parathyroidectomy for the treatment of primary hyperparathyroidism? Int J Surg. 2015;15:55–60.
11. Garas G, Arora A, Tolley N. Robotic surgery of the parathyroid glands. In: Grillone GA, Jalisi S, editors. Robotic surgery of the head and neck a comprehensive guide. New York: Springer; 2015. p. 133–46.
12. Chung WY. Pros of robotic transaxillary thyroid surgery: its impact on cancer control and surgical quality. Thyroid. 2012;22(10):986–7.
13. Arora A, Garas G, Sharma S, Muthuswamy K, Budge J, Palazzo F, Darzi A, Tolley N. Comparing transaxillary robotic thyroidectomy with conventional surgery in a UK population: a case control study. Int J Surg. 2016;27:110–7.
14. Kang SW, Jeong JJ, Yun JS, Sung TY, Lee SC, Lee YS, Nam KH, Chang HS, Chung WY, Park CS. Robot-assisted endoscopic surgery for thyroid cancer: experience with the first 100 patients. Surg Endosc. 2009;23(11):2399–406.
15. Foley CS, Agcaoglu O, Siperstein AE, Berber E. Robotic transaxillary endocrine surgery: a comparison with conventional open technique. Surg Endosc. 2012;26(8):2259–66.
16. Garas G, Okabayashi K, Ashrafian H, Shetty K, Palazzo F, Tolley N, Darzi A, Athanasiou T, Zacharakis E. Which hemostatic device in thyroid surgery? A network meta-analysis of surgical technologies. Thyroid. 2013;23(9):1138–50.
17. Mownah OA, Pafitanis G, Drake WM, Crinnion JN. Contemporary surgical treatment of primary hyperparathyroidism without intraoperative parathyroid hormone measurement. Ann R Coll Surg Engl. 2015;97(8):603–7.
18. Soyder A, Unubol M, Omurlu IK, Guney E, Ozbas S. Minimally invasive parathyroidectomy without using intraoperative parathyroid hormone monitoring or gamma probe. Ulus Cerrahi Derg. 2015;31(1): 9–14.
19. Stavrakis AI, Ituarte PH, Ko CY, Yeh MW. Surgeon volume as a predictor of outcomes in inpatient and outpatient endocrine surgery. Surgery. 2007;142(6):887–899; discussion 887–99.
20. Athanasiou T, Patel V, Garas G, Ashrafian H, Shetty K, Sevdalis N, Panzarasa P, Darzi A, Paroutis S. Mentoring perception and academic performance: an Academic Health Science Centre survey. Postgrad Med J. 2016;92(1092):597–602.

12 Robot-Assisted Neck Surgery

Hyung Kwon Byeon and Yoon Woo Koh

12.1 Introduction

Conventional surgeries for various surgically treatable neck tumors adopted the transcervical approach to "open up" the surgical field which were sometimes unfavorable for the patient since the resulting scars were perceived disfiguring and the surgeries also caused various postoperative morbidities. The neck is the most easily recognized and exposed area, and the psychosocial impact may be even more displeasing if a large incisional scar has been created due to neck dissection for head and neck cancer with cervical metastasis. Furthermore, conventional transcervical approach-based surgeries often require large amount of normal tissue dissection just for the purpose of surgical access which could lead to prolonged postoperative recovery and various degrees of functional deterioration.

Consequently in order to reduce the extent of surgical trauma and minimize these surgery-related morbidities, numerous surgical approaches from a distant port have been developed. These so-called remote-access surgeries were founded upon the technological advances of endoscopy and surgical robotics. Based on the early attempts of robotic facelift thyroidectomies by Terris et al. [1–5] and the authors' extensive surgical experience on former endoscopic and robotic gasless transaxillary thyroidectomy [6, 7], we have extrapolated the application of the RA approach to nearly all aspects of head and neck surgery with the aid of the robotic system (Da Vinci Si Robotic System; Intuitive Surgical Inc., Sunnyvale, CA) [8–17]. The authors have seen the promising role of RA approach from its versatile applications.

H.K. Byeon, MD, PhD • Y.W. Koh, MD, PhD (✉)
Department of Otorhinolaryngology, Yonsei University College of Medicine, Seoul, South Korea
e-mail: EWELL@yuhs.ac; ywkohent@gmail.com

Z. Gil et al. (eds.), *Atlas of Head and Neck Robotic Surgery*, DOI 10.1007/978-3-319-49578-1_12

12.2 Fundamental Concept

The modified facelift (MFL) incision when performing conventional parotidectomy forms the basis for RA incision. The only difference between the MFL and RA incision is the existence of the preauricular limb (Fig. 12.1). Most of the time this robotic procedure can be conducted with the RA incision; however, if there is a necessity for extended access or if a parotidectomy is simultaneously performed at the same side, the MFL incision can be made. Since the surgical access port is remotely placed, common procedures of working space creation and pre-robotic gross dissection are universally applied to all RA robotic neck surgeries.

12.2.1 Universal Surgical Sequence

First, a RA incision is made and an appropriate working space is established (Figs. 12.2 and 12.3).

Next, a self-retaining retractor (L & C Bio, Seongnam-si, Korea) is placed to maintain the working space and then certain surgical steps of gross dissection under the naked eye are conducted beforehand, to move on to the robotic dissection. Recently, this procedure can also be done at the surgeon's robotic console with the help of the upgraded da Vinci Xi system, since an extra robotic instrumental arm can be inserted through the RA port (Fig. 12.4).

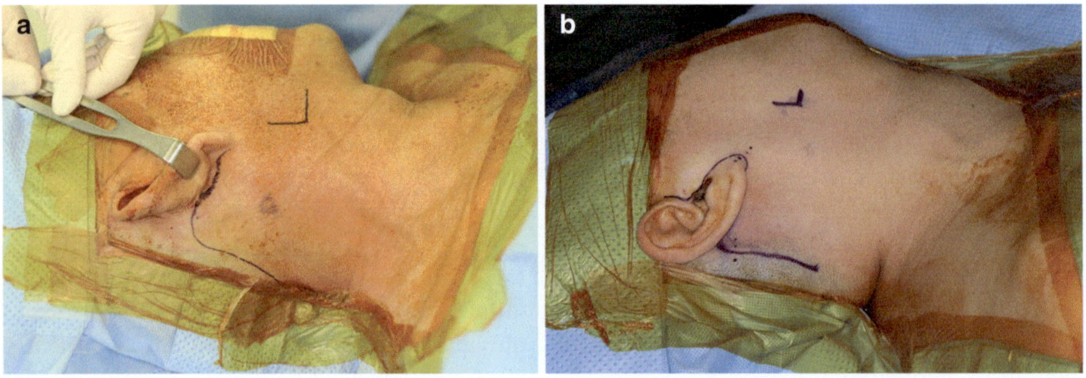

Fig. 12.1 The position of the patient is supine with the head rotated to the contralateral side of the approach just as you would perform a parotidectomy. The neck, however, is relaxed in its natural position and not extended with shoulder rolls. (**a**) Retroauricular incision. (**b**) Modified facelift incision

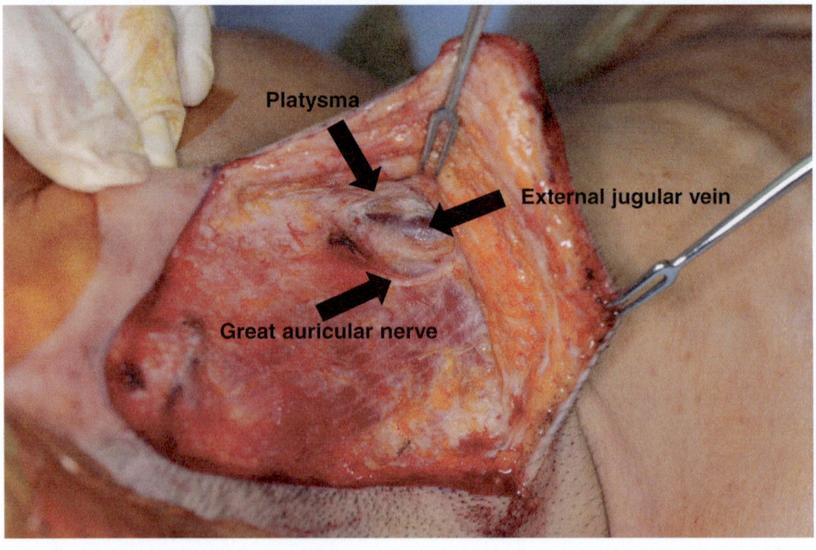

Fig. 12.2 A subplatysmal skin flap is elevated leaving the great auricular nerve and the external jugular vein on the SCM fascia (Operative photograph of right-sided approach)

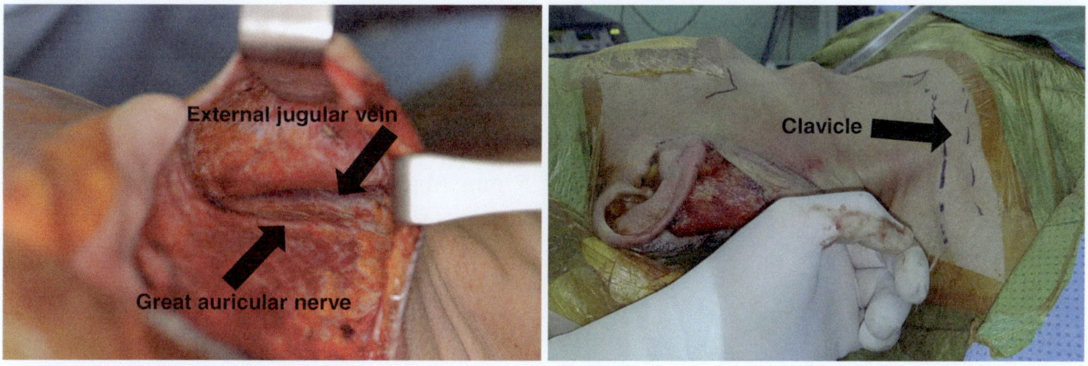

Fig. 12.3 The skin-subplatysmal flap is elevated so that it reaches the clavicle inferiorly, midline of the anterior neck medially, and the inferior border of the mandible superiorly. The posterior extent of the working space can be either made anterior or posterior to the SCM border depending on the type of robotic neck procedure

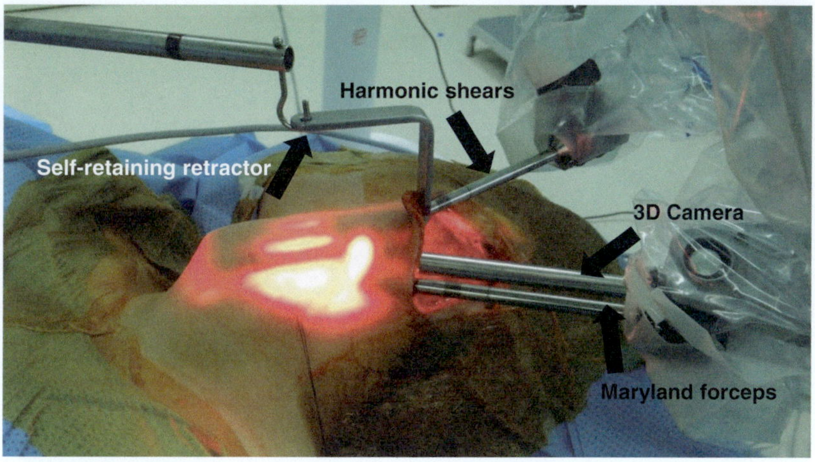

Fig. 12.4 After completion of working space creation and gross dissection, the robotic arms are docked to commence robotic dissection. A facedown 30° dual endoscope is placed at the center, and two robotic instrument arms each equipped with 5 mm Maryland forceps and 5 mm Harmonic curved shears are inserted at either side (Operative photograph of left-sided approach)

12.3 Surgical Technique

12.3.1 Robotic Surgery of Benign Neck Mass

Almost all cases of benign neck mass can be competently removed by the RA approach. Here, three commonly performed surgical procedures are addressed in detail.

12.3.1.1 Robot-Assisted Sistrunk's Operation (Fig. 12.5)

Following the docking of the robotic arms, the midline of the neck is recognized by dividing the fibroadipose tissue at the anterior neck using a 5 mm Maryland forceps and a 5 mm spatula monopolar cautery (Figs. 12.6 and 12.7).

Further mobilization of the contralateral side of the hyoid bone is done and resected also with the bone cutter. The thyroglossal duct should be traced further beyond the hyoid bone, and eventually the main mass together with the resected hyoid bone is removed en bloc through the RA port.

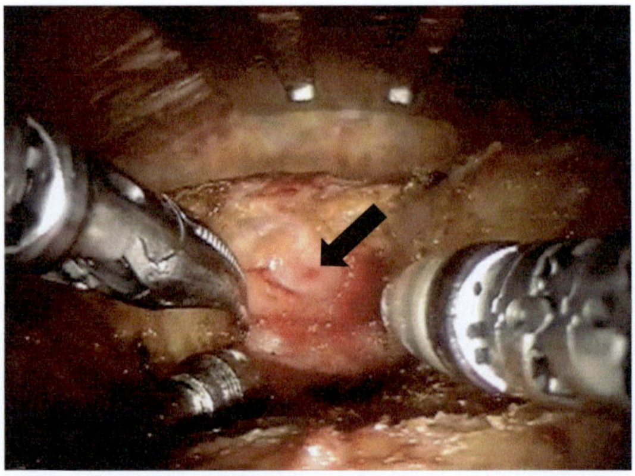

Fig. 12.5 After subplatysmal skin flap elevation through the RA incision and establishment of the working space, the robotic arms are introduced. Contour of the thyroglossal duct cyst lesion (*arrow*) can be readily visualized beneath the strap muscles (Operative photograph of left-sided approach)

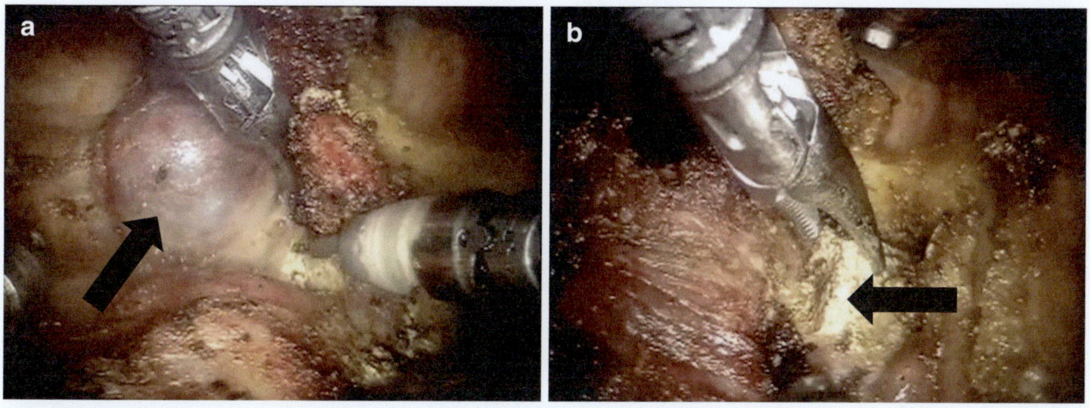

Fig. 12.6 The cystic lesion is carefully dissected and mobilized, and the contour of the hyoid bone is identified and skeletonized. (**a**) *Arrow*: thyroglossal duct cyst. (**b**) *Arrow*: ipsilateral hyoid bone (Operative photograph of left-sided approach)

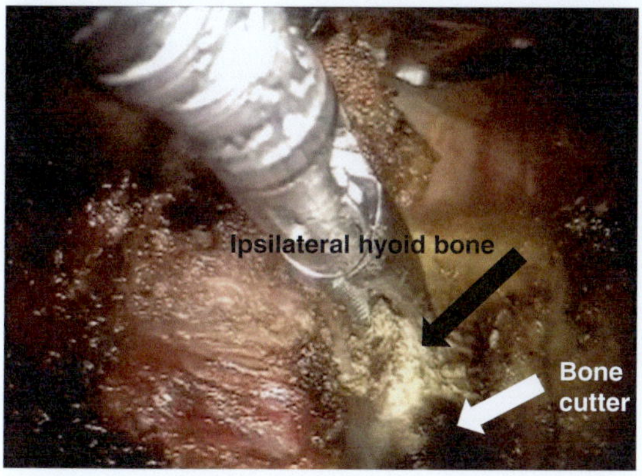

Fig. 12.7 Once the ipsilateral side of the hyoid bone is sufficiently mobilized, a conventional bone cutter is directly inserted through the RA port by the patient-side assistant, and the bone is cut

12.3.1.2 Robot-Assisted Neurogenic Tumor Excision

The subplatysmal skin flap is elevated, and sufficient area of working space is created before the robotic docking. Generally, for the removal of neurogenic tumors a Metzenbaum scissors (PK™ Dissecting Forceps) is used for the enucleation of the tumor (Fig. 12.8).

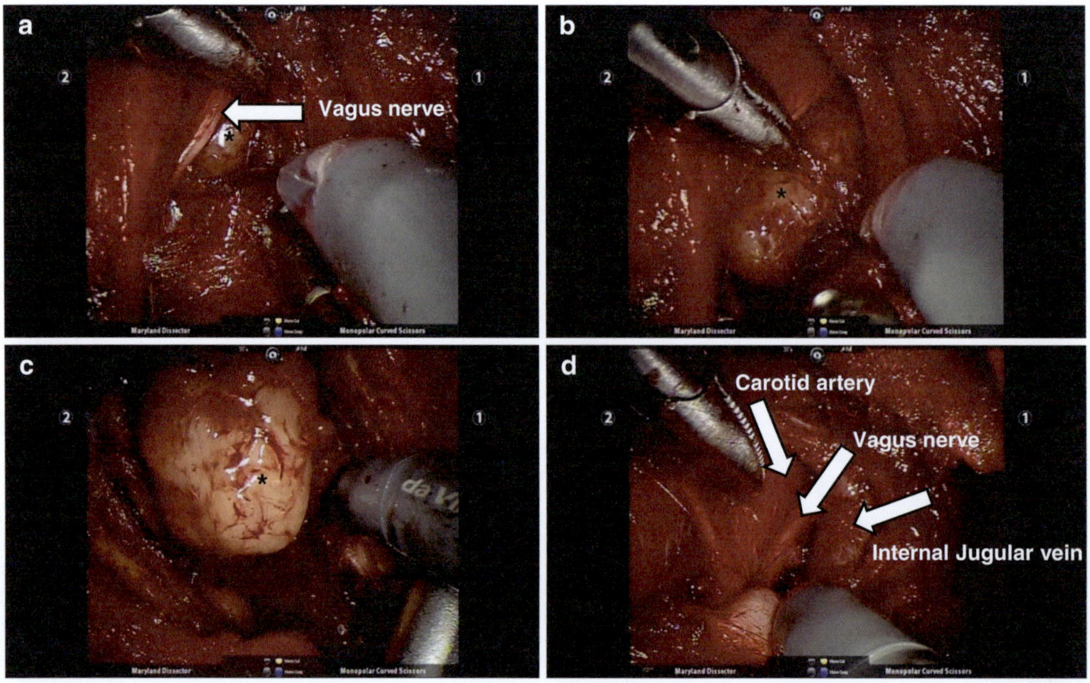

Fig. 12.8 Removal of vagal schwannoma. (Right-sided approach). (**a**) The neurogenic tumor is usually located in close proximity to the carotid sheath so dissection must be cautiously done when exposing the tumor. Special attention must be paid to prevent any injuries to other nerves around the carotid sheath. (**b**, **c**) Using the dissecting forceps, the true capsule of the neurogenic tumor (*asterisk*) is revealed, and the tumor is enucleated to minimize postoperative neural damage. (**d**) Post-removal surgical view with clear visualization of vital structures of the carotid sheath

12.3.1.3 Robot-Assisted Submandibular Gland Excision

After creating a sufficient area of working space, a self-retaining retractor is placed to maintain the height for robotic arms docking (Figs. 12.9 and 12.10).

Further subcapsular dissection is performed around the superior border of the SMG to proceed the dissection to the anterior portion of the gland (Fig. 12.11).

Care must be taken not to violate the tumor itself during the dissection. Interaction of the robotic surgeon with the patient-side assistant surgeon is important. The traction and countertraction manipulation should be well coordinated by appropriate handling of the Yankauer suction tip or endoscopic dissector held by the assistant. This surgical technique of robot-assisted submandibular gland resection is considered a key, fundamental procedure for robot-assisted neck dissection (RAND), so it is recommended for a beginning surgeon to experience a sufficient number of these procedures before attempting RAND.

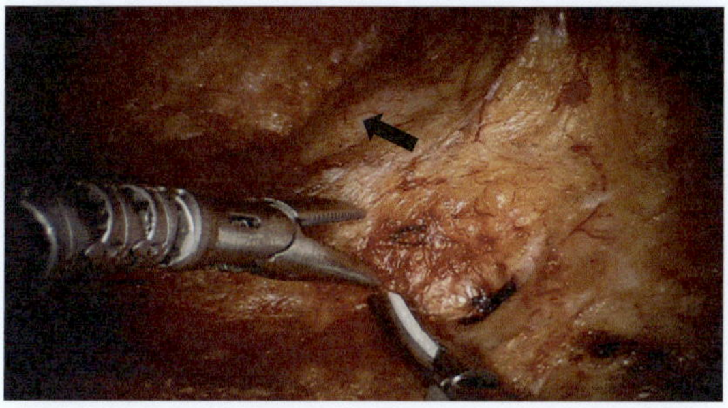

Fig. 12.9 Once the robotic arms are all introduced, the contour of the submandibular gland (*arrow*) can be clearly delineated from the surgeon's console (Left-sided approach)

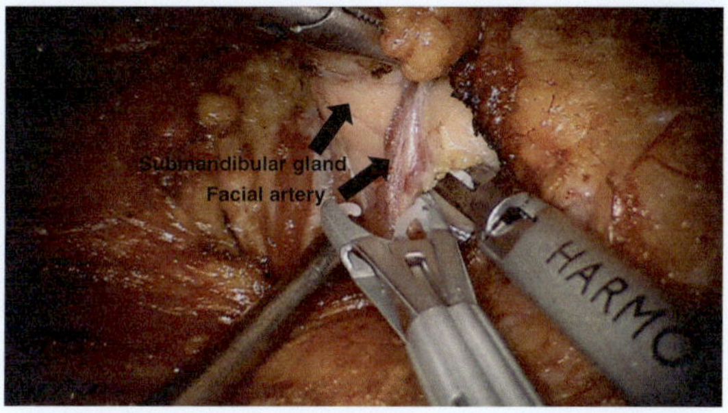

Fig. 12.10 The robotic dissection is commenced at the lower border of the submandibular gland. Subcapsular dissection is continued with Harmonic curved shears or monopolar cautery until the proximal portion of the facial artery is identified. The vessel can be ligated either by Harmonic curved shears or Hem-o-lok ligation system (Teleflex Inc., Research Triangle Park, NC) (Left-sided approach)

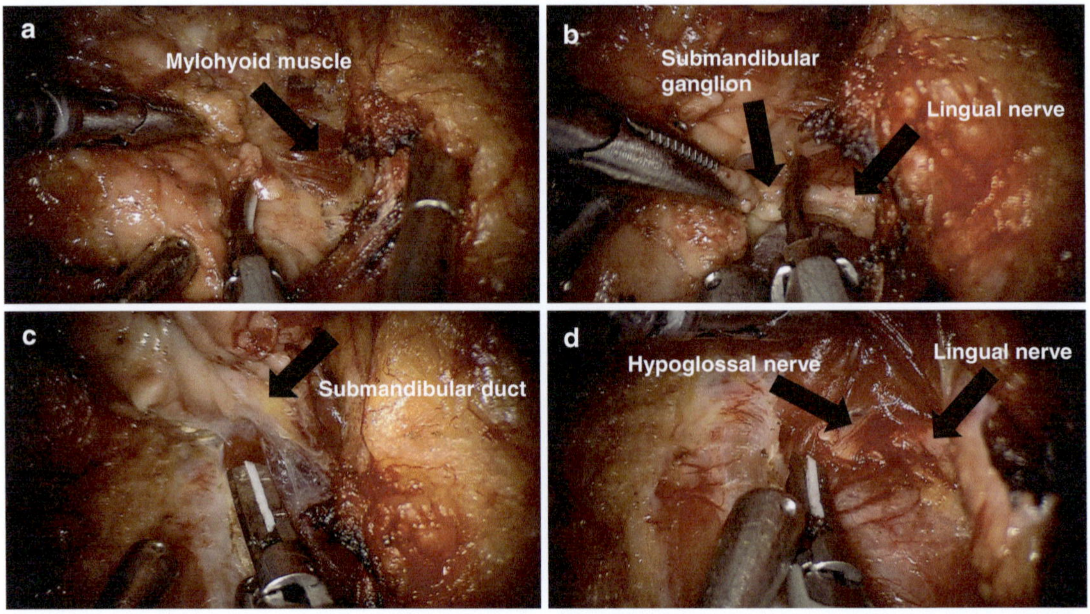

Fig. 12.11 (**a**) The specimen is retracted posteriorly to identify the mylohyoid muscle located at the anterior aspect of the submandibular gland. (**b**, **c**) The posterior border of the mylohyoid muscle is dissected, and posterior retraction of the submandibular gland is maintained to reveal the Wharton's duct and submandibular ganglion. These anatomical structures are ligated after confirming the intact course of the lingual nerve and hypoglossal nerve. (**d**) Surgical view after submandibular gland removal showing intact lingual nerve and hypoglossal nerve (Left-sided approach)

12.3.2 Robot-Assisted Neck Dissection

The procedure of RAND can be equally applied to both cN0 or cN+ necks in head and neck cancer. For the RAND in cN+ necks, main vital neurovascular anatomical structures such as spinal accessory nerve, internal jugular vein, and sternocleidomastoid muscle must be preserved considering that the main purpose of RAND is to minimize postoperative morbidities. Therefore, in any cases where this is not feasible, the authors recommend conventional open neck dissection rather than RAND. Careful, prudent selection of patients for therapeutic RAND must therefore be carried out beforehand, with close examinations of preoperative imagings.

Here, the RAND procedure is specified in detail with emphasis on two distinct operations: selective neck dissection (levels I–III) and comprehensive neck dissection (levels I–V). Other types of neck dissection can be performed by selective modifications of these two procedures.

12.3.2.1 Selective Neck Dissection (Levels I–III)

Pre-robotic Procedure

Certain amount of dissection is conducted under naked eye beforehand, prior to robotic dissection. Generally, the dissection is followed according to the conventional neck dissection procedure (Figs. 12.12, 12.13, and 12.14).

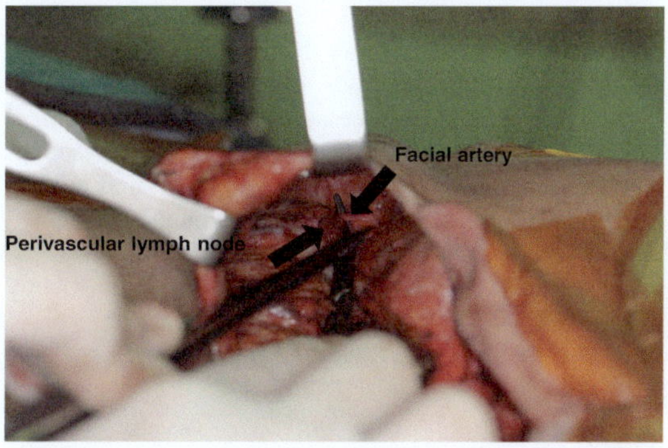

Fig. 12.12 First, level Ib dissection is performed. The marginal branch of the facial nerve is identified by visualizing the facial vessels around the mandibular notch. The nerve is handled with extreme care while dissection of the perifacial lymph nodes is done. After ligation of facial artery and vein, the lymphoadipose tissues inferior to the parotid tail are dissected (Left-sided approach)

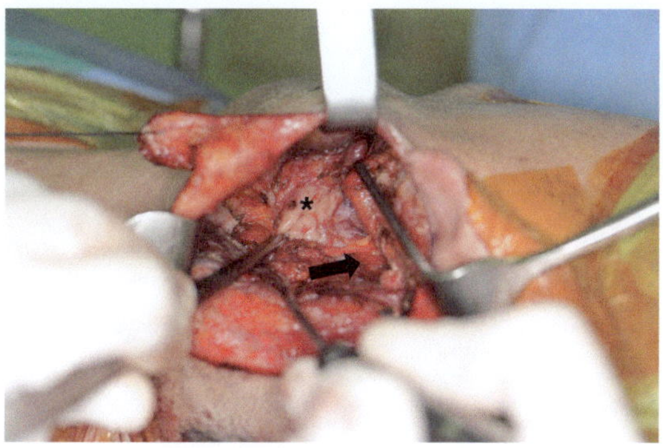

Fig. 12.13 Dissection is continued to the inferior border of submandibular gland (*asterisk*), revealing the posterior belly of digastric muscle (*arrow*) below (Left-sided approach)

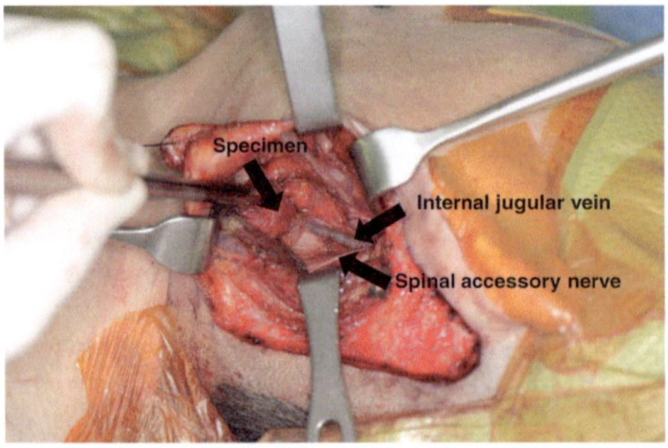

Fig. 12.14 Dissection along the anterior border of sternocleidomastoid muscle leads to exposure of the internal jugular vein. The spinal accessory nerve is then identified where it crosses the internal jugular vein and is sequentially skeletonized, to remove the fibrofatty tissues of level IIb. Next levels IIa and III are continuously dissected toward the carotid sheath. Here, the specimen can be either removed or pushed aside to continue the robotic dissection (*Left*-sided approach)

Robotic Dissection (Figs. 12.15, 12.16, 12.17, and 12.18)

Next the direction of dissection is turned to levels II and III, around the carotid sheath. The inferior extent of the dissection is the omohyoid muscle, and the medial extent is the midline strap muscles. The specimen is then removed en bloc.

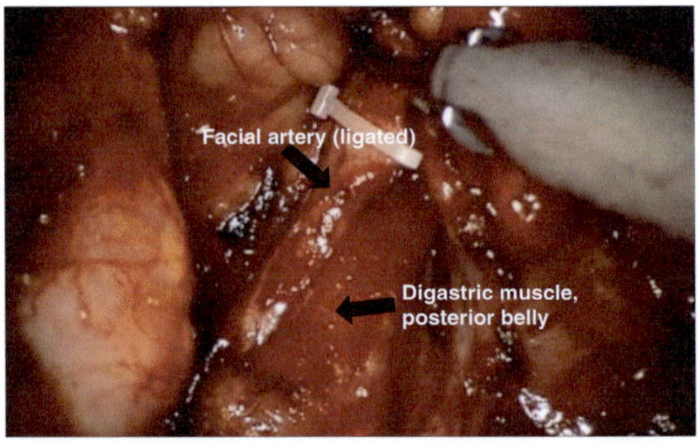

Fig. 12.15 The robotic dissection is commenced at level I. After recognizing the posterior belly of the digastric muscle, the previously dissected proximal facial artery at the posterior portion of the submandibular gland is ligated with Harmonic curved shears or Hem-o-lok ligation system (Right-sided approach)

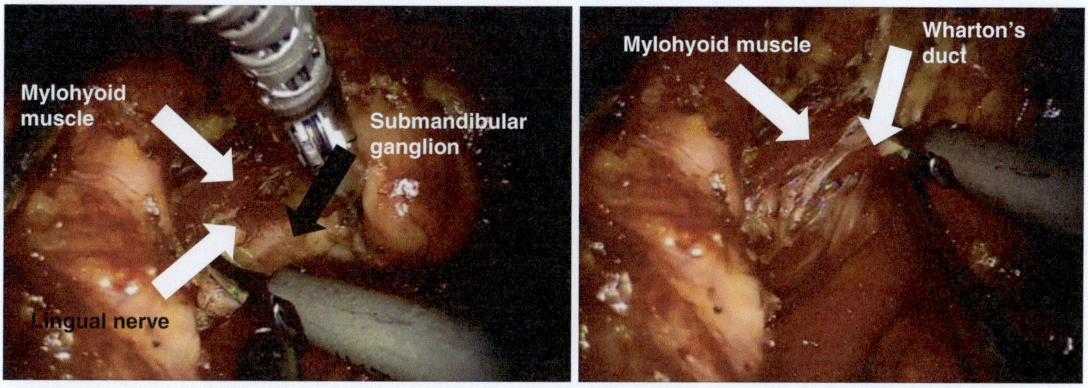

Fig. 12.16 Dissection is then continued anteriorly to identify the mylohyoid muscle and the underlying submandibular ganglion and Wharton's duct which are consequently sealed off (Right-sided approach)

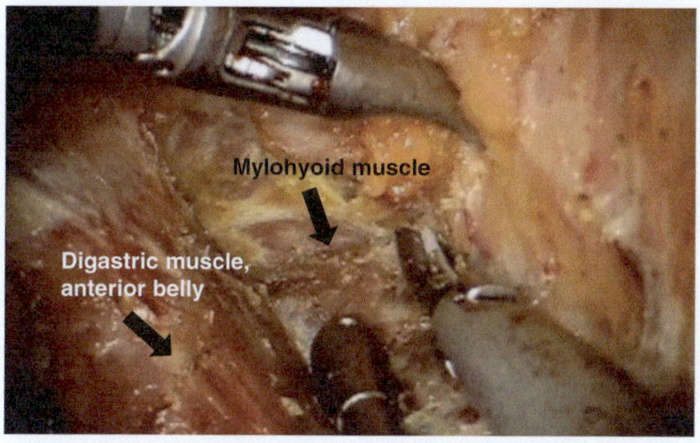

Fig. 12.17 The specimen is then retracted posteriorly, and the dissection moves on to level Ia between the anterior bellies of right and left digastric muscles (Right-sided approach)

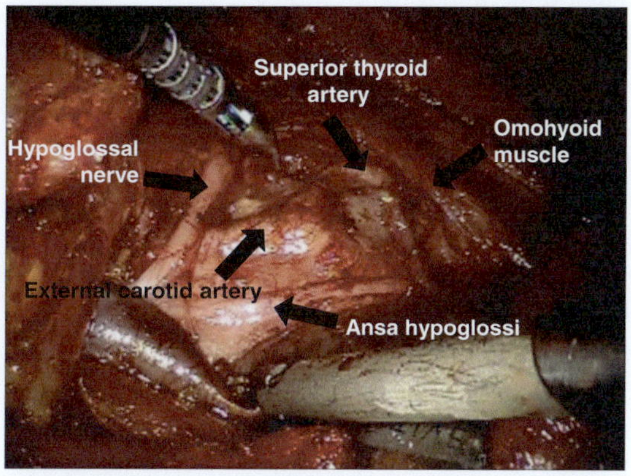

Fig. 12.18 Postsurgical view. The resulting postsurgical field is irrigated and thoroughly checked for any bleeding points, and a closed suction drain is inserted posterior to the hairline, and then the skin is closed with simple interrupted sutures (Right-sided approach)

12.3.2.2 Modified Radical Neck Dissection (Levels I–V or II–V)

Pre-robotic Procedure

The RA incision and skin-subplatysmal flap is elevated similarly; however, when creating the working space, the flap should be sufficiently elevated beyond the posterior border of the sternocleidomastoid muscle to meet the trapezius muscle so that levels IV and V are properly addressed. When level I is omitted in the procedure, the skin flap does not have to be as high up as to the inferior margin of the mandible. It would only increase the chance of direct/indirect marginal mandibular nerve injury.

After placing the self-retaining retractor, gross dissection is initiated at the appropriate level according to the type of neck dissection (levels I–V or II–V)

For the comprehensive dissection of level I–V, the dissection starts at level Ib by identifying the marginal branch of facial nerve as described previously for the selective neck dissection of levels I–III. When conducting the neck dissection of levels II–V, the dissection is commenced at level II with identification of the inferior border of the submandibular gland.

Dividing the fascia at the inferior border of submandibular gland, the dissection is proceeded posteriorly to release the parotid tail. Likewise, the posterior belly of digastric muscle is identified below the submandibular gland, and it is followed posteriorly to locate the internal jugular vein. Next, the spinal accessory nerve is identified, and the fascia at the anterior border of the sternocleidomastoid muscle is opened up. The dissection is continued medially visualizing the carotid sheath and as far inferior as possible to level IV (Figs. 12.19 and 12.20).

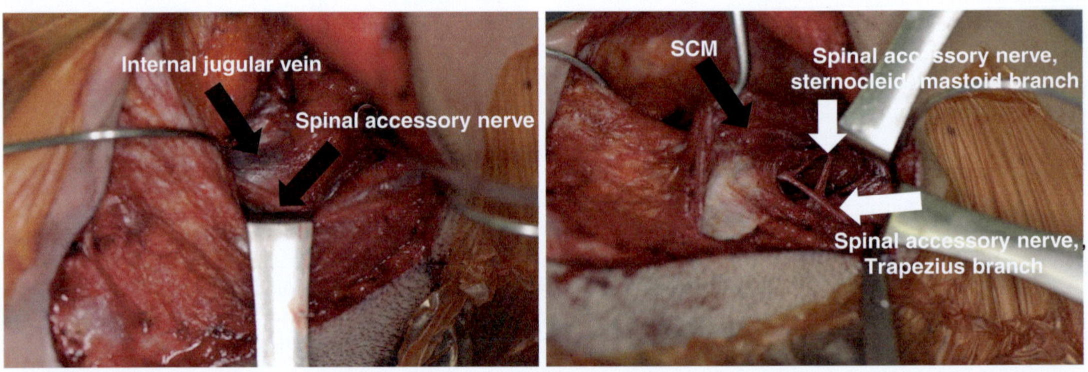

Fig. 12.19 The course of spinal accessory nerve is traced and skeletonized from its exit near the skull base to its entry at the trapezius muscle (Right-sided approach)

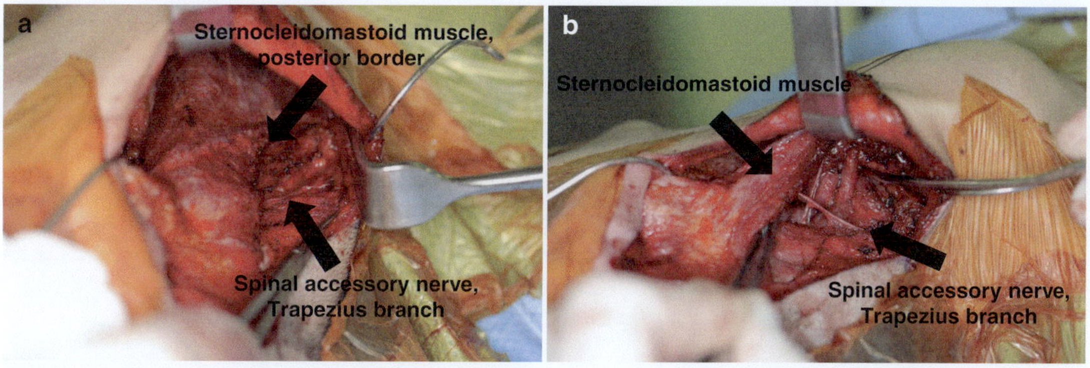

Fig. 12.20 (**a**) The next step is releasing the fascia at the posterior border of the sternocleidomastoid muscle so that the muscle can be lifted upward with a retractor. The lymph nodes tissue covering levels IIb and Va is collectively dissected and driven toward the lateral aspect of the carotid sheath at levels IIa and upper III. Here, some portion of levels IIa and III are further dissected under direct vision. (**b**) Next, the self-retaining retractor is readjusted so that the sternocleidomastoid muscle is elevated and maintained together with the skin flap. Before the robotic docking, the dissected specimen is usually taken out to obtain an optimal surgical view from the robotic console (Right-sided approach)

Robotic Dissection (Figs. 12.21, 12.22, 12.23, and 12.24)

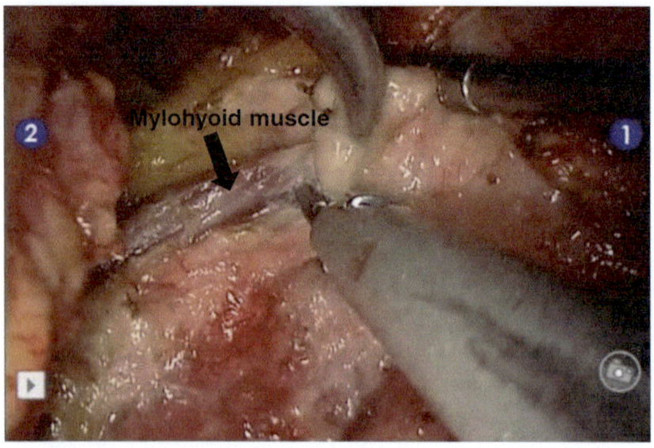

Fig. 12.21 If level I dissection is included in the operation, the robotic arms are aligned so that they maintain a parallel axis to the inferior margin of the mandible. Level I dissection is carried out as previously described for the selective neck dissection of levels I–III (Right-sided approach)

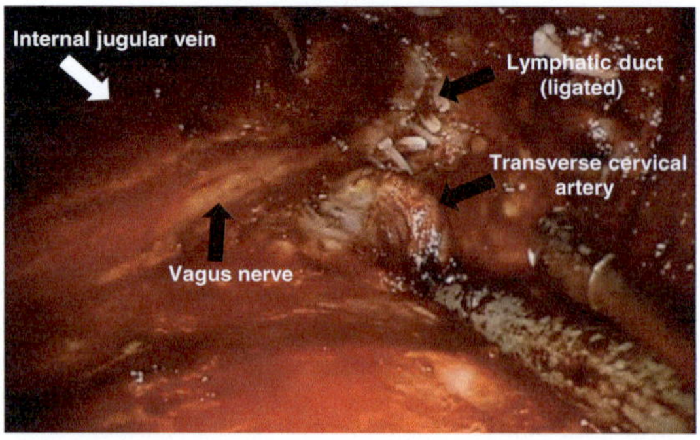

Fig. 12.23 When dissecting the area around the internal jugular vein near the clavicle, the lymphatic or thoracic duct should be routinely checked and ligated using hemoclips or Hem-o-lok ligation system even it has not been violated, to prevent the possibility of future chyle leakage (Right-sided approach)

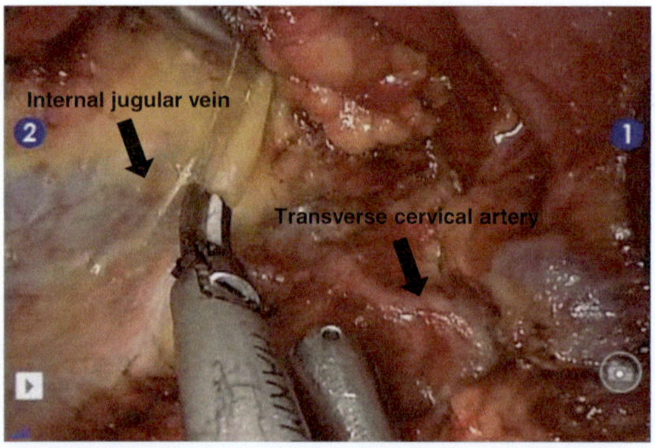

Fig. 12.22 The transverse cervical artery and the phrenic nerve running underneath this vessel can be identified during the dissection of levels Vb and inferior IV. The dissection is continued medially until it meets the carotid sheath (*Right*-sided approach)

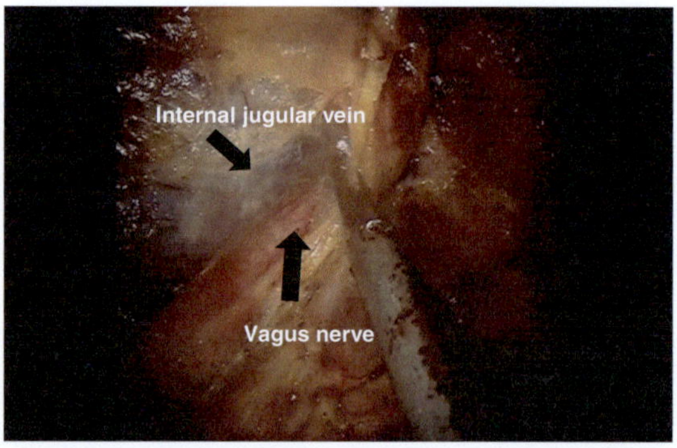

Fig. 12.24 The dissection is directed superiorly, identifying the vagus nerve, carotid artery, and internal jugular vein and carefully preserving the structures. During carotid sheath dissection, appropriate maneuvers must be provided by the assistant surgeon to maintain an appropriate traction-counter traction force balance to aid the dissection procedure. The branches of internal jugular vein are ligated with harmonic curved shears or Hem-o-lok ligation system

To begin levels IV and V dissection, the robotic arms should be repositioned so that the axis is in a cephalocaudal direction, facing toward the clavicle. The previously dissected tissue of level Va is grasped with the robot, and dissection is conducted superiorly to inferiorly. As the level of dissection reaches level Vb, the specimen is retracted medially, and the dissection continues to meet the omohyoid muscle which is consequently cut.

After completion of the dissection, the final neck specimen is delivered through the RA port. The postsurgical bed is irrigated and bleeding control done, before placing a closed suction drain. The surgical wound is then sutured with simple interrupted sutures.

12.4 Surgical Considerations

Generally, the Harmonic curved shears-mounted robotic arm is placed at the surgeon's dominant hand and the Maryland forceps at the nondominant hand. In terms of difficulty, there is no significant difference between a right-sided and a left-sided surgery; however, the dominant-sided surgery may be more comfortable to perform for the robotic surgeon.

12.5 Potential Postoperative Complications

Possible complications of this robotic RA surgery include:

- Nerve injury
  - Lingual nerve injury
  - Hypoglossal nerve injury
  - Marginal mandibular branch of facial nerve injury (mouth corner deviation)
  - Vagus nerve injury (vocal cord palsy)
  - Sympathetic nerve injury (Horner's syndrome)
  - Spinal accessory nerve injury (spinal accessory nerve syndrome)
  - Phrenic nerve injury
- Bleeding/hematoma
- Seroma
- Chyle leakage (lymphatic/thoracic duct injury)
- Wound infection, dehiscence
- Ischemia or necrosis of skin flap

The potential complications are similar to those from a conventional open neck operation. Mouth corner deviation may result from various degree of injury of the marginal branch of the facial nerve. The surgeon should pay special attention when dissecting around level I to avoid direct/indirect injury to the facial nerve. Main causes of indirect injury to the marginal mandibular nerve are thermal energy generated by surgical instruments and traction made by external retractors. Most indirect injuries of the facial nerve cause temporary mouth corner deviation which generally resolves within 2–3 months after the operation.

The surgical field from the RA port is relatively narrow, so there is a higher chance of major neurovascular structure injuries. A comprehensive knowledge and familiarizing the local surgical anatomy and a sufficient amount of surgical experience are prerequisites to minimize such complications.

Occasionally skin problems such as ischemic change or necrosis may occur at the RA skin flap. These consequences can be avoided by limiting the upper end of the flap to the level of the external auditory meatus and avoiding an acute angle of the skin curvature when designing the incision. Hair loss can occur along the skin incision within the hairline, but this can be minimized by beveling the incision at this portion.

12.6 Further Applications

Robot-assisted neck surgery via RA approach can be applied virtually to all surgeries for lesions located in the neck. Other benign neck mass such as parapharyngeal tumor, branchial cleft cyst, and lipoma can be removed, and thyroidectomy can also be performed via RA approach, with the aid of the robotic system. Hypopharyngeal tumors can also be removed robotically by the RA approach after exposing the tumor via lateral pharyngotomy. Moreover, free flap reconstruction is feasible with the robot inserted from the RA port.

It is expected that this surgical technique will continuously evolve even more with the technological refinements regarding the robotic system. Already, the introduction of the upgraded da Vinci Xi system (Intuitive Surgical Inc., Sunnyvale, CA) has enabled inserting an extra robotic instrumental arm through the RA port, thereby minimizing the role of the assistant surgeon. Furthermore, unlike the former procedure, the robotic dissection can be now be conducted right after the working space creation, since an extra robotic arm will provide more comfortable dissection and sustained retraction. Most recently, there are expectations that there will emerge a multi-instrument-mounted, "single-port" robotic system which will take the robotic neck surgery to the next level. Not only would the RA robotic surgery be easier to learn and practice, but the surgical skill itself could be further refined by placing a smaller incision.

References

1. Singer MC, Seybt MW, Terris DJ. Robotic facelift thyroidectomy: I. Preclinical simulation and morphometric assessment. Laryngoscope. 2011;121:1631–5.
2. Terris DJ, Singer MC, Seybt MW. Robotic facelift thyroidectomy: II. Clinical feasibility and safety. Laryngoscope. 2011;121:1636–41.
3. Terris DJ, Singer MC, Seybt MW. Robotic facelift thyroidectomy: patient selection and technical considerations. Surg Laparosc Endosc Percutaneous Technol. 2011;21:237–42.
4. Terris DJ, Singer MC. Qualitative and quantitative differences between 2 robotic thyroidectomy techniques. Otolaryngol Head Neck Surg. 2012;147:20–5.
5. Terris DJ, Singer MC. Robotic facelift thyroidectomy: facilitating remote access surgery. Head Neck. 2012;34:746–7.
6. Koh YW, Park JH, Kim JW, et al. Endoscopic hemithyroidectomy with prophylactic ipsilateral central neck dissection via an unilateral axillo-breast approach without gas insufflation for unilateral micropapillary thyroid carcinoma: preliminary report. Surg Endosc. 2010;24:188–97.
7. Koh YW, Kim JW, Lee SW, Choi EC. Endoscopic thyroidectomy via a unilateral axillo-breast approach without gas insufflation for unilateral benign thyroid lesions. Surg Endosc. 2009;23:2053–60.
8. Koh YW, Choi EC. Robotic approaches to the neck. Otolaryngol Clin N Am. 2014;47:433–54.
9. Kim CH, Byeon HK, Shin YS, et al. Robot-assisted Sistrunk operation via a retroauricular approach for thyroglossal duct cyst. Head Neck. 2014;36:456–8.
10. Koh YW, Chung WY, Hong HJ, et al. Robot-assisted selective neck dissection via modified face-lift approach for early oral tongue cancer: a video demonstration. Ann Surg Oncol. 2012;19:1334–5.
11. Kim CH, Chang JW, Choi EC, et al. Robotically assisted selective neck dissection in parotid gland cancer: preliminary report. Laryngoscope. 2013;123:646–50.
12. Shin YS, Choi EC, Kim CH, et al. Robot-assisted selective neck dissection combined with facelift parotidectomy in parotid cancer. Head Neck. 2014;36:592–5.
13. Kim CH, Koh YW, Kim D, et al. Robotic-assisted neck dissection in submandibular gland cancer: preliminary report. J Oral Maxillofac Surg. 2013;71:1450–7.
14. Lee HS, Kim WS, Hong HJ, et al. Robot-assisted supraomohyoid neck dissection via a modified facelift or retroauricular approach in early-stage cN0 squamous cell carcinoma of the oral cavity: a comparative study with conventional technique. Ann Surg Oncol. 2012;19:3871–8.
15. Kim WS, Byeon HK, Park YM, et al. Therapeutic robot-assisted neck dissection via a retroauricular or modified facelift approach in head and neck cancer: a comparative study with conventional transcervical neck dissection. Head Neck. 2015;37:249–54.
16. Park YM, Lee WJ, Yun IS, et al. Free flap reconstruction after robot-assisted neck dissection via a modified face-lift or retroauricular approach. Ann Surg Oncol. 2013;20:891–8.
17. Byeon HK, Holsinger FC, Tufano RP, Chung HJ, Kim WS, Koh YW, Choi EC. Robotic total thyroidectomy with modified radical neck dissection via unilateral retroauricular approach. Ann Surg Oncol. 2014 Nov;21(12):3872–5.

Transoral Robotic Resection of Parapharyngeal Space Tumors

13

Moran Amit, Irit Duek, and Ziv Gil

13.1 Introduction

Parapharyngeal space tumors (PPSTs) account for only 0.5% of head and neck neoplasms. However, many types of tumors can involve this region. The relationship of these tumors to the styloid process, i.e., prestyloid and poststyloid, aids in their classification. Prestyloid PPSTs deflect the internal carotid artery (ICA) posteriorly and are most commonly benign salivary gland tumors; poststyloid tumors push the ICA anteriorly and are most commonly paragangliomas and nerve sheath tumors (Fig. 13.1). These tumors are most commonly managed by surgical resection via transcervical or transmandibular approaches. The efficacy and limitations of these approaches are well established [1–3]. Very large PPSTs, or those that are located high at the base of the skull, often require combined approaches, which may include mandibulotomy or infratemporal fossa approaches. Since the latter carries a considerable risk for morbidity, there is increasing interest in the use of the da Vinci surgical robotic system (Intuitive Surgical, Sunnyvale, CA). This system obviates the need for a mandibulotomy to approach the oropharynx [4–6] and enables a transoral approach to resect PPSTs [7]. The da Vinci robotic apparatus provides high magnification three-dimensional (3D) visual access to lateral-based structures and enables direct angular visualization and instrumentation at and around structures. The 5 mm robotic-guided arms enable an assistant to introduce additional instruments into the operating field to aid retraction, suction, and cauterization. This approach is expected to reduce tumor spillage and morbidity, to shorten the length of hospital stay, and to achieve early

The original version of this chapter was revised. The spelling of the second author's name was corrected. An erratum to this chapter can be found at DOI 10.1007/978-3-319-49578-1_22

M. Amit, MD, PhD
The Laboratory for Applied Cancer Research, Department of Otolaryngology Head and Neck Surgery, the Head and Neck Center, Rambam Healthcare Campus, Clinical Research Institute at Rambam, Rappaport Institute of Medicine and Research, The Technion, Israel Institute of Technology, Haifa, Israel

I. Duek, MD
Department of Otolaryngology Head and Neck Surgery, the Head and Neck Center, Rambam Healthcare Campus, Clinical Research Institute at Rambam, Rappaport Institute of Medicine and Research, The Technion, Israel Institute of Technology, Haifa, Israel

Z. Gil, MD, PhD (✉)
The Laboratory for Applied Cancer Research, Department of Otolaryngology Head and Neck Surgery, the Head and Neck Center, Rambam Healthcare Campus, Clinical Research Institute at Rambam, Rappaport Institute of Medicine and Research, The Technion, Israel Institute of Technology, Haifa, Israel

Department of Otolaryngology, Rambam Medical Center, The Technion, Israel Institute of Technology, Haifa 66036, Israel
e-mail: ziv@baseofskull.org

Z. Gil et al. (eds.), *Atlas of Head and Neck Robotic Surgery*, DOI 10.1007/978-3-319-49578-1_13

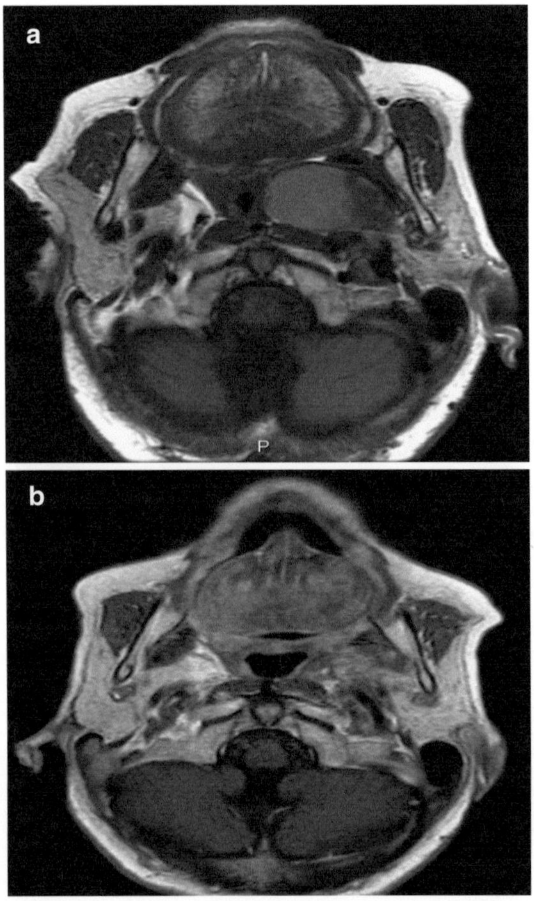

Fig. 13.1 Axial T1-weighted with gadolinium magnetic resonance images of a 78-year-old patient with prestyloid parapharyngeal pleomorphic adenoma; (**a**) preoperative, (**b**) 2 months postoperative

reinstatement of quality of life. A recent meta-analysis presented the utility of TORS as a single or combined approach for PPST in nearly 50 patients with minimal surgical morbidity [8]. In this chapter, we describe the indications and surgical technique of TORS for resection of PPST.

13.2 Surgical Anatomy

The parapharyngeal space (PPS) is a potential space lateral to the oropharynx. The PPS is shaped like an inverted teepee, extending from the skull base superiorly to the greater cornu of the hyoid bone inferiorly. The PPS is bound medially by the superior pharyngeal constrictors and laterally by the medial pterygoid muscle, mandibular ramus, and deep lobe of the parotid gland. The anterior border of the PPS is the pterygomandibular raphe and the pterygoid fascia. Posteriorly, the PPS extends to the cervical vertebrae and prevertebral muscles. An important landmark in the PPS is a fascial band extending from the styloid process to the tensor veli palatini. This structure further divides the PPS to an anteromedial compartment (i.e., prestyloid) and a posterolateral (i.e., poststyloid) compartment. The prestyloid compartment contains the retromandibular portion of the deep lobe of the parotid gland, adipose tissue, and lymph nodes associated with the parotid gland. The poststyloid compartment contains vital structures like the internal carotid artery, the internal jugular vein, CNs IX–XII, and the sympathetic chain.

13.3 Preoperative Evaluation

Patients should be assessed for cranial neuropathies, breathing disturbances, and trismus. Physical examination should include palpation of the neck and the parotid gland in search of lymph node metastases. Cranial nerves are evaluated. Mouth opening might be limited due to extension of the tumor into the pterygopalatine fossa. Mouth opening is particularly important since relative contraindications to TORS include inadequate oral exposure and limited cervical spine mobility. The extent of the oropharyngeal mass should be evaluated with flexible fiber optic evaluation of the oropharynx.

Imaging should include magnetic resonance imaging (MRI); however, contrast computerized tomographic (CT) scans are acceptable. Visualization of a vascular flow void on an MRI study is usually sufficient for the diagnosis of a vascular tumor such as a paraganglioma, but magnetic resonance angiography (MRA) may be added for a more precise diagnosis. If a malignant tumor is suspected, radiological staging is completed using a positron emission tomography-CT hybrid (PET-CT) for assessing the presence of regional and distant metastases. Surgeons must be acutely aware of a more medial position of the carotid artery as it passes through the PPS.

Preoperative tissue evaluation with fine needle aspiration (FNA) biopsy should be obtained, particularly in the setting of a suspected salivary gland malignancy or an enlarged lymph node. When radiographic studies are diagnostic of a vascular lesion, biopsy is not recommended. Awareness of the potential pathologies that might be encountered is important, and imaging should precede FNA, to avoid potential bleeding.

13.4 Operative Technique

13.4.1 Patient Positioning

The patient is placed in a supine position and is nasally intubated via the contralateral nostril. The operating table should be positioned with the patient's head away from the ventilator to allow space for the robotic cart to fit under the bed. The patient should be positioned in the patient supine with a horizontally oriented shoulder roll. The patient's arms do not need to be tucked for TORS; however, if a transcervical approach is expected, both arms should be tucked. Sterile draping is not required if TORS is done alone.

Suspension pharyngoscopy using the Feyh-Kastenbauer (FK) laryngeal retractor (Gyrus AMI, Southborough, MA) is performed, and the patient is placed in suspension. A 2-0 silk suture through the anterior tongue is placed for retraction to maximize exposure; gauze is positioned between the teeth and tongue to avoid tongue laceration. The patient's eyes are protected with Opti-Guard® safety goggles.

13.4.2 Robot Setup

The da Vinci Surgical System (Intuitive Surgical, Inc., Sunnyvale, CA) is docked diagonally to the patient's bed. The bed should be lowered to accommodate the robotic arms. A 0° 8°mm camera is installed and inserted to the mouth. The robotic arm ipsilateral to the lesion is installed with a 5 mm monopolar cautery with a spatula tip. Maryland dissector forceps is installed in the arm contralateral to the tumor. The robotic arms are positioned so that instrument tips are within the field of view of the endoscope with minimal angulation. As such, they are approximately parallel to the optical arm, minimizing collision with each other.

An assistant is positioned at the head of the bed. The assistant must be familiar with endoscopic techniques since he will be working off of the screen rather than by direct visualization. Moreover, the assistant must be familiar with the robot to troubleshoot device failures and interference of the arms. The assistant is equipped with a Yankauer suction, bipolar diathermy and LigaSure™ 5 mm blunt tip 23 cm for vessel sealing, atraumatic grasping, and blunt dissection. The latter enables cutting independent of sealing.

13.4.3 Dissection

The procedure is initiated with an incision over the prominent aspect of the mass, through the oropharyngeal mucosa, from superior to inferior. In case there is no prominence at the oropharynx, an inverted L-shaped incision is used along the lateral aspect of the anterior tonsillar pillar (Fig. 13.2). Next, dissection is undertaken through the submucosal muscle layer (Fig. 13.3). Traction and countertraction are important for dissecting through the superior constrictor musculature. Dissection through the superior constrictor muscles with the tip of the Bovie cautery eventually leads to an identification of the mass capsule (Fig. 13.4). At this stage, a well-defined plane is identified, and dissection proceeds along the mass (Fig. 13.5). As mucosal flaps are developed, lateral retraction of the anterior tonsillar pillar using pillar retractor or a suture increases exposure to the parapharyngeal space. The palate can be retracted anteriorly using a soft rubber catheter placed in the nose.

The Maryland dissector is used to gently grasp the superior constrictor musculature and pull it medially, and a combination of Bovie electrocautery and blunt dissection is used to further define the capsule. At this stage, the parapharyngeal fat may be visualized. The assistant can help with blunt dissection and retraction of soft tissues. When the anteromedial aspect of the mass is defined, a higher magnification can be used to appreciate its size and extent. If accessible, the inferior aspect of the mass is grasped and pulled medially to assist with the lateral dissection (Fig. 13.6). In case of a benign cystic mass, it can be decompressed at this stage, to facilitate its mobilization within the narrow confines of the oral cavity and to address the remaining superior-lateral attachments. The more cephalad medial pterygoid muscle may be visualized, and further lateral dissection should be avoided to minimize exposure of the carotid artery.

During this portion of the resection, branches of the external carotid artery traversing the PPS are encountered and should be clipped or cauterized. After the superior and lateral attachments are removed, the assistant retracts the tumor medially. If a tumor's inferior aspect is fully visualized, inferior dissection is completed and the lesion is removed (Fig. 13.7). The remaining cavity is copiously irrigated with 37 °C saline, hemostasis is confirmed before and after the robotic arms are removed, and the incision is closed primarily with 2-0 Vicryl sutures.

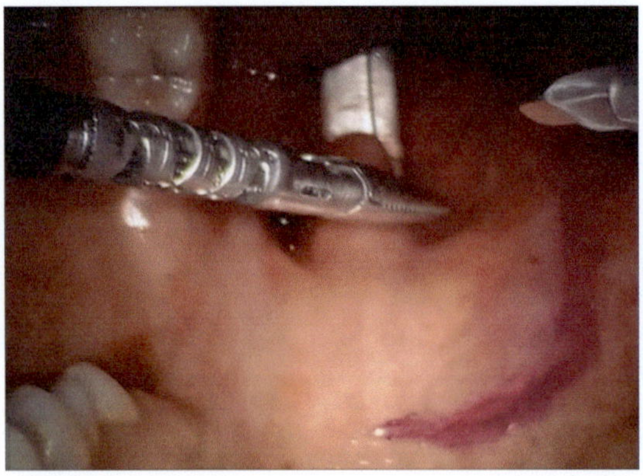

Fig. 13.2 Inverted L-shaped incision over anterior pillar mucosa

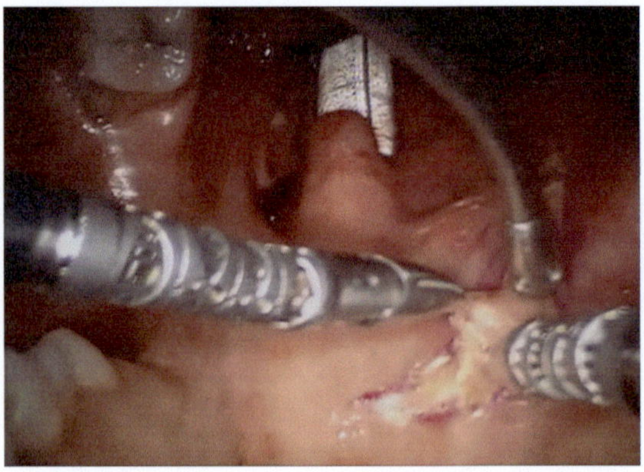

Fig. 13.3 Raising submucosal flaps at the palatoglossal fold

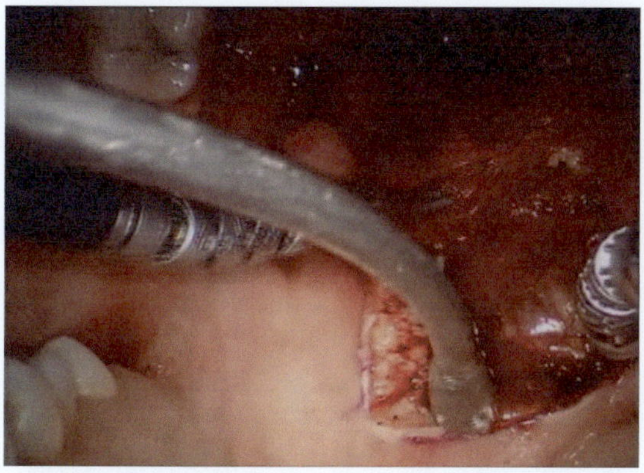

Fig. 13.4 Exposure of the superomedial aspect of the tumor

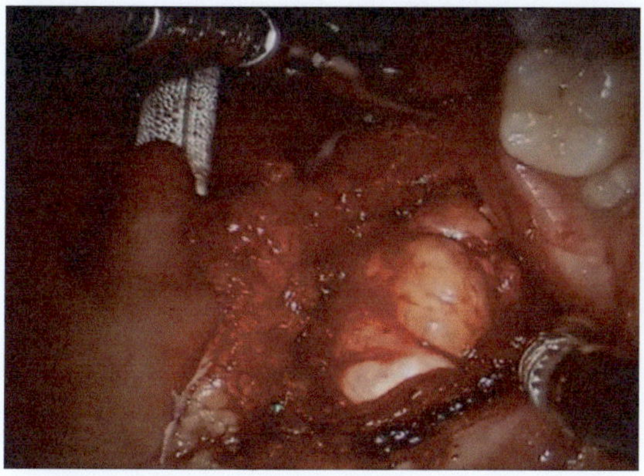

Fig. 13.5 Anterior tumor exposure

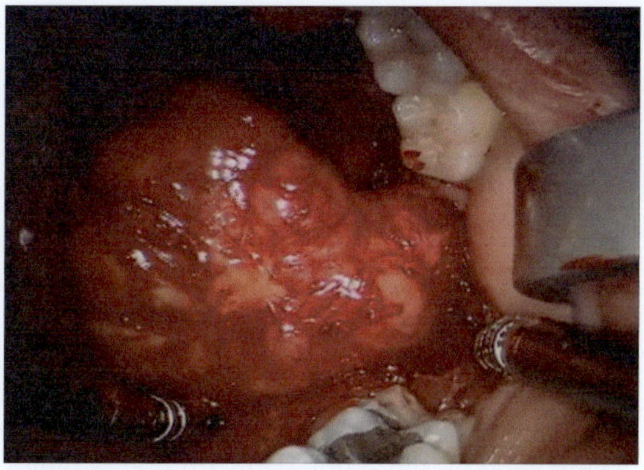

Fig. 13.6 After inferomedial release, the tumor is medially retracted

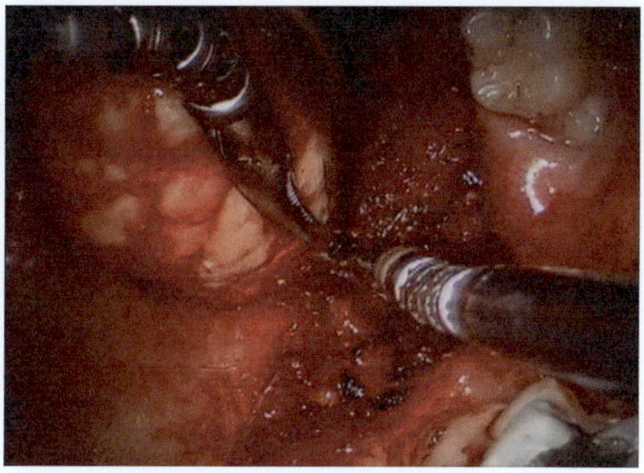

Fig. 13.7 Lateral dissection at the parapharyngeal space. During this portion of the resection, branches of the external carotid artery traversing the PPS are encountered and should be clipped or cauterized

13.5 Combining the Transcervical Endoscopic with the Transoral Robotic Approach

While the transoral robotic approach to the PPS is feasible and safe, it carries limitations, such as exposure of the lateral and posterior aspects of the PPS. With such approach, the PPS tumor is situated between the robotic arm and the carotid artery. Since PPS tumors (pleomorphic adenomas, carcinomas, and schwannomas) cannot be manipulated by the robot, TORS requires finger dissection and separation of the tumor from the mouth or neck, especially in large PPS tumors. The traditional finger dissection, whether performed from the neck or the mouth, increases the risk of neurovascular injury and tumor spillage. To overcome these limitations, the authors utilize a combined approach with transcervical endoscopic dissection of the lesion through a small skin incision, followed by transoral robotic removal of the tumor (unpublished data). The technique enables release of the lesion from the neurovascular structures and muscles and safe peroral removal of the intact tumor using the da Vinci robotic system (Intuitive Surgical, Inc., Sunnyvale, CA).

The indications for this approach are (1) high small pleomorphic adenomas, (2) large pleomorphic adenomas of the PPS, and (3) symptomatic PPS schwannomas. Tumors with a large poststyloid extent or in close proximity to the carotid artery should be dissected under direct visualization to avoid vascular injuries. Combining the transcervical endoscopic technique with the transoral robotic approach allows for precise inferolateral dissection along the carotid artery as it passes through the PPS.

The procedure starts with the transcervical endoscopic dissection. The patient is positioned supine with a horizontally oriented shoulder roll in place. The patient's head is turned away from the operative side, and the table is rotated with the operative side away from the anesthesia machine. At this stage, no muscle relaxation is administered to facilitate CN XI identification. Along a transverse skin crest, 4 cm below the mandible, perform a 2.5 cm skin incision (Fig. 13.8). A superior subplatysmal flap is elevated to the level of the mandible (Fig. 13.9). In some cases, the submandibular gland should be excised to enhance exposure (Fig. 13.10). The posterior belly of the digastric muscle is identified, and dissection is performed along the medial aspect of the sternocleidomastoid muscle until the accessory nerve is identified (Fig. 13.11). Next, the hypoglossal nerve is identified and mobilized, and the internal jugular vein, common carotid artery, and vagus nerve are identified. The posterior belly of the digastric and stylohyoid muscles are then divided, and the styloid process with the stylomandibular ligament is divided to improve exposure.

At this stage, a 0° endoscope (KARL STORZ, Tuttlingen Germany) is delivered through the tunnel into the depth of the surgical incision (Fig. 13.12). The medial pterygoid muscle is visualized and dissected along its length to access the post-styloid space, while preserving the ascending pharyngeal artery and the hypoglossal nerve (Fig. 13.13). At this step, dissection along the inferolateral aspect of the tumor capsule is performed, to expose and define its upper limit (Fig. 13.14). The dissection is performed in parallel and anteriorly to the internal carotid artery superiorly up to its attachment to the skull base, avoiding the hypoglossal nerve (Fig. 13.15). After releasing the tumor (Fig. 13.16), the wound is irrigated and covered with moist gauze. Complete circumferential dissection is achieved with the complementary TORS approach described above. During the transoral resection, an assistant might apply external pressure on the tumor via a cervical wound to enhance tumor visualization. After resection, the cervical wound is irrigated and hemostasis is confirmed. The wound is closed over a suction drain with a 4-0 absorbable subcutaneous suture and a 5-0 nylon interrupted skin suture.

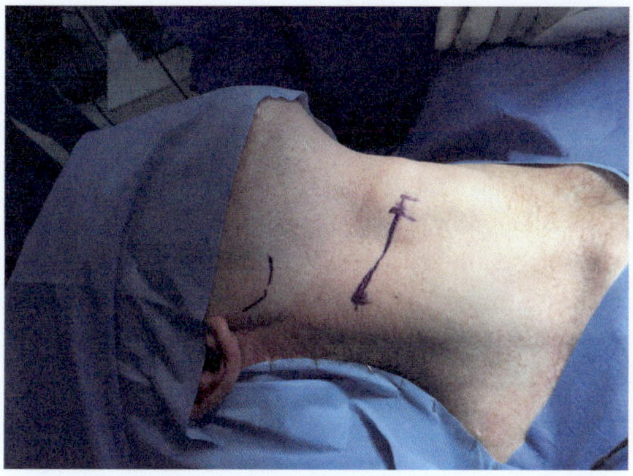

Fig. 13.8 The patient is placed in a supine position with his neck extended and rotated to the contralateral side. A 3 cm skin incision is made along a transverse skin crest, approximately 4 cm below the mandible

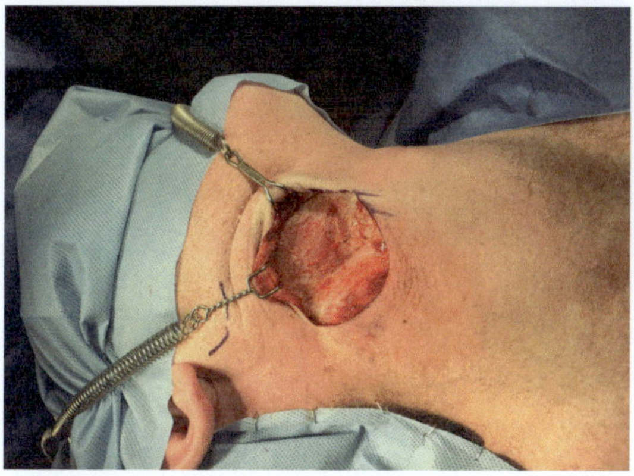

Fig. 13.9 A superior subplatysmal flap is elevated to the level of the mandible

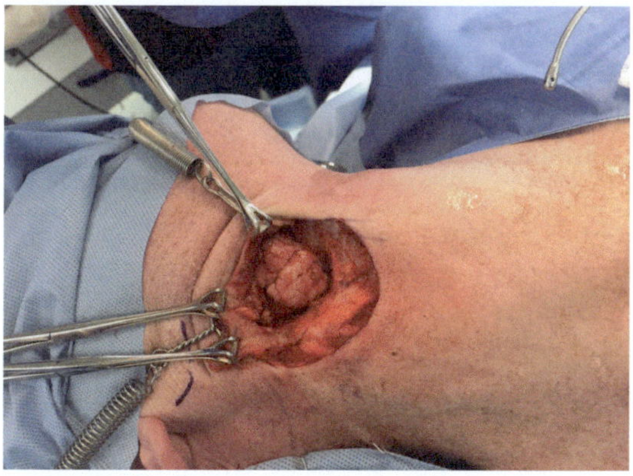

Fig. 13.10 The submandibular gland is exposed. It should be excised to enhance exposure after identifying facial vessels, hypoglossal nerve, and lingual nerve

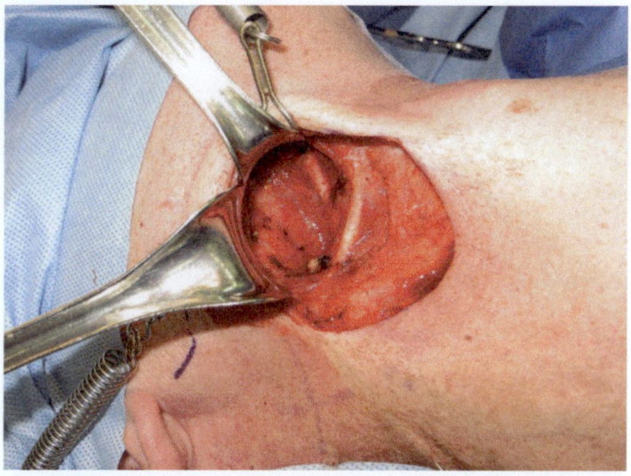

Fig. 13.11 The posterior belly of the digastric muscle, the medial aspect of the sternocleidomastoid muscle, the accessory nerve, the hypoglossal nerve, and the lingual nerve are identified and preserved

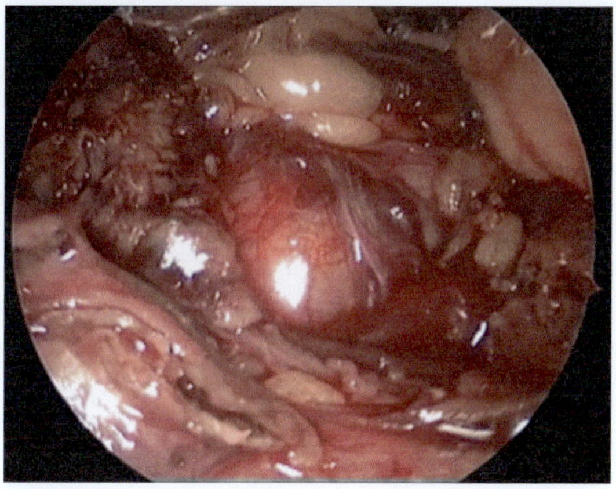

Fig. 13.12 A 0° endoscope is introduced into the depth of the surgical incision.

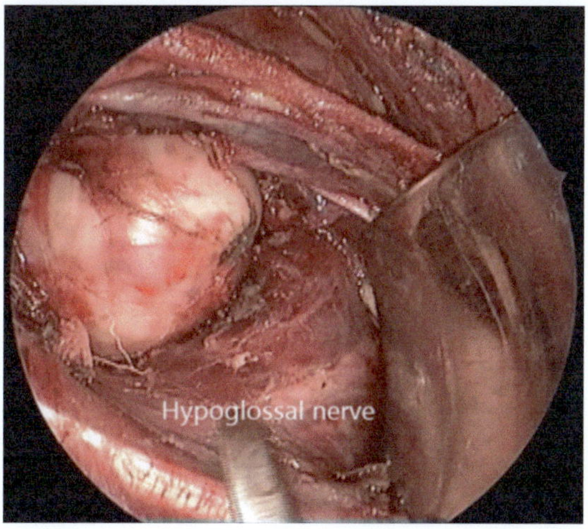

Fig. 13.13 The dissection is performed in parallel and anteriorly to the internal carotid artery, superiorly up to its attachment to the skull base, avoiding the tumor

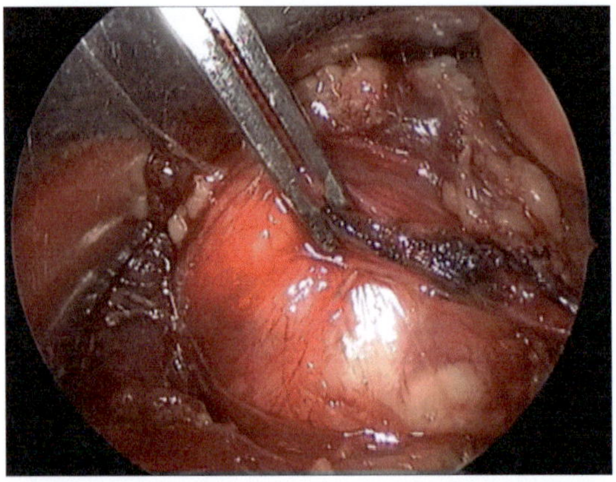

Fig. 13.14 The tumor, still tethered by surrounding tissues, is released circumferentially at the extracapsular plane

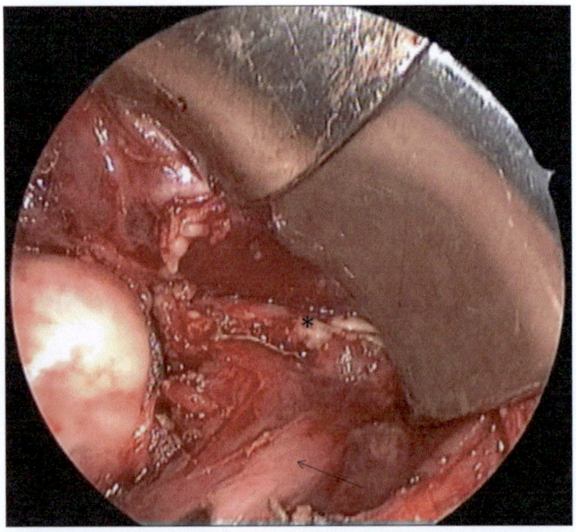

Fig. 13.15 Hypoglossal nerve (*black arrow*) and lingual nerve (*black asterisk*) are identified and preserved

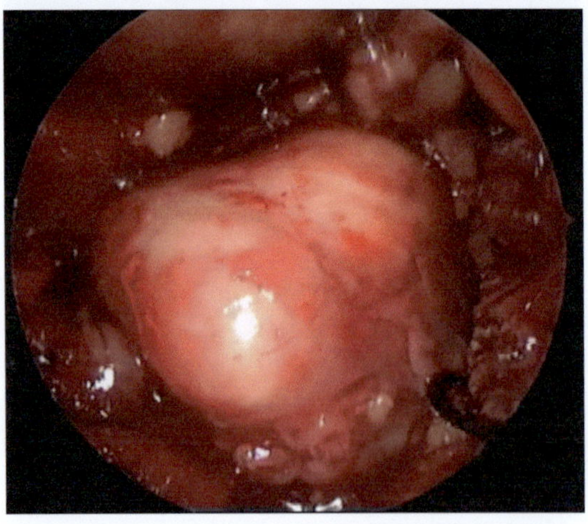

Fig. 13.16 The tumor inferolateral aspect is completely dissected at its capsule, to expose and define its surrounding limits

13.6 Postoperative Management

The patient is extubated and immediately transferred to the postsurgery care unit before transfer to the ward. Prophylactic antibiotic treatment is not indicated in the postoperative period. For pain control, patients are treated with nonsteroidal anti-inflammatory drugs (diclofenac 75 mg intramuscularly or orally) once daily or with tramadol 40–100 mg if requested by the patient or considered necessary by the nurses. Patients begin an oral diet on the following day and are discharged 1 or 2 days after the surgery. If drains are placed, they are removed on postoperative day 1 or 2.

13.7 Discussion

The complex 3D architecture of the PPS and various structures passing within it constitute the more challenging aspects in head and neck surgery. The technique described here provides safe dissection within this area. Tremor filtration, angled instrumentation, and increased freedom of instrument movement are ideal when approaching the PPS. Compared with conventional techniques, TORS allows for more delicate handling of tissues, hence healthy tissue preservation. The improved optics with 3D visualization of TORS, including the use of a stereo-optic 0° or 30°camera, enable identification of the important structures that are at risk and locate them in their 3D context prior to excision. As an individual's experience with the robotic technique increases, the need for identification of some structures may diminish under certain circumstances and shorten surgical time. Increased surgical precision enables precise resection with clear surgical margins and the potential sparing of adjuvant treatment in some patients.

Conclusions

Robotic surgery is rapidly becoming integrated into transoral head and neck surgery. As surgical robotics advances, instruments will become smaller and less expensive, and the technology will become available at peripheral medical centers. These advances will improve treatment of tumors in the parapharyngeal space, with minimal morbidity and excellent functional and cosmetic outcomes.

References

1. Chang SS, Goldenberg D, Koch WM. Transcervical approach to benign parapharyngeal space tumors. Ann Otol Rhinol Laryngol. 2012;121(9):620–4.
2. Linkov G, Morris LG, Shah JP, Kraus DH. First bite syndrome: incidence, risk factors, treatment, and outcomes. Laryngoscope. 2012;122(8):1773–8.
3. Presutti L, Molteni G, Malve L, Marchioni D, Ghidini A, Tassi S, et al. Parapharyngeal space tumors without mandibulotomy: our experience. Eur Arch Otorhinolaryngol: Off J Eur Fed Otorhinolaryngol Soc. 2012;269(1):265–73.
4. Villanueva NL, de Almeida JR, Sikora AG, Miles BA, Genden EM. Transoral robotic surgery for the management of oropharyngeal minor salivary gland tumors. Head Neck. 2013;36:28.
5. Lin HS, Rowley JA, Badr MS, Folbe AJ, Yoo GH, Victor L, et al. Transoral robotic surgery for treatment of obstructive sleep apnea-hypopnea syndrome. Laryngoscope. 2013;123(7):1811–6.
6. Vicini C, Dallan I, Canzi P, Frassineti S, Nacci A, Seccia V, et al. Transoral robotic surgery of the tongue base in obstructive sleep Apnea-Hypopnea syndrome: anatomic considerations and clinical experience. Head Neck. 2012;34(1):15–22.
7. FDA. December 2012 510(k) Clearances 2012. Available from: http://www.accessdata.fda.gov/cdrh_docs/pdf12/K123463.pdf.
8. Chan JY, Tsang RK, Eisele DW, Richmon JD. Transoral robotic surgery of the parapharyngeal space: a case series and systematic review. Head Neck. 2015;37(2):293–8.

Robotic Surgery of the Skull Base

14

Michael E. Kupferman and Ehab Hanna

14.1 Introduction

In the past several years, transnasal endoscopic approaches have been increasingly used for surgical access and treatment of neoplastic and benign lesions of the anterior and central skull base. Endoscopic surgery is used with increasing frequency for surgical resection of tumors of the sinonasal tract, such as inverted papilloma, angiofibroma, osteomas, and other benign fibro-osseous lesions, and in selected patients with malignant sinonasal tumors [1–5]. Endoscopic approaches are also becoming popular for transsphenoidal access to the sella turcica and are considered by many centers as the preferred surgical approach for treatment of pituitary adenomas [6–9]. More recently, there has been an emerging trend to expand the use of transnasal endoscopic approaches in the surgical treatment of suprasellar, petroclival, infratemporal, and other intracranial skull base tumors [10–14].

The increasing popularity of these endoscopic skull base approaches may be attributed to a larger trend toward more "minimally invasive" techniques across all surgical disciplines. The main advantage of transnasal endoscopic skull base approaches is providing more direct access to the anterior and central skull base while avoiding craniofacial incisions and extensive bone removal commonly used in open surgical approaches. Also, the wider angle of vision and angled lenses increases the range of the endoscopic visual surgical field compared with the "line of sight" visual field gained by surgical loupes or microscopes.

One major disadvantage of transnasal endoscopic approaches is the inability to provide a truly watertight dural closure and reconstruction. Current techniques of endoscopic skull base reconstruction, such as tissue grafts, mucosal flaps, and tissue sealants, provide adequate reconstruction of limited skull base defects, such as a post-traumatic cerebrospinal fluid leak [15, 16]. However, for larger dural defects, these endoscopic techniques have higher cerebrospinal fluid leak rates compared with traditional reconstructive techniques used in open surgery, such as the vascularized pericranial flap [10].

While the application of robotic technology to surgery has rapidly expanded over the last 5 years, one of the least studied but fertile areas for application of surgical robotics in the head and neck is for minimally invasive skull base surgery. Certain advantages that these novel systems offer are the ability to perform bimanual surgery in confined cavities with instrumentation that exceeds the capabilities of the human hand, providing the surgeon with a 3D view of the surgical field. Significant advances in surgical robotics have been made [17], although a role for robotic-based applications in skull base surgery has not been completely defined.

M.E. Kupferman, MD (✉) • E. Hanna, MD
Department of Head and Neck Surgery,
MD Anderson Cancer Center, 1515 Holcombe Blvd,
Unit 1445, Houston, TX 77030, USA
e-mail: mekupfer@mdanderson.org

Z. Gil et al. (eds.), *Atlas of Head and Neck Robotic Surgery*, DOI 10.1007/978-3-319-49578-1_14

14.2 Techniques

14.2.1 Approach to the Anterior Cranial Fossa

The feasibility of using the surgical robot to access the anterior and central skull base has been demonstrated in a cadaver model [18]. Caldwell-Luc incisions and wide anterior maxillary antrostomies followed by wide middle meatal antrostomies are the entry points for the surgical arms (Fig. 14.1a). Sufficient access can be obtained without compromising the infraorbital nerves (Fig. 14.1b), and a posterior septectomy provides a common bilateral surgical field. The robotic endoscope is then placed into the patient's nare and the right and left surgical arms introduced through the respective maxillary sinuses (Fig. 14.1c). Anterior and posterior ethmoidectomies are performed, and sphenoidotomies provide exposure to the planum sphenoidale, sella turcica, and parasellar regions (Fig. 14.2a, b). With current technology, this would be best performed using traditional transnasal endoscopic techniques prior to docking the robotic patient cart. In addition, current robotic instrumentation does not include a drill, although prototypes are under preclinical investigation. Therefore, removal of the anterior skull base bone would likewise be best performed without robotic assistance. Access to the anterior cranial fossa is provided by sharp dissection of the anterior skull base and incision of the dura (Fig. 14.3a–c). The dual robotic arms can be used for primary repair of the dura [19]. This approach provides excellent access to the anterior and central skull base, including the cribriform plate, fovea ethmoidalis, medial orbits, planum sphenoidale, nasopharynx, pterygopalatine fossa, and clivus. The most significant advantage of this approach is the ability to perform two-handed tremor-free endoscopic closure of dural defects. To date, this approach remains investigational in nature due to the lack of bone-cutting instrumentation, as discussed at the end of this chapter.

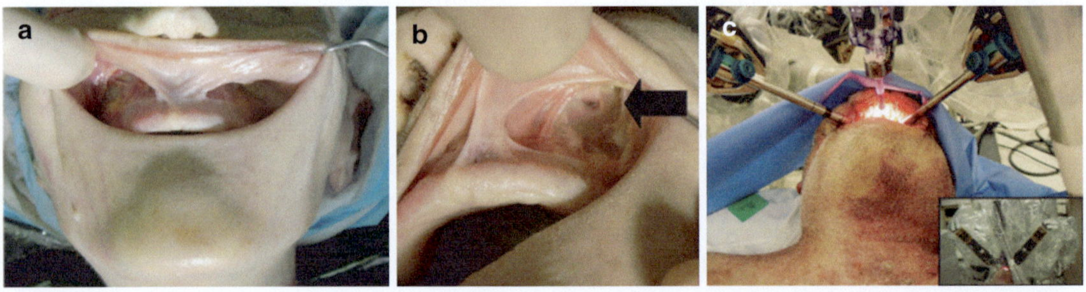

Fig. 14.1 (**a**) Sublabial incisions with bilateral exposure of the face of the maxilla. (**b**) Identification and preservation of the infraorbital nerve (*arrow*). (**c**) Docking of the camera (*C*) and the robotic arms via maxillary antrotomies

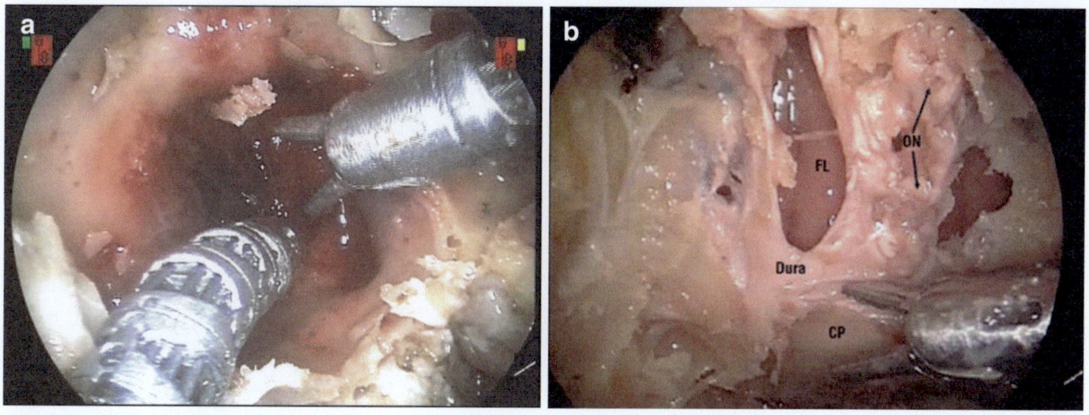

Fig. 14.2 (**a**) Dissection of the posterior wall of the sphenoid sinus. (**b**) The cribriform plate (CP) is removed bilaterally, and the cut edges of the olfactory nerves (ON) are shown; the dura is incised or resected to expose the inferior surface of the frontal lobes (FL) intracranially

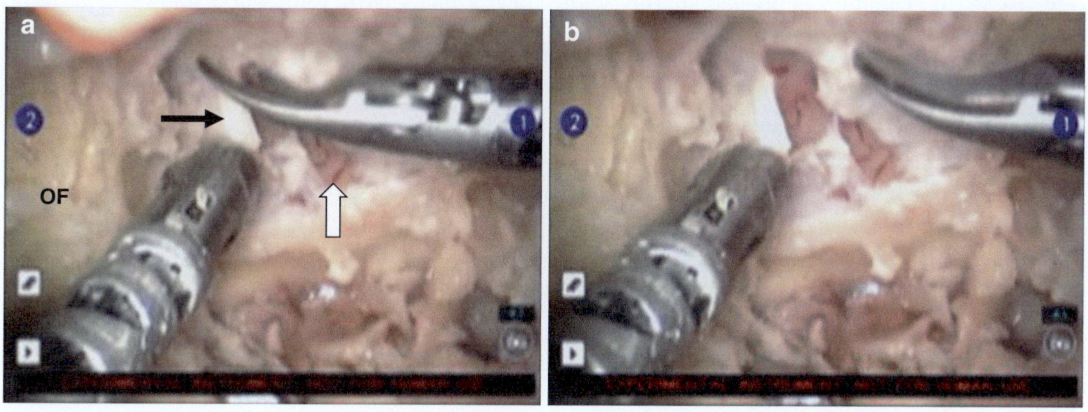

Fig. 14.3 (**a**) Resection of the cribriform plate (CP) and (**b**, **c**) incision of the dura (*black arrow*) with the robotic instrumentation after complete exposure of medial orbital walls (OF—orbital fat) and sphenoid sinus (S). The frontal lobe is visible (*white arrow*)

14.2.2 Approach to the Pituitary Fossa

While the transnasal endoscopic approach to the pituitary fossa has become a widely utilized technique for surgical resection [20, 21], robotic surgery in this anatomic location may provide unique advantages over the four-handed technique. The feasibility of a robotic approach to the pituitary fossa has been described by the authors and remains investigational [22].

Similar to the approach to the anterior cranial fossa, access involves creating bilateral maxillary antrostomies and docking the robotic arms and camera, as described above. An anterior sphenoidotomy is then performed and the sellar floor removed to expose the dura of the pituitary fossa (Fig. 14.4a, b). The dura is opened sharply with the robotic scissors to allow for exploration of the pituitary gland (Fig. 14.5a). Blunt and sharp dissection may be then performed to excise the pituitary gland after the optic chiasm and hypothalamus are exposed (Fig. 14.5b). Dissection of the lateral wall of the sphenoid sinus may also be performed with high-speed drills and fine rongeurs to access the cavernous sinus. Using this technique access to the central skull base, including the planum sphenoidale, the pituitary gland, cavernous carotid, mammillary bodies, and optic chiasm, can be achieved (Fig. 14.5c).

A transcervical approach to the skull base in canine and cadaver models has been previously described. Access to the sphenoid, clivus, sella, and suprasellar anterior fossa can be obtained by placing a 30 degree robotic endoscope transorally and placing the right and left robotic arms through the lateral pharyngeal walls via a transcervical technique, posterior to the submandibular gland [23].

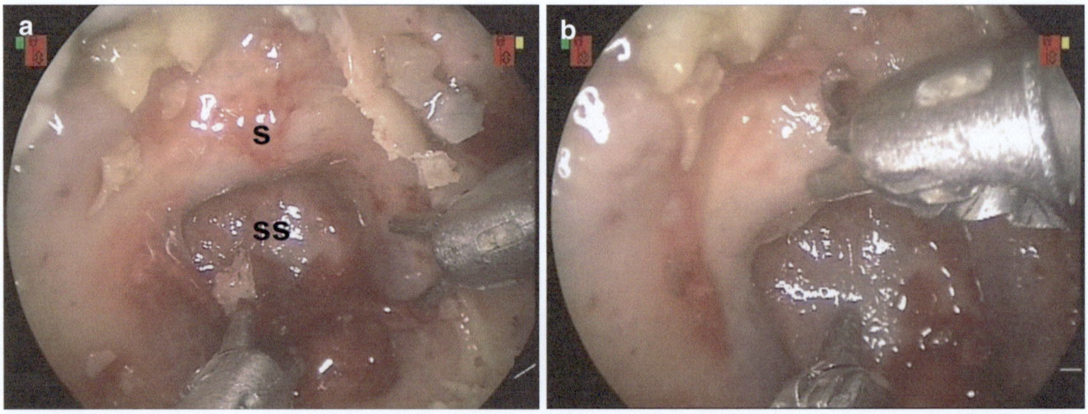

Fig. 14.4 (**a**) Exposure of the anterior face of the sella (*s* sella, *ss* sphenoid sinus). (**c**) Entry into the pituitary fossa

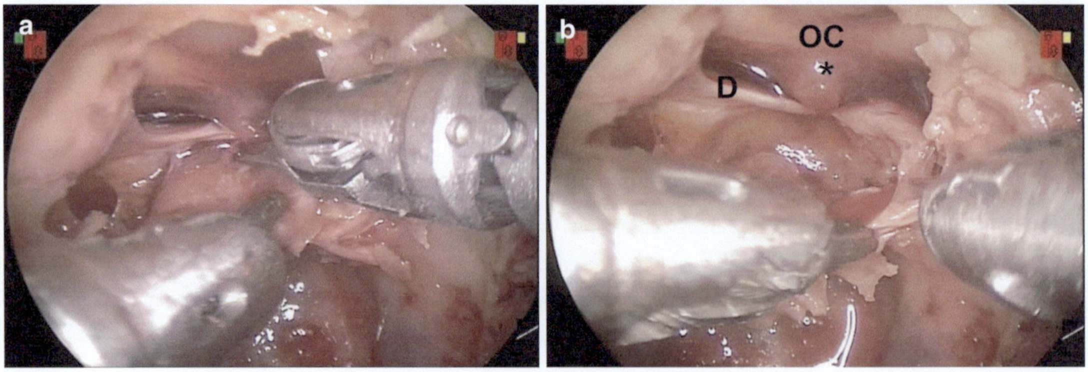

Fig. 14.5 (**a**) Resection of the pituitary gland. (**b**) Transected pituitary stalk and exposure of the optic chiasm (* pituitary stalk, *D* diaphragma sellae, *OC* optic chiasm). (**c**) Visualization of the mammillary bodies (MB)

14.2.3 Approach to the Nasopharynx

Robotic surgery of the nasopharynx is perhaps the only anatomic site of the skull base that is most amenable to surgical dissection with current iterations of surgical robotics. The feasibility of robotic resection of nasopharyngeal lesions in a cadaver was first described in 2008 [24], and subsequent case reports of surgical management of nasopharyngeal cancers have been published in the literature [25].

A Dingman retractor is utilized to expose the oral cavity, and the soft palate is divided under direct visualization—lateral retraction of the divided palate is achieved with Vicryl suture (Fig. 14.6a). The da Vinci robot is then docked at the head of the bed, and the robotic arms are positioned into the oral cavity. Typically, a 30 degree endoscope providing a superiorly oriented view of the oropharynx and nasopharynx is utilized. Using the Maryland forceps and the spatula cautery, the nasopharynx soft tissue may then be progressively degloved (Fig. 14.6b) between the carotid arteries and Eustachian tubes (Fig. 14.6c) laterally and the skull base and prevertebral musculature posteriorly. Once the tumor is resected, the palate is closed in three layers with absorbable suture. The advantage of this technique is that it allows for en bloc excision of nasopharyngeal lesions and may offer the advantage of decreased morbidity compared to either re-irradiation or open surgical approaches for recurrent nasopharyngeal carcinoma. Further study is necessary to delineate the optimal surgical indications.

14.2.4 Approach to the Infratemporal Fossa

Both preclinical studies and case reports addressing the infratemporal fossa and parapharyngeal space via robotic approaches have been described [26, 27]. Dissection is performed through the lateral pharyngeal wall to access the parapharyngeal space. Using the 30 degree endoscope directed superiorly, the parapharyngeal space can be carefully explored to identify the neurovascular contents—jugular vein, internal carotid, and CN IX, X, XI, and XII. To gain exposure superiorly and laterally (to the infratemporal fossa), the styloid musculature can be resected and pterygoid muscles partially released. This approach may be best suited for well-circumscribed benign lesions.

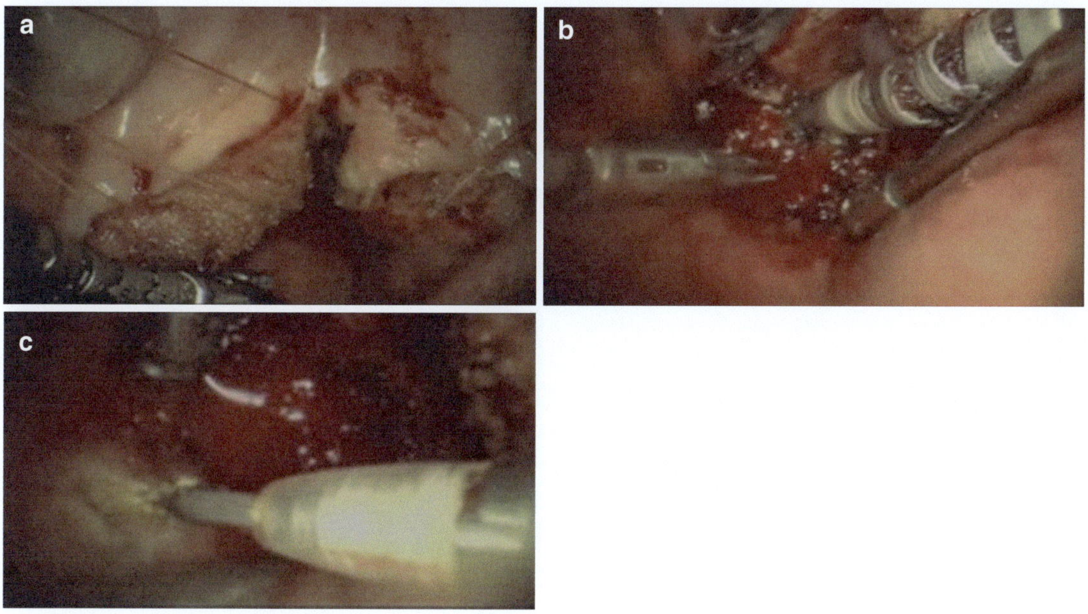

Fig. 14.6 (**a**) Exposure of the nasopharynx is achieved with a palatal split incision. (**b**) Incisions in the superior and inferior aspects of the nasopharynx commence the posterior dissection. (**c**) Incision through the Eustachian tube commences the lateral dissection

14.2.5 Skull Base Reconstruction

Perhaps the most significant limitation of current transnasal endoscopic techniques is the inability to reconstruct dural defects with a sutured watertight dural closure. Options for repair of the skull base include free mucosal grafts, fascia lata grafts, pedicled mucosal grafts, and biological materials [15, 16, 28–30]. While each has advantages and disadvantages, only the pedicled mucoperiosteal grafts are vascularized [31], a necessary component of any reconstruction in patients undergoing postoperative irradiation or in previously irradiated patients. One of the major drawbacks of the endoscopic approach is the inability to perform a suture-based reconstruction of the dura using currently available technology, an approach that is easily undertaken with a pericranial flap through the transcranial approach. We previously reported the feasibility of an endonasal robotic surgical dural reconstruction to address this problem in skull base surgery.

Repair of the skull base defect can be performed robotically with two distinct techniques. First, repair of the dura may be primarily reconstructed with both continuous and interrupted suture technique (Fig. 14.7a). Additionally, harvested sinonasal mucoperiosteal graft can be sutured into dural defects with both running and interrupted suture techniques (Fig. 14.7b). While these techniques have been demonstrated in cadaver models, their application in human use has yet to be realized.

A balanced analysis of where robotic surgery may lie on the spectrum of surgical modalities suggests that robotic-assisted skull base surgery offers unique advantages that are lacking in either microscopic or transnasal endoscopic techniques. These can be divided in four major areas: optical, ergonomic, dissection, and reconstructive. The following is a discussion of how endoscopic robotic surgery can overcome some of the limitations of these other techniques and where robotic surgery has limitations.

14.2.5.1 Optical Limitations

The two-dimensional visualization provided by single-channel optical systems in current endoscopes lacks the depth perception of 3D vision provided by the binocular optical systems used in standard microsurgery. During endoscopic surgery, depth perception relies more on tactile than on visual cues. Visual depth perception is particularly important when operating on critical intracranial neurovascular structures, especially when working in a deep and limited space. The 5 mm robotic endoscope has a dual-channel optical system coupled with a dual charge-coupled device, which allows for 3D visualization of the surgical field at the surgeon's console. This "binocular endoscope" allows the surgeon to have the combined benefit of a wider angle of vision and the depth perception of 3D visualization.

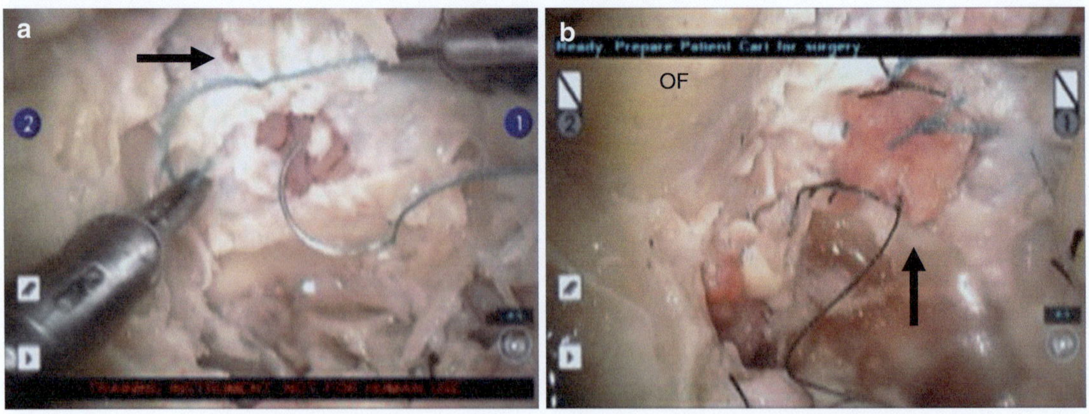

Fig. 14.7 (**a**) Primary repair of a dural defect (*arrow*) with polyglactin suture (Ethicon). (**b**) Repair of a large dural defect with a mucosal graft (*white arrow*)

14.2.5.2 Ergonomic Limitations

Current endoscopic techniques have several ergonomic limitations. Bimanual surgery is only feasible if the endoscope is held by an assistant or a mechanical holder. A surgical assistant is preferred because of the constant need to adjust the position (depth and angle) of the endoscope during endoscopic surgery. This not only limits the direct control of the endoscope by the primary surgeon but also requires the assistance of a relatively experienced endoscopic surgeon who can seamlessly follow the primary surgeon in every step of the operation.

Also, both surgeons have to work within the confined space provided by the nostrils, which in some cases limits ergonomic freedom. In addition, as the surgical field gets deeper, longer instruments are needed, and, with lack of proper arm support, precision may be limited by fine tremor, especially when using fine instrumentation for delicate dissection of critical neurovascular structures. The robotic system has four arms, all of which are controlled by the primary surgeon sitting at the console. One arm, the camera port, holds the endoscope; two arms hold right- and left-hand instruments; and a fourth "spare" arm may be dedicated for retraction or a third instrument. This allows the primary surgeon simultaneous direct control of the endoscope and the instrumentation, an advantage not feasible with non-robotic endoscopic techniques. Another advantage of the "endowrist" technology used in the da Vinci robotic instrumentation is its ability to provide movement at the instrument tip with 7° of freedom and 90° of articulation and motion scaling. This allows the surgeon, who sits comfortably at the console with an adjustable arm, support to perform precise tremor-free movement in a deep and confined space, with working angles usually not achievable with non-robotic instruments.

14.2.5.3 Dissection Limitations

In its current iteration, the da Vinci robotic system is designed exclusively for soft tissue surgery, while the paranasal sinuses and skull base are bony anatomic structures. Access to tumors in these domains requires bone-cutting instrumentation, including rongeurs, osteotomes, and drills. The exquisitely tuned internal pulley system within the robotic arms is not engineered for the stress forces that bony dissection requires. In our experience, use of the robotic dissecting instruments led to rapid deterioration in the functionality and life-span of the equipment (unpublished data). Moreover, prototype bone-cutting instrumentation, including robotically controlled drills and rongeurs, has yet to be commercialized (unpublished data). While an entirely endonasal approach has been developed by the authors, its broad implementation has yet to be undertaken (unpublished data). Further optimization of the robotic instrumentation will be required before skull base surgery can be effectively performed with the novel technology.

14.2.5.4 Reconstructive Limitations

The most significant limitation of current transnasal endoscopic techniques is the inability to suture and provide watertight dural closure or reconstruction of dural defects. Endoscopic repair of dural defects relies on nonvascularized fat, mucosal or allogeneic grafts, or vascularized septal or nasal rotational mucosal flaps. These reconstructions are then covered with fibrin sealants and supported by either absorbable or nonabsorbable packing. While these methods may provide adequate reconstruction of minor dural tears or defects, their ability to provide safe and reliable reconstruction of larger dural defects remains to be seen. Preliminary results suggest that these methods have a higher cerebrospinal fluid leak rate compared with the more standard dural reconstruction using pedicled (axial) flaps, such as the pericranial flap or microvascular free flaps. Adequate and reliable dural reconstruction is critical in minimizing the morbidity of skull base resections, particularly in patients who received or will undergo high-dose radiation therapy. As described above, robotic-assisted surgery allows for successful and precise endoscopic suturing of the dura. This may drastically impact the utility and safety of endoscopic surgery of intracranial intradural lesions of the skull base.

Conclusion

While still in the developmental stages, robotic applications to skull base surgery are forthcoming. Transantral robotic surgery provides stereoscopic endoscopic access to the anterior skull base and pituitary fossa and allows for two-handed endoscopic manipulation and reconstruction. Traditional suture and reconstructive techniques can be implemented in this confined surgical site with the use of robotic technology. These advantages may expand the indications of minimally invasive endoscopic approaches to the skull base. Future development and refinement of endonasal robotic instrumentation is critical before applying these techniques in the clinical setting.

References

1. Hanna E, DeMonte F, Ibrahim S, Roberts D, Levine N, Kupferman M. Endoscopic resection of sinonasal cancers with and without craniotomy: oncologic results. Arch Otolaryngol Head Neck Surg. 2009;135(12):1219–24.
2. Lund V, Howard DJ, Wei WI. Endoscopic resection of malignant tumors of the nose and sinuses. Am J Rhinol. 2007;21(1):89–94.
3. Nicolai P, Battaglia P, Bignami M, et al. Endoscopic surgery for malignant tumors of the sinonasal tract and adjacent skull base: a 10-year experience. Am J Rhinol. 2008;22(3):308–16.
4. Suriano M, De Vincentiis M, Colli A, Benfari G, Mascelli A, Gallo A. Endoscopic treatment of esthesioneuroblastoma: a minimally invasive approach combined with radiation therapy. Otolaryngol Head Neck Surg. 2007;136(1):104–7.
5. Shipchandler TZ, Batra PS, Citardi MJ, Bolger WE, Lanza DC. Outcomes for endoscopic resection of sinonasal squamous cell carcinoma. Laryngoscope. 2005;115(11):1983–7.
6. Anand VK, Schwartz TH, Hiltzik DH, Kacker A. Endoscopic transphenoidal pituitary surgery with real-time intraoperative magnetic resonance imaging. Am J Rhinol. 2006;20(4):401–5.
7. Schwartz TH, Stieg PE, Anand VK. Endoscopic transsphenoidal pituitary surgery with intraoperative magnetic resonance imaging. Neurosurgery. 2006;58(1 Suppl):ONS44–ONS51; discussion ONS44–51.
8. Sethi DS, Leong JL. Endoscopic pituitary surgery. Otolaryngol Clin N Am 2006;39(3):563–583, x.
9. Teo C. Application of endoscopy to the surgical management of craniopharyngiomas. Childs Nerv Syst. 2005;21(8–9):696–700.
10. Kassam A, Carrau RL, Snyderman CH, Gardner P, Mintz A. Evolution of reconstructive techniques following endoscopic expanded endonasal approaches. Neurosurg Focus. 2005;19(1):E8.
11. Kassam A, Snyderman CH, Mintz A, Gardner P, Carrau RL. Expanded endonasal approach: the rostrocaudal axis. Part I. Crista galli to the sella turcica. Neurosurg Focus. 2005;19(1):E3.
12. Kassam AB, Gardner P, Snyderman C, Mintz A, Carrau R. Expanded endonasal approach: fully endoscopic, completely transnasal approach to the middle third of the clivus, petrous bone, middle cranial fossa, and infratemporal fossa. Neurosurg Focus. 2005;19(1):E6.
13. Kassam AB, Snyderman C, Gardner P, Carrau R, Spiro R. The expanded endonasal approach: a fully endoscopic transnasal approach and resection of the odontoid process: technical case report. Neurosurgery 2005;57(1 Suppl):E213; discussion E213
14. Solari D, Magro F, Cappabianca P, et al. Anatomical study of the pterygopalatine fossa using an endoscopic endonasal approach: spatial relations and distances between surgical landmarks. J Neurosurg. 2007;106(1):157–63.
15. Basu D, Haughey BH, Hartman JM. Determinants of success in endoscopic cerebrospinal fluid leak repair. Otolaryngol Head Neck Surg. 2006;135(5):769–73.
16. Locatelli D, Rampa F, Acchiardi I, Bignami M, De Bernardi F, Castelnuovo P. Endoscopic endonasal approaches for repair of cerebrospinal fluid leaks: nine-year experience. Neurosurgery 2006;58(4 Suppl 2):ONS-246–ONS-256; discussiom ONS-256–247.
17. Weinstein GS, O'Malley Jr BW, Snyder W, Hockstein NG. Transoral robotic surgery: supraglottic partial laryngectomy. Ann Otol Rhinol Laryngol. 2007;116(1):19–23.
18. Hanna EY, Holsinger C, DeMonte F, Kupferman M. Robotic endoscopic surgery of the skull base: a novel surgical approach. Arch Otolaryngol Head Neck Surg. 2007;133(12):1209–14.
19. Kupferman ME, Demonte F, Levine N, Hanna E. Feasibility of a robotic surgical approach to reconstruct the skull base. Skull Base: Off J N Am Skull Base Soc [et al]. 2011;21(2):79–82.
20. Cappabianca P, Cavallo LM, de Divitiis O, Solari D, Esposito F, Colao A. Endoscopic pituitary surgery. Pituitary. 2008;11(4):385–90.
21. Liu JK, Weiss MH, Couldwell WT. Surgical approaches to pituitary tumors. Neurosurg Clin N Am. 2003;14(1):93–107.
22. Kupferman M, Demonte F, Holsinger FC, Hanna E. Transantral robotic access to the pituitary gland. Otolaryngol Head Neck Surg. 2009;141(3):413–5.
23. O'Malley Jr BW, Weinstein GS. Robotic anterior and midline skull base surgery: preclinical investigations. Int J Radiat Oncol Biol Phys. 2007;69(2 Suppl):S125–8.

24. Ozer E, Waltonen J. Transoral robotic nasopharyngectomy: a novel approach for nasopharyngeal lesions. Laryngoscope. 2008;118(9):1613–6.
25. Wei WI, Ho WK. Transoral robotic resection of recurrent nasopharyngeal carcinoma. Laryngoscope. 2010;120(10):2011–4.
26. McCool RR, Warren FM, Wiggins 3rd RH, Hunt JP. Robotic surgery of the infratemporal fossa utilizing novel suprahyoid port. Laryngoscope. 2010;120(9): 1738–43.
27. O'Malley Jr BW, Weinstein GS. Robotic skull base surgery: preclinical investigations to human clinical application. Arch Otolaryngol Head Neck Surg. 2007;133(12):1215–9.
28. Hadad G, Bassagasteguy L, Carrau RL, et al. A novel reconstructive technique after endoscopic expanded endonasal approaches: vascular pedicle nasoseptal flap. Laryngoscope. 2006;116(10):1882–6.
29. Leong JL, Citardi MJ, Batra PS. Reconstruction of skull base defects after minimally invasive endoscopic resection of anterior skull base neoplasms. Am J Rhinol. 2006;20(5):476–82.
30. Mehta RP, Cueva RA, Brown JD, et al. What's new in skull base medicine and surgery? Skull Base Committee Report. Otolaryngol Head Neck Surg. 2006;135(4):620–30.
31. Kassam ABMD, Carrau RLMD, Snyderman CHMD, et al. Endoscopic reconstruction of the cranial base using a pedicled nasoseptal flap. Neurosurgery 2008;63(1) Operative Neurosurgery Supplement(1): ONS44–S53.

The Utilization of Transoral Robotic Surgery in the Pediatric Patient

15

Prasad John Thottam and Deepak K. Mehta

15.1 Introduction

Transoral robotic surgery (TORS) was first described in head and neck cancer cases in adults and, over time, expanded into treatment for adult obstructive sleep apnea (OSA). As the technology involving this technique and its associated instrumentation has improved, its utilization has expanded. More recently, through a series of publications, there has been an evolving interest in the treatment of pediatric airway ailments.

TORS in the pediatric population was first described in 2007, and in the past 8 years, only a few articles have been produced on this topic. The topics published began with feasibility and developed into examinations of surgical results [1]. To date, TORS has been described in the pediatric population for palatine tonsillectomy, oropharyngeal reconstruction, laryngeal cleft repair, lingual tonsillectomy, and base of tongue reduction/resection [1–6]. Recently it has been shown to be both feasible and effective in the treatment of refractory OSA when surgically addressing BOT and lingual hypertrophy [2].

The small size of the pediatric oral cavity can often limit the view and maneuverability of manual instrumentation in this patient population. This is where the three-dimensional endoscopic view, two active instrumentation arms, and the increased dexterity/rotational capability can be of great assistance for a more complete and effective surgery. Needless to say, as technology further develops and instrumentation becomes even smaller, the scope of surgical options will increase. Currently, the youngest patient managed through TORS in our practice or published was 15 months of age [6]. Unfortunately, the prolonged robotic docking time, cost, and sparse data are currently limitations to this technique.

P.J. Thottam, DO, FAAP (✉)
Michigan State University, East Lansing, MI, USA

Beaumont Children's Hospital, Royal Oak, MI, USA

Oakland University-William Beaumont, Royal Oak, MI, USA

Michigan Pediatric Ear, Nose and Throat Associates, Royal Oak, MI, USA
e-mail: pthottam@gmail.com

D.K. Mehta, MD
Baylor College of Medicine, Houston, TX, USA

Aerodigestive Center, Texas Children's Hospital, Houston, TX, USA

Z. Gil et al. (eds.), *Atlas of Head and Neck Robotic Surgery*, DOI 10.1007/978-3-319-49578-1_15

15.2 General Robotic Setup

1. Anesthesia
   (a) General
   (b) Laser-protected oral or nasal intubation
2. Patient and robotic unit positioning (Fig. 15.1)
   (a) Shoulder roll placed.
   (b) Operating table positioned 90–180° from anesthesiologist.
   (c) Oral retractor positioned and secured on surgical stand or supported on patient's chest with or without towels.
      (i) Dingman, Crowe-Davis, and McIvor retractors can be used for oral exposure including BOT.
      (ii) It is the authors' opinion that the Feyh-Kastenbauer (F-K) retractor is the most versatile and is good for hypopharynx and larynx exposure.
   (d) Surgical assistant is positioned at patient's head.
   (e) Robotic unit is positioned at patient's right side.
      (i) Transorally a 12 mm video endoscope (0 or 30°) with a laterally placed instrumentation (5 mm) and cautery.

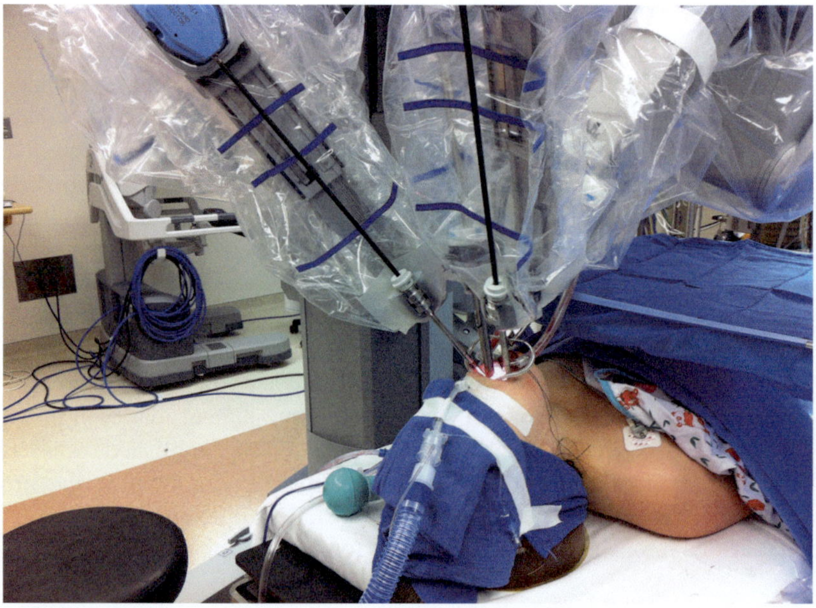

Fig. 15.1 Oral cavity access in pediatric patient for lingual tonsillectomy and base of tongue reduction

15.3 Procedures Performed

1. TORS of the lingual tonsil and base of tongue
    - (a) Surgical procedure
        - (i) McIvor or Dingman retractor is placed using a flat tongue blade.
        - (ii) 5 mm spatula cautery and Maryland forceps are utilized.
        - (iii) 30 degree 12 mm video endoscope provides a superior view of region.
        - (iv) Care is taken to place the distal aspect of the tongue blade at the circumvallate papillae in order to expose the base of tongue and lingual tonsillar tissue.
        - (v) The lingual tonsillar tissue is taken in two specimen sections starting from midline and moving laterally.
            1. This improves visualization and enables the two specimens to be taken en bloc.
        - (vi) The muscular aspect of the base of tongue is removed in similar medial to lateral fashion.
            1. Care is taken not to extend deep into the base of tongue laterally in order to avoid the lingual artery.
        - (vii) Area is irrigated and allowed to heal by secondary intention.
    - (b) Complications
        - (i) Intraoperative:
            1. Hemorrhage
            2. Dental trauma
            3. Accidental extubation/loss of airway
        - (ii) Postoperative
            1. Pain
            2. Dehydration
            3. Bleeding
                - (a) Minor bleed
                - (b) Lingual artery hemorrhage
            4. Infection
2. TORS for the treatment of laryngeal cleft
    - (a) Surgical procedure
        - (i) Patient is intubated for TORS-directed laryngeal cleft repair.
        - (ii) Patient is suspended and the larynx is secured transorally using the F-K retractor.
        - (iii) 5 mm spatula cautery and Maryland forceps are utilized.
        - (iv) 0 degree 12 mm video endoscope provides a good view of the supraglottis and glottis.
        - (v) The supraglottic interarytenoid region is isolated.
        - (vi) Cautery is utilized on coagulation setting of four to incise the interarytenoid mucosa beginning at the deepest center portion of the cleft and moving laterally (Fig. 15.2).
        - (vii) Submucosal flaps are elevated and dissected using Maryland forceps.
        - (viii) Both the esophageal and laryngeal sides of the cleft are elevated.
        - (ix) At least two sutures are placed: one on the esophageal side and one on the laryngeal aspect using 4-0 or 5-0 polydioxanone (PDS) suture (Fig. 15.3).
            1. Care is taken to begin within the defect to ensure that both knots are buried.

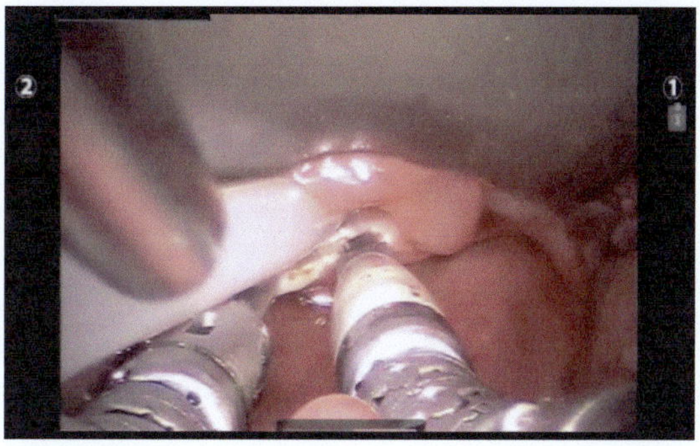

Fig. 15.2 Electrocautery used to create open edges of interarytenoid space

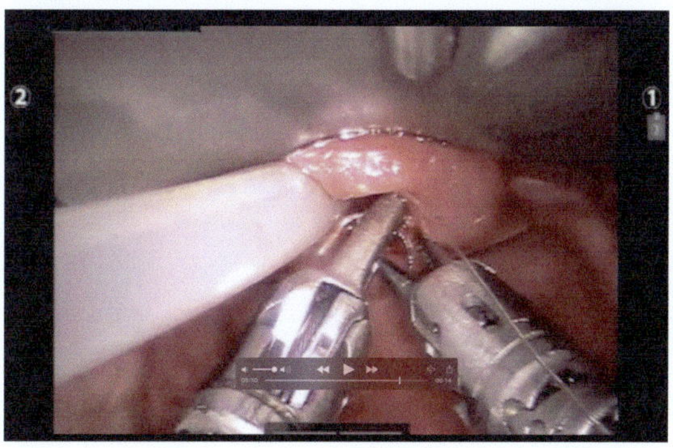

Fig. 15.3 Maryland forceps utilized to place suture to repair cleft

(b) Complications
  (i) Intraoperative
    1. Accidental extubation/loss of airway
    2. Accidental laryngeal or esophageal injury
    3. Dental trauma
  (ii) Postoperative
    1. Pain
    2. Dehydration
    3. Bleeding
    4. Infection
    5. Suture dehiscence post-repair
    6. Granulation formation at site of repair
    7. Esophageal stricture
    8. Supraglottic stenosis
    9. Dysphagia (aspiration or penetration)

15.4 Discussion

With a well-established role in adult otolaryngology, TORS in pediatric head and neck surgery is evolving, and its uses are broadening. To date, efficacy data is primarily limited to the above described procedures and oropharyngeal stenosis.

When examining TORS for BOT resection and lingual tonsillectomy, it is argued that in certain patients the ease of dissection and superior view allows for a more accurate and complete resection with limited increased risk [2, 5]. A recent examination of TORS for pediatric BOT and lingual tonsil surgery reported a greater than 50 % reduction in obstructive apnea-hypopnea index (O-AHI) score postoperatively [2]. In the same study, the majority of patients were discharged on postoperative day 1, and no intraoperative complications were reported [2]. This data, though limited by patient population size, is indeed promising as TORS further develops.

Laryngeal cleft surgery is often tedious and difficult for the pediatric otolaryngologist who is limited by patient oral cavity size, visualization, instrument rotation, human tremor, and the need to protect the patient's airway. TORS has been described as an option for these surgeries [6]. The ability to have a suitable view of the interarytenoid region and laryngeal cleft while maintaining airway safety through intubation is a noted benefit to these procedures. Recently Leonardis and colleagues described their experience with TORS-assisted LC repair in the pediatric population [6]. In this particular study, five patients were examined; all were extubated without complication and all passed subsequent 4-week postoperative swallowing examinations, demonstrating successful results [6]. The authors cited visualization, increased range of motion, and filtration of surgeon tremor as potential benefits in their experience [6].

For the treatment of pharyngeal stenosis, similar limitations, as previously described in the pediatric population, remain true with the addition of a more limited view secondary to scar tissue and contracture. In a case series published, TORS technology was utilized for access to significant nasopharyngeal stenosis in an 8-year-old child [7]. Through the use of TORS visualization and operative instrumentation, scar division, flap elevation, and proper nasopharyngeal port creation were achieved [7]. This report, though limited, does demonstrate the expanding utilization of this technology.

Conclusion

In the pediatric population, limitations exist secondary to child size and associated access. Studies on this subject are sparse, but published data has demonstrated feasibility and promising outcomes without excessive complications when compared to traditional surgical technique [1–3, 5, 6]. Though this chapter focuses primarily on TORS directed at lingual, BOT, and laryngeal cleft surgical options, TORS has been reported to be successful for the treatment of pharyngeal stenosis and other oropharyngeal pathology in the pediatric population [7].

References

1. Rahbar R, Ferrari LR, Borer JG, Peters CA. Robotic surgery in the pediatric airway: application and safety. Arch Otolaryngol-Head Neck Surg. 2007;133:46–50. discussion 50
2. Thottam PJ, Govil N, Duvvuri U, Mehta D. Transoral robotic surgery for sleep apnea in children: is it effective? Int J Pediatr Otorhinolaryngol. 2015;79:2234–7.
3. Watters K, Ferrari L, Rahbar R. Minimally invasive approach to laryngeal cleft. Laryngoscope. 2013;123:264–8.
4. Faust RA, Rahbar R. Robotic surgical technique for pediatric laryngotracheal reconstruction. Otolaryngol Clin N Am. 2008;41:1045–51. xi
5. Leonardis RL, Duvvuri U, Mehta D. Transoral robotic-assisted lingual tonsillectomy in the pediatric population. JAMA Otolaryngol Head Neck Surg. 2013;139:1032–6.
6. Leonardis RL, Duvvuri U, Mehta D. Transoral robotic-assisted laryngeal cleft repair in the pediatric patient. Laryngoscope. 2014;124:2167–9.
7. Byrd JK, Leonardis RL, Bonawitz SC, Losee JE, Duvvuri U. Transoral robotic surgery for pharyngeal stenosis. Int J Med Robot Comput Assist Surg: MRCAS. 2014;10:418–22.

Robotic Reconstructive Surgery

16

Amir E. Ibrahim, Karim A. Sarhane, and Jesse C. Selber

The management of oropharyngeal and base of tongue cancers remains a challenging endeavor. The high incidence of morbidity following the traditional surgical method to resect such tumors (lip and mandible splitting, Fig. 16.1) has led to the use of primary chemoradiation therapy as an alternative treatment [1, 2]. However, toxicity rates following this approach were considerably high (acute mucositis, xerostomia, and long-term swallowing dysfunction), and there was no improvement in functional status [3]. Thus, driven by the desire to offer a less morbid alternative to both traditional surgical resection and chemoradiation, transoral robotic surgery (TORS) using the da Vinci Surgical System was developed. This approach showed great success in resecting pharyngeal and laryngeal malignant lesions, achieving similar survival rates as compared to primary chemoradiation therapy, but with improved functional and aesthetic outcomes as it obviated the need for lip and mandible splitting [4–6]. This minimally invasive technique however left a challenging defect to reconstruct. The reconstructive challenge is that the cylinder of the oropharynx remains almost entirely closed, severely restricting its access when planning to inset and contour vascularized tissue. This anatomic region (between the uvula and the epiglottis) is particularly difficult to approach without a mandibulotomy or a wide pharyngotomy. As such, the senior author developed a minimally invasive robotic reconstructive approach, known as transoral robotic *reconstructive* surgery (TOR*R*S) [7], to address the defects created after TORS. In this chapter we discuss the clinical application of transoral robotic *r*econstructive surgery (TOR*R*S).

A.E. Ibrahim, MD
Division of Plastic Surgery, Department of Surgery, American University of Beirut Medical Center, Beirut, Lebanon

K.A. Sarhane, MD, MSc
Department of Surgery, University of Toledo Medical Center, Toledo, OH, USA

J.C. Selber, MD, MPH, FACS (✉)
Department of Plastic Surgery, University of Texas M.D. Anderson Cancer Center, Unit 1488, 1400 Pressler Street, Houston, TX 77030, USA
e-mail: jcselber@mdanderson.org

Z. Gil et al. (eds.), *Atlas of Head and Neck Robotic Surgery*, DOI 10.1007/978-3-319-49578-1_16

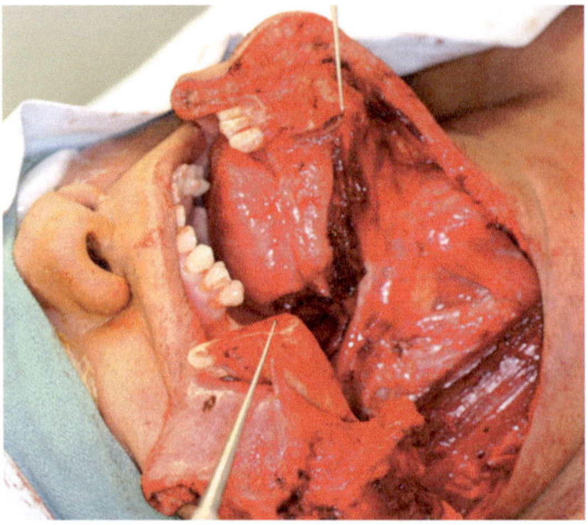

Fig. 16.1 Traditional surgical approach to oropharyngeal tumors (lip splitting and mandibulotomy). This technique is associated with disfigurement and with an increased risk of osteoradionecrosis and fracture at the mandibulotomy site after adjuvant radiotherapy

16.1 The Ascent of TOR*R*S

The defects created after TORS require meticulous reconstructive techniques to preserve normal anatomy and ensure good functional outcomes. Small defects, such as those at the base of tongue, can heal by secondary intention with good functional outcomes, and hence do not require reconstruction. Those in the tonsillar area and those extending to the soft palate, however, require vascularized tissue coverage as they result in carotid sheath exposure, oro- or pharyngocutaneous fistulas, and a potential for velopharyngeal incompetence. Some of these defects can be satisfactorily reconstructed with facial artery musculomucosal (FAMM) flaps, buccal rotation flaps, and pharyngeal flaps. Bonawiz et al. reported successful reconstruction of defects of the soft palate in five patients who underwent combined robotic-assisted resection of malignant lesions with immediate FAMM flap reconstruction [8]. Also, Selber reported the use of the robot to reconstruct a defect of the soft palate, tonsillar pillar, and pharyngeal wall with a FAMM flap in one patient in his case series describing robotic reconstruction [9].

Defects resulting from larger tumor resections are more complex and often extend from the tip of the tongue all the way to the epiglottis, involving a significant pharyngeal component and a pharyngotomy. The reconstructive challenge created by these minimally invasive resections is that the cylinder of the oropharynx remains almost entirely closed, severely restricting access to oropharyngeal anatomy as plastic surgeons attempt to inset and contour vascularized tissue. The anatomic region between the uvula and the epiglottis is very difficult to approach without a mandibulotomy or a wide pharyngotomy. Preserving a competent velopharyngeal sphincter, a watertight seal between the pharynx and neck, and adequate sensations and volume in the tongue base are necessary to optimize the physiological function of the oropharynx and minimize functional deficits [10, 11]. To achieve these goals, transoral robotic *reconstructive* surgery (TOR*R*S) [12], whether using free flaps, local flaps, or primary closure, seems to be a logical approach. This technique appears to be a superior option in some cases and also holds great promise in expanding the indications for minimally invasive resection procedures. Combining transoral robotic flap inset with a manual approach through the existing pharyngotomy defect is also feasible. It is worth noting that although a pharyngotomy was created, it is much smaller than the wide pharyngotomies traditionally required for accessing such tumors as access to the upper pharynx is achieved robotically rather than through the neck. The senior author has thoroughly documented the value of TOR*R*S for challenging defects of the head and neck and has demonstrated both feasibility [13] and effectiveness [9] of this reconstructive method. More recently, Song et al. reported their experience with free flap robotic reconstruction of oropharyngeal defects after robotic extirpation and also showed the feasibility of this new reconstructive approach in insetting flaps at a deep portion of the oropharynx without the need to perform a traditional mandibulotomy [10].

In addition, by taking this approach, plastic surgeons are able to provide a reliable reconstructive support for the head and neck surgeon to robotically resect larger, deeper, and more complex tumors that would be very challenging to reconstruct through traditional methods.

16.2 Indications and Preoperative Evaluation

Clear-cut indications for the application of TOR*R*S are still not well defined. Reports describing its use have elaborated so far on its feasibility, safety, and extent of applicability; no clear instructions incorporating patient and tumor factors have yet been put forth. Longfield et al. proposed recently an algorithm for the use of TOR*R*S based on tumor site, tumor extent, and patient-specific factors [14]. This can be used a structural scheme to which future recommendations can be incorporated.

16.2.1 Tumor Site

Tumor site is most probably the most important factor affecting the feasibility of a transoral robotic approach for resection and reconstruction.

Oral cavity lesions are accessible manually and would not benefit from TORS. An exception however is large retromolar trigone lesions. Tumors in this area are adjacent to the base of tongue (BOT), tonsil, and mandibular ramus. A robotic approach in this setting would be a good option for both resection and reconstruction. Local flaps such as the FAMM flap, buccal fat pad flap, and buccal and pharyngeal mucosal transposition flaps can be used. Free flaps are rarely used. The area is very restricted for flap inset, and also this would entail dissecting and exposing the neck to the oropharynx. So unless there is an indication for free tissue transfer (such as prior radiation or resections), avoiding such method is advocated.

On the other hand, tumors located within the oropharynx (tonsil, BOT, soft palate) benefit significantly from transoral robotic resection and reconstruction. It is true that these tumors were resected by alternative methods for many years [15, 16]; however, limited dexterity and visualization have always been a major disadvantage. With the ascent of robotic technology, improved visualization and more precise instrumentation have allowed the resection of more complex and invasive tumors. Defects created by such large resections (where critical structures—carotid sheath or bone—are exposed) are best addressed using robotic free flap reconstruction [9, 17]. Free flap options include radial forearm and anterolateral thigh flaps, and recipient vessels include either the superior thyroid artery or the facial artery.

For soft palate tumors, free flaps or palatoplasties are usually performed. In select cases, similar functional outcomes may be obtained with a prosthetic obturator [18, 19].

For tumors extending to the supraglottic larynx, reconstruction is guided by the extent of hypopharyngeal involvement and whether the lesion is above or below the hyoid bone. In patients with a large oral opening, the supra- and infrahyoid areas can be directly attained, and TORS might not be required. Free tissue transfer is also not feasible in this area. In case the defect is large enough to require free flap reconstruction [20], a tracheostomy is needed and will most likely be done through the flap itself. This increases the risk of airway compromise if partial dehiscence occurs.

16.2.2 Tumor Extent

As noted previously, small tumors (i.e., T1 and T2) can be allowed to heal by secondary intention; this approach is safe and results in satisfactory functional outcomes. As for larger lesions (i.e., T3, T4) or for posterior T2 tumors, or when the carotid sheath is exposed, or a surgical fistula is created, or velopharyngeal compromise is anticipated to occur, vascularized tissue is required to reconstruct the normal anatomy and optimize functional outcomes. Some of these lesions may also undergo "hybrid" resections, i.e., combining a transoral approach with a small pharyngotomy. This is usually followed by a "hybrid" reconstruction, where TOR*R*S is performed, and the deepest inset is completed through the neck.

16.2.3 Prior Therapy

Neck irradiation compromises both the local micro- and macrovasculature, making local flaps undesirable for reconstruction. Also, prior neck irradiation increases the odds for receiving adjuvant radiation therapy. In such cases, free tissue transfer is advocated (even when the defects are small enough not to require coverage). This type of reconstruction brings in healthy vascularized tissue ensuring a durable form of coverage and allowing for re-irradiation [10, 13].

16.2.4 Patient Factors

Patient performance status constitutes the major determinant for any type of surgery. As obesity rates are increasing [21], medical comorbidities such as diabetes and vascular diseases are becoming more common among all age groups. Such conditions compromise perfusion and wound healing and thus increase the risk of dehiscence, infections, and other wound complications. Tight glycemic control in the pre- and postoperative period is essential.

More frequent than obesity, however, head and neck cancer patients are malnourished and suffer from chronic cachexia and muscle wasting. In addition to these factors, significant smoking history and poor cardiopulmonary status may also compromise the operative course of such patients by making them susceptible to the adverse effects of long operative times and general anesthesia. It is also important to consider the other preoperative patient variables that were notoriously associated with poor postoperative performance, such as anemia [22, 23], coronary or peripheral vascular disease, dysphagia, or a history of recurrent aspirations.

16.3 Surgical Technique

16.3.1 Patient Setup

TOR*R*S is usually combined with TORS (during which patient positioning has already been performed). Patients are usually placed in the supine position and supported with a shoulder roll to provide adequate neck extension. A doughnut gel pad is used for occipital scalp protection. Both upper and lower extremities are well padded to prevent nerve injury, especially for overweight and obese patients [24]. TED stockings and sequential compressing devices are also applied to the lower extremities in an effort to minimize deep vein thrombosis.

16.3.2 Robotic Setup

The setup for the robotic portion is similar for all TOR*R*S cases [9]. First, an optical window is created in the mouth. When the tongue base is not involved, a Dingman retractor is placed in the mouth to create a stable interdental opening and provide lingual retraction; other retractors have also been tested for this use and were employed clinically [25]. When reconstruction of the base of tongue is however required, the tongue must remain mobile. A cheek retractor is placed to maintain a stable frame, a mouth prop is used to create a wide interdental opening, and a suture is placed at the tip of the tongue for manipulation (Fig. 16.2).

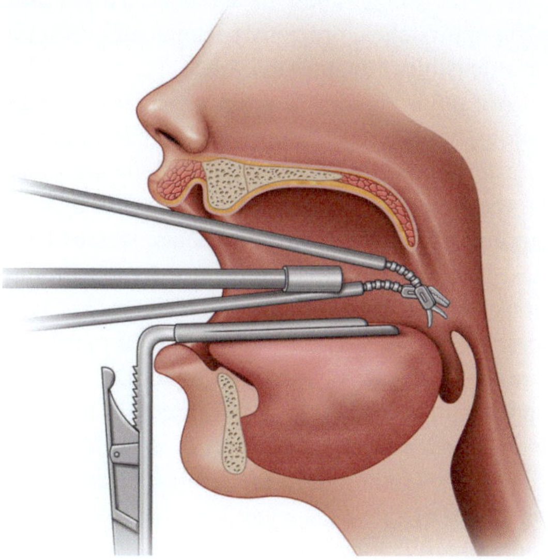

Fig. 16.2 Representative illustration of the robotic setup for oropharyngeal surgery. A Dingman oral retractor is used to keep the mouth open. Two robotic arms and an endoscope are used to operate

16.3.3 Robotic Docking

The exact location and position of the patient side cart depends on the location of the defect. Since the robotic arms function best when the working area is lined up with the base and when the arms are working back toward it, it is recommended to position the robot at 45° from the foot of the right side of the operating table for defects located in the right tonsillar area. Whereas when the defect is in the left tonsillar area, 45° from the foot of the left side is preferred. For central or posterior pharyngeal defects, either of these two positions is acceptable. In any case, the patient side cart should be against the base of the bed, in order to bring it as close as possible to the mouth. When operating on the palate, it would be more convenient to bring the robot in from the head of the bed.

In all of these settings, the two robotic arms are aligned around a point converging at the target anatomy in the oropharynx. The shoulders of the three arms should be angled at 90°, and the arms should form approximately 45° angle with the endoscope.

16.3.4 Robotic Flap Inset

Following flap elevation, inset within the mouth is performed using two 8 mm needle drivers and 4.0 or 3.0 Vicryl sutures. Two needle drivers are preferable to a needle driver and grasper because it is sometimes necessary to place sutures with both arms of the robot (depending on the angle and location within the oral cavity). The suture is trimmed to approximately 3 in. in length, in order to avoid extra suture material in the mouth. Interrupted sutures are placed and tied using human arms. Economy of motion is important because small movements at the tips of the instruments correspond to large movements more proximally. Excursion of the robotic arms is limited by the area within the mouth retractor. On occasion, when the space is too restricted, such as in the glossopharyngeal sulcus, sutures can be placed robotically, taking advantage of the improved visualization and dexterity, and then tied down blindly by hand.

16.3.5 Robotic-Assisted Microvascular Anastomosis

Once the robotic portion of the inset is performed, the arms can be removed from the mouth, instruments changed, and then placed back in proximity to the neck vessels. Arms n° 1 and 2 are equipped with Black Diamond Microneedle drivers, rather than the larger jawed needle drivers used during the inset. A third arm equipped with a "fine tissue forceps" attachment serves as a stationary assistant, and the surgeon is able to toggle back and forth between arms n° 1 and 3, depending on which one is being used to position the vessel and which is being used to saw. 9.0 nylon sutures are commonly used for the anastomosis.

Robotic microvascular anastomosis is a promising technique. The facial artery is the most utilized recipient artery. It courses beneath the hypoglossal nerve and underneath the digastric sling, often high under the body of the mandible. If the patient has tracheostomy, the space available to perform the anastomosis may be confined. The robot's precision and visualization in restricted spaces address such issues and permit microanastomosis to be performed with much more confidence. The robot actually adds precision and a high definition 3D vision to any type of microanastomosis (whether in a challenging environment or not). This made the robotic platform inherently more precise than the human hand in any micro-setting.

Due to lack of haptic or tactile feedback, careful attention to visual cues is vital, particularly when it comes to setting down the knot. It is important to maintain equal slack in both ends of the suture, and to minimize movement of the anastomosis while tying (as this represents a differential in applied tension), and to only pull until the air in the knot disappears. These measures are essential to minimize vessel trauma. Due to poorly designed robotic microsurgical instruments with broad and flat tips and with diamond dust coating (Diamond Microneedle drivers), attention is needed to avoid inadvertent cutting of the suture.

16.4 TOR*RS* Advantages and Disadvantages

TOR*RS* benefits from the all advantages offered by the robotic platform (enhanced precision, improved dexterity, enhanced hand-eye coordination, ergonomic positioning, and smooth patient recovery). These have rendered many surgical approaches, previously technically difficult or unfeasible, now possible.

Although rapidly developing, TOR*RS* technology has not yet achieved its full potential due to a few limitations. These limitations are those of the general robotic platform which include among others, technical constraints, lack of haptics, size of the devices, instrumentation limitations, lack of flexibility of certain energy devices, and problems with multi-quadrant surgery. Another important question affecting broader application of robotic-assisted surgery is learning curve. When operating the robot, a comprehensive understanding of its mechanics, kinetics, and operative dynamics is a major prerequisite; basic functionality alone is not enough [26]. Moreover, for robotic microsurgery, considering its technical complexity and the consequences of its failure, advanced teaching modules and robust learning assessment tools are needed to ensure a solid training and safe use [27].

16.5 Conclusion

Adapting the robotic platform for the resection (TORS) and reconstruction (TOR*R*S) of head and neck malignancies seems a very advantageous approach in terms of both oncologic and functional outcomes. TOR*R*S allowed access to the difficult anatomy of the oropharynx and achieved the goals of reconstruction, which are preservation of a competent velopharyngeal sphincter, a watertight seal between the pharynx and neck, and adequate sensation and volume in the tongue base. Widespread application of this beneficial technology is dependent on minimizing cost and implementing training programs. Currently, most residency programs in the United States have not yet placed enough emphasis on robotic surgery training. Developing competency to perform robotic procedures is left to individual hospitals. Students, residents, and fellows should make every effort to keep up and follow all the new innovations in robotic surgery as this technology is most likely to reshape the way head and neck surgery is practiced.

16.6 Case Examples

Case 1

A 74-year-old male, with a history of T2 N1 M0 right tonsillar squamous cell carcinoma treated with primary radiation therapy in the distant past, developed subsequently a T2 N0 M0 left tonsillar squamous cell carcinoma (Fig. 16.3). He underwent transoral robotic resection. The defect included the posterior tonsillar pillar, a portion of the soft palate, and a portion of the posterior pharynx. The overall defect was small, but the carotid sheath was exposed, and there was a concern for velopharyngeal incompetence. Hence, a left-sided, inferiorly based facial artery musculomucosal (FAMM) flap was planned. The flap extended from the ipsilateral retromolar trigone to the frenulum of the gingivobuccal sulcus. It was passed over the third molar and into the defect to reconstruct the posterior tonsillar pillar (Fig. 16.4). A Dingman retractor was used to maintain an interdental opening and to retract the cheeks and tongue. Inset of the flap was performed robotically. Absorbable sutures were used. A bite block was placed to protect the pedicle.

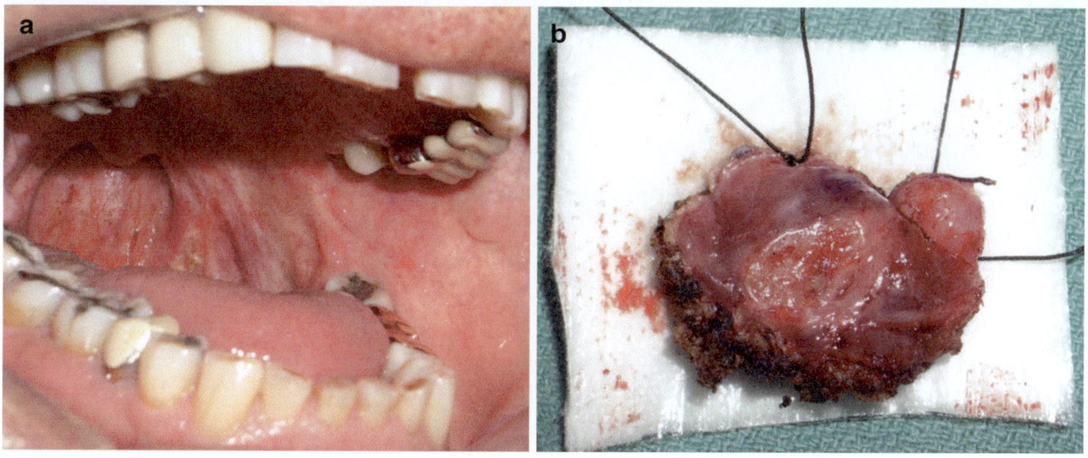

Fig. 16.3 Left tonsillar cancer (**a**). Resected specimen using TORS (**b**)

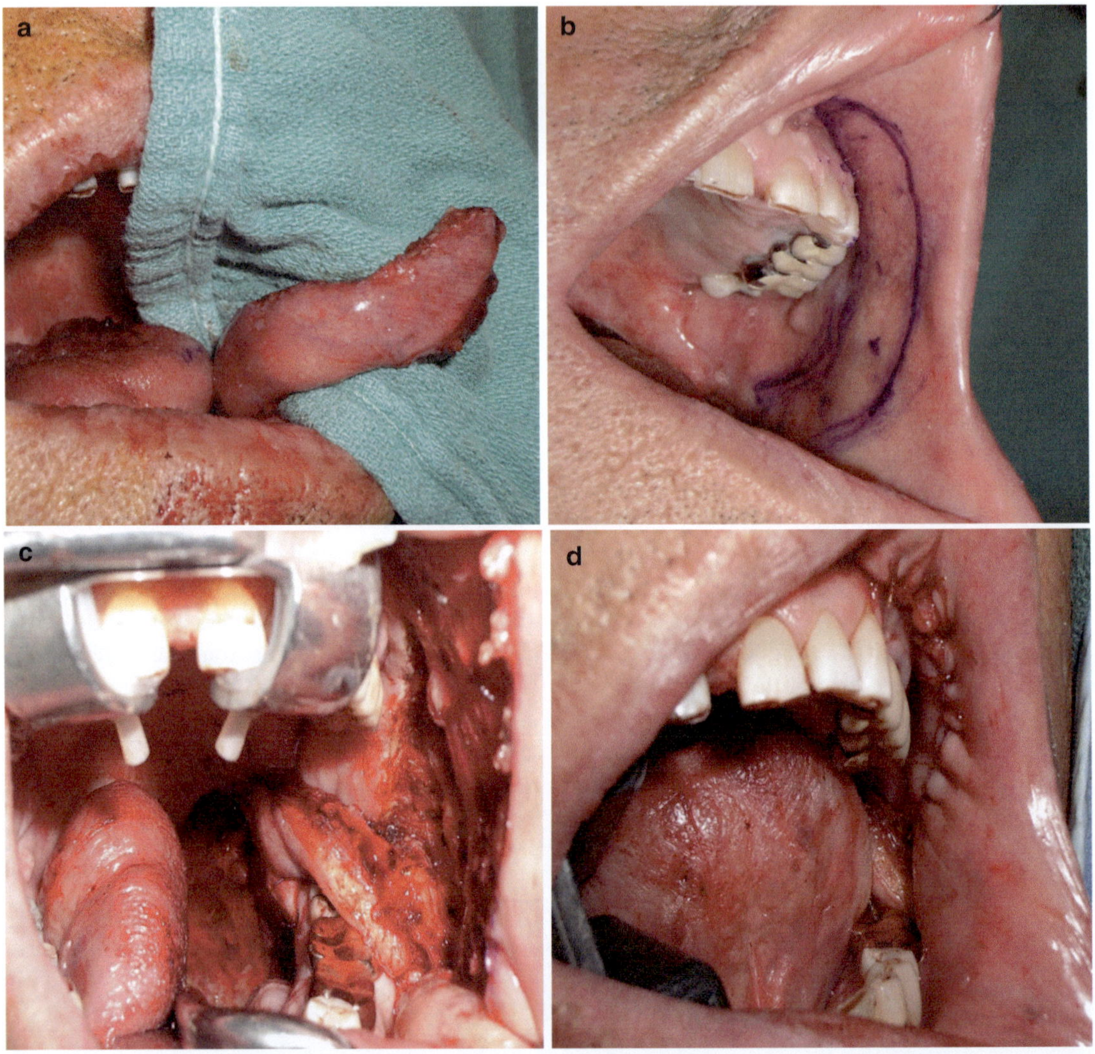

Fig. 16.4 Left facial artery musculomucosal (FAMM) flap planned to reconstruct a defect created after resecting a left tonsillar cancer. TORRS enhances visualization and dexterity during flap inset. (**a**, **b**) Flap design and harvest. (**c**) Flap transposition to the surgical defect. (**d**) Donor-site closure

Case 2

A 62-year-old man presented with a recurrent T3 N1 M0 left posterolateral pharynx squamous cell carcinoma following radiation therapy in the past. He underwent transoral robotic resection with a small lateral pharyngotomy and a left neck dissection (Fig. 16.5). Although the pharyngotomy was small (~15 cm^2), a large portion of the pharynx (~50 cm^2) was resected from the epiglottis to the soft palate. A 6 × 9 cm radial forearm flap was used (Fig. 16.6). The upper pharyngeal component was inset robotically, and the remainder of the inset was performed through the pharyngotomy. The patient side cart, which was already in place from the robotic resection and inset, was adjusted, and the robotic arterial anastomosis carried out successfully (Fig. 16.7). The venous anastomosis was then coupled under loupe magnification. The patient was decannulated, discharged within a week, and passed a modified barium swallow study 3 weeks postoperatively (Fig. 16.8). His speech and swallowing are normal, and he is tolerating a regular diet not needing any tube feeding (Fig. 16.9).

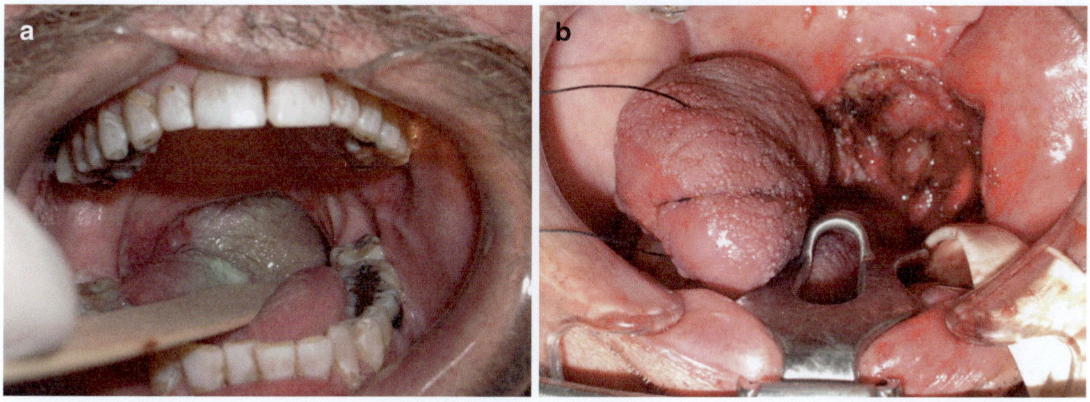

Fig. 16.5 (**a**) Recurrent left squamous cell carcinoma of the anterior tonsillar pillar. (**b**) Surgical defect after robotic resection

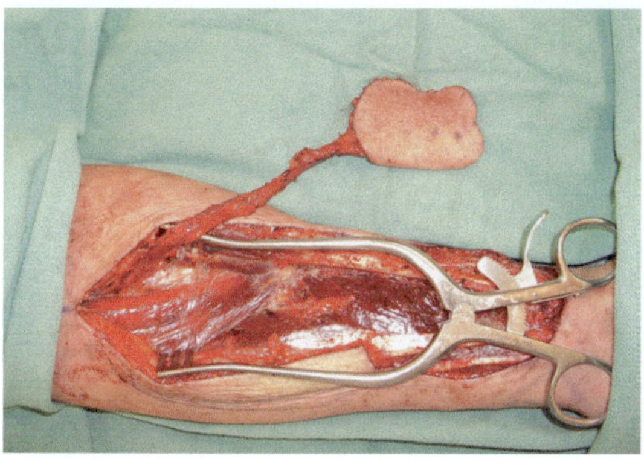

Fig. 16.6 A radial forearm fasciocutaneous free flap was harvested in preparation for robot-assisted *inset*

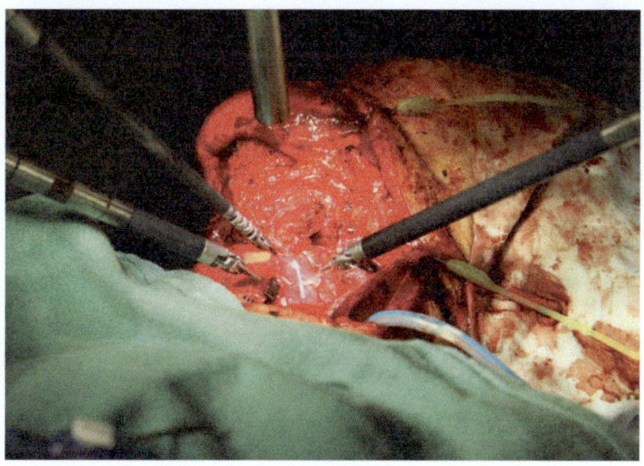

Fig. 16.7 Robotic microvascular anastomosis of the radial artery to the left facial artery

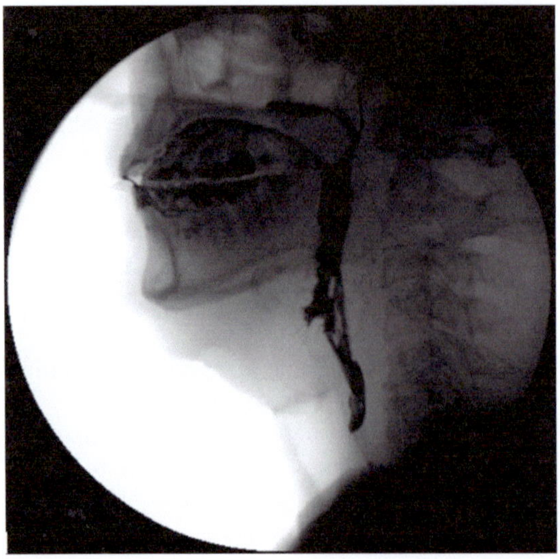

Fig. 16.8 Modified barium swallow following TORRS of the oropharynx using a radial forearm free flap; no evidence of leakage or aspiration

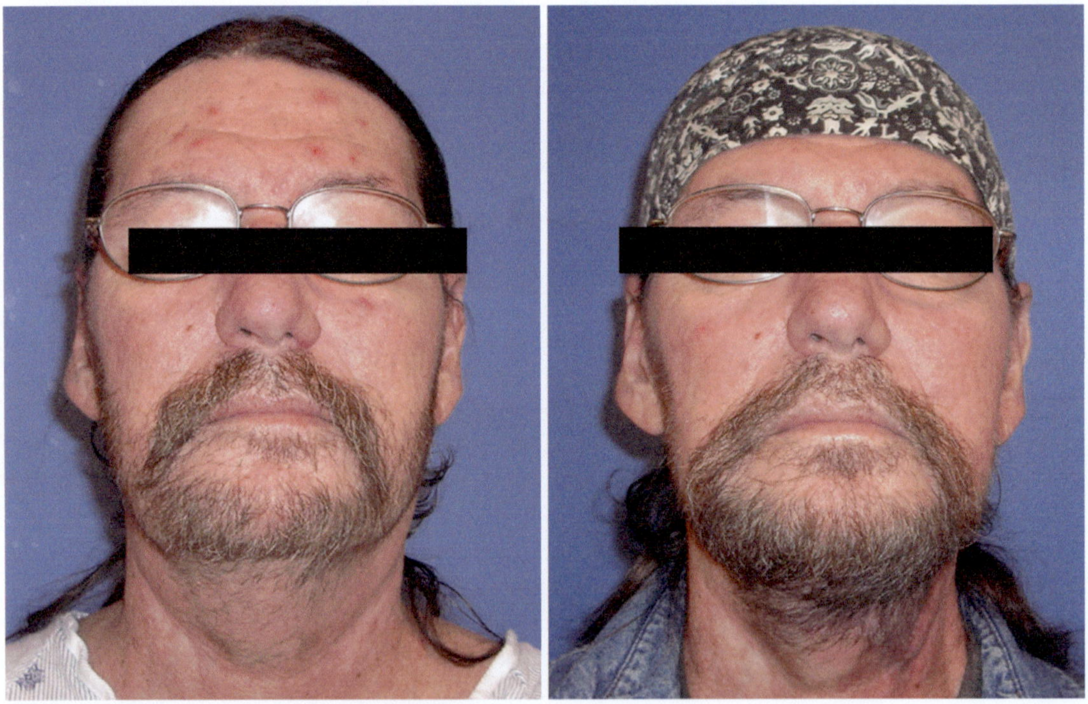

Fig. 16.9 Pre- and postoperative appearance following TORS and TORRS of a left oropharyngeal cancer. The use of the robot provided improved visualization and surgical manipulation while obviating the need for lip and mandible splitting

References

1. Machtay M, Moughan J, Trotti A, Garden AS, Weber RS, Cooper JS, et al. Factors associated with severe late toxicity after concurrent chemoradiation for locally advanced head and neck cancer: an RTOG analysis. J Clin Oncol [Internet]. 2008 [cited 2013 Dec 17];26(21):3582–9. Available from: http://www.ncbi.nlm.nih.gov/pubmed/18559875.
2. Walvekar RR, Li RJ, Gooding WE, Gibson MK, Heron D, Johnson JT, et al. Role of surgery in limited (T1-2, N0-1) cancers of the oropharynx. Laryngoscope [Internet]. 2008 [cited 2013 Dec 30];118(12):2129–34. Available from: http://www.ncbi.nlm.nih.gov/pubmed/18948826.
3. Nguyen NP, Vos P, Smith HJ, Nguyen PD, Alfieri A, Karlsson U, et al. Concurrent chemoradiation for locally advanced oropharyngeal cancer. Am J Otolaryngol [Internet]. 2007 [cited 2013 Dec 31];28(1):3–8. Available from: http://www.ncbi.nlm.nih.gov/pubmed/17162122.
4. Weinstein GS, O'malley BW, Hockstein NG. Transoral robotic surgery: supraglottic laryngectomy in a canine model. Laryngoscope [Internet]. 2005 [cited 2013 Nov 5];115(7):1315–1319. Available from: http://www.ncbi.nlm.nih.gov/pubmed/15995528.
5. Genden EM, Desai S, Sung C-K. Transoral robotic surgery for the management of head and neck cancer: a preliminary experience. Head Neck [Internet]. 2009 [cited 2013 Nov 6];31(3):283–9. Available from: http://www.ncbi.nlm.nih.gov/pubmed/18972413.
6. Dowthwaite SA, Franklin JH, Palma DA, Fung K, Yoo J, Nichols AC. The role of transoral robotic surgery in the management of oropharyngeal cancer: a review of the literature. ISRN Oncol. 2012;2012:945162.
7. Selber JC, Sarhane KA, Ibrahim AE, Holsinger FC. Transoral robotic reconstructive surgery. Semin Plast Surg [Internet] Thieme Medical Publishers; 2014 [cited 2014 May 6];28(01):35–8. Available from: http://www.ncbi.nlm.nih.gov/pubmed/24872777.
8. Bonawitz SC, Duvvuri U. Robotic-assisted FAMM flap for soft palate reconstruction. Laryngoscope [Internet]. 2013 [cited 2013 Dec 31];123(4):870–4. Available from: http://www.ncbi.nlm.nih.gov/pubmed/23529879.
9. Selber JC. Transoral robotic reconstruction of oropharyngeal defects: a case series. Plast Reconstr Surg [Internet]. 2010 [cited 2013 Nov 6];126(6):1978–87. Available from: http://www.ncbi.nlm.nih.gov/pubmed/21124136.
10. Song HG, Yun IS, Lee WJ, Lew DH, Rah DK. Robot-assisted free flap in head and neck reconstruction. Arch Plast Surg [Internet]. 2013 [cited 2013 Nov 6];40(4):353–358. Available from: http://www.pubmedcentral.nih.gov/articlerender.fcgi?artid=3723995&tool=pmcentrez&rendertype=abstract.
11. DeAlmeida JR, Park RCW, Genden EM. Reconstruction of transoral robotic surgery defects: principles and techniques. J Reconstr Microsurg [Internet]. 2012 [cited 2013 Dec 22];28(7):465–72. Available from: http://www.ncbi.nlm.nih.gov/pubmed/22744899
12. Selber J. Discussion: Robotic-assisted FAMM flap for soft palate reconstruction. Laryngoscope. 2014. doi:10.1002/lary.23579. [Epub ahead of print]
13. Selber JC, Robb G, Serletti JM, Weinstein G, Weber R, Holsinger FC. Transoral robotic free flap reconstruction of oropharyngeal defects: a preclinical investigation. Plast Reconstr Surg [Internet]. 2010 [cited 2013 Nov 6];125(3):896–900. Available from: http://www.ncbi.nlm.nih.gov/pubmed/20195117.
14. Longfield EA, Holsinger FC, Selber JC. Reconstruction after robotic head and neck surgery: when and why. J Reconstr Microsurg [Internet]. 2012 [cited 2013 Nov 5];28(7):445–50. Available from: http://www.ncbi.nlm.nih.gov/pubmed/22399257.
15. Holsinger FC, McWhorter AJ, Ménard M, Garcia D, Laccourreye O. Transoral lateral oropharyngectomy for squamous cell carcinoma of the tonsillar region: I. Technique, complications, and functional results. Arch Otolaryngol Head Neck Surg [Internet]. 2005 [cited 2013 Dec 17];131(7):583–91. Available from: http://www.ncbi.nlm.nih.gov/pubmed/16027280.
16. Laccourreye O, Hans S, Ménard M, Garcia D, Brasnu D, Holsinger FC. Transoral lateral oropharyngectomy for squamous cell carcinoma of the tonsillar region: II. An analysis of the incidence, related variables, and consequences of local recurrence. Arch Otolaryngol Head Neck Surg [Internet]. 2005 [cited 2013 Dec 17];131(7):592–9. Available from: http://www.ncbi.nlm.nih.gov/pubmed/16027281.
17. Genden EM, Kotz T, Tong CCL, Smith C, Sikora AG, Teng MS, et al. Transoral robotic resection and reconstruction for head and neck cancer. Laryngoscope [Internet]. 2011 [cited 2013 Dec 31];121(8):1668–74. Available from: http://www.ncbi.nlm.nih.gov/pubmed/21792953.
18. Rieger J, Bohle Iii G, Huryn J, Tang JL, Harris J, Seikaly H. Surgical reconstruction versus prosthetic obturation of extensive soft palate defects: a comparison of speech outcomes. Int J Prosthodont [Internet]. 2009 [cited 2013 Dec 17];22(6):566–72. Available from: http://www.ncbi.nlm.nih.gov/pubmed/19918590.
19. Marsh JL, Wray RC. Speech prosthesis versus pharyngeal flap: a randomized evaluation of the management of velopharyngeal incompetency. Plast Reconstr Surg [Internet]. 1980 [cited 2013 Dec 17];65(5):592–4. Available from: http://www.ncbi.nlm.nih.gov/pubmed/7367500.
20. Mukhija VK, Sung C-K, Desai SC, Wanna G, Genden EM. Transoral robotic assisted free flap reconstruction. Otolaryngol Head Neck Surg [Internet]. 2009 Jan [cited 2013 Nov 6];140(1):124–5. Available from: http://www.ncbi.nlm.nih.gov/pubmed/19130975.
21. Atiyeh B, Sarhane K. Overweight and obesity: a true global epidemic. In: Atiyeh BS, editor. Body contouring following bariatric surgery and massive weight loss post-bariatric body contouring. Sharjah: Bentham Science Publishers; 2012. p. 3.

22. Sarhane K, Flores J, Cooney C, Abreu F, Lacayo M, Baltodano P, et al. Preoperative anemia and postoperative outcomes in immediate breast reconstructive surgery: a critical analysis of 10,958 patients from the ACS-NSQIP database. Plast Reconstr Surg GO [Internet]. 2013;1(5):e30. Available from: http://journals.lww.com/prsgo/pages/articleviewer.aspx?year=2013&issue=08000&article=00001&type=Fulltext
23. Hill JB, Patel A, Del Corral G A, Sexton KW, Ehrenfeld JM, Guillamondegui OD, et al. Preoperative anemia predicts thrombosis and free flap failure in microvascular reconstruction. Ann Plast Surg [Internet]. 2012 [cited 2012 Nov 5];69(4):364–7. Available from: http://www.ncbi.nlm.nih.gov/pubmed/22964664.
24. Sarhane K, Kobeissy F. Anesthetic management in body contouring surgery. J Anesth Clin Res [Internet]. 2012 [cited 2013 Jul 26];3(e106). Available from: http://www.omicsonline.org/2155-6148/2155-6148-3-e106.php?aid=8335.
25. O'Malley BW, Weinstein GS, Snyder W, Hockstein NG. Transoral robotic surgery (TORS) for base of tongue neoplasms. Laryngoscope [Internet]. 2006 [cited 2013 Nov 5];116(8):1465–72. Available from: http://www.ncbi.nlm.nih.gov/pubmed/16885755.
26. Selber J, Pederson J. Robotic muscle harvest. Telemicrosurgery. Paris: Springer; 2012.
27. Selber JC, Alrasheed T. Robotic microsurgical training and evaluation. Semin Plast Surg [Internet]. 2014 [cited 2015 Jul 13];28(1):5–10. Available from: http://www.pubmedcentral.nih.gov/articlerender.fcgi?artid=3946019&tool=pmcentrez&rendertype=abstract.

Robotic Otology

17

Pooneh Roshani Tabrizi, Reza Monfaredi, Wen P. Liu, Russell H. Taylor, Kevin Cleary, and Diego Preciado

17.1 Introduction

Otologic surgery is an attractive otolaryngologic field for the implementation of robotic systems as a means to improve surgical outcome. In particular, given the physical millimetric restrictions in surgical access to inner ear sites and the microscopic anatomical elements within the middle ear space, surgical precision is of paramount importance during these cases.

The introduction of the otologic microscope to the field during the 1950s led to a revolution in otologic surgery [1], effectively making a myriad of previously unthinkable surgical maneuvers physically possible. The breakthrough of microscopic visualization coupled with the use of the high powered dental-type burrs, along with continuous suction and irrigation in place of the mallet, gouge, and rongeur forceps, gave rise to a whole new field of surgical hearing restoration. Examples include different tympanoplasty and stapes surgical techniques, mastoidectomy with safe facial recess drilling, cochleostomy, labyrinthectomy, and improved cholesteatoma extirpation, just to name a few. More recently, endoscopic otologic surgery has become a popular and burgeoning alternative to traditional binocular microscopic approaches [2]. Many advantages relative to the microscope are reported. For one, there is a dramatically improved field of view with comparable or improved magnification of the middle ear space. The endoscopes allow for visualization "around corners," clefts, and recesses. No longer are areas of the middle ear "hidden" from view. In fact, a whole realm of middle ear anatomy is being defined due to the improvement in optics conferred by the endoscope [3]. Regardless of microscopic or endoscopic visualization, precision in terms of optics and magnification are crucial factors for otologic surgery.

A second aspect of otologic surgery, attractive for robotic applications, is that the anatomical components of the ear, housed within the confines of the temporal bone, are fixed in bone and as such are highly predictable and stable in terms of the limits of their location and limits of dissection. With increasing resolution of temporal bone imaging ostensibly resulting in improved segmentation of middle ear structures, it is becoming increasingly feasible to preprogram the location and physical extent of critical landmarks into complete or partial automation systems for otologic surgery, including robotics. As an example, for cochlear implantation (CI), there are critical structures that need to be avoided, and an accurate path has to be opened through the bone to expose and enter

P.R. Tabrizi, PhD • R. Monfaredi, PhD • W.P. Liu, PhD
R.H. Taylor, PhD • K. Cleary, PhD
D. Preciado, MD, PhD (✉)
Sheikh Zayed Institute for Pediatric Surgical Innovation, Children's National Health System, 111 Michigan Av NW, Washington, DC 20010, USA
e-mail: dpreciad@cnmc.org

Z. Gil et al. (eds.), *Atlas of Head and Neck Robotic Surgery*, DOI 10.1007/978-3-319-49578-1_17

the cochlea at a specific and precise location, relative to the round window. Appropriate cochleostomy placement is critical to allow for scala tympani cochlear electrode array insertion. Recent studies, however, suggest that a significant proportion of cochlear implant surgeons do not adequately position the cochleostomy anterior inferior to the round window, into the scala tympani [4, 5]. Arguably, this is attributed to the fact that less experienced surgeons are more likely to have inadequate exposure of the round window through the facial recess. This is in part likely due to a fear of injuring the facial nerve, causing some to leave the bone overlying the nerve undrilled, incompletely opening the facial recess and obscuring the round window view. Other potential factors that contribute to an inadequate cochleostomy placement include variable round window anatomy, a poor angle of visualization approach, and a lack of understanding of cochlear anatomy. These factors are especially prevalent in cases involving very young or otitis-prone children with poorly pneumatized mastoids, in complicated revision cases, or in cases with complex or absent bony landmarks. Indeed, increasingly precise surgical robotic systems capable of providing either immediate intraoperative feedback of temporal bone anatomy or further automating temporal bone surgery could potentially be revolutionary. This is true not only in cochlear implantation but in other otologic procedures, such as those requiring hearing preservation to remove cerebellopontine angle tumors, petrous apex approaches, and labyrinthectomy.

Despite these attractive characteristics for the usage of robotic systems in otologic surgery, as of yet no such system has been implemented for widespread clinical use. Perhaps the most amount of progress has been made in the development of a fully automated CI robot, but clinical acceptance and implementation remains to be seen. This chapter will review work done in the field of otologic robotic surgery and articulate advantages of these efforts along with potential current limitations or roadblocks to widespread surgical utilization.

17.2 Definitions

17.2.1 Robot

The term "robot" was coined by the Czech playright Karel Capek in 1921 [6]. The word "robot" is from the Czech word "robota" which means forced labor [6]. Since that time, robots have developed for a variety of applications such as manufacturing, surgery, rehabilitation, aerospace functions, home service, military purposes, rescue missions, inspection, sports, and entertainment.

17.2.2 DOF

An object has n degrees of freedom (DOF) if its configuration can be minimally specified by n parameters [7]. A rigid body in three-dimensional space would normally have six DOFs, three translational (up and down, left and right, forward and backward) and three rotational (roll, yaw, and pitch). A human arm has seven controllable DOFs in total; three DOF are provided by the shoulder, one by the elbow, and three by the wrist [6].

17.3 History of Robotics Including Medical Robotics

The first application of robot in the surgery field was in a neurosurgical procedure in 1985 [8]. This robot was named the PUMA 560 and applied to improve the position accuracy of a needle for the computerized tomography (CT)-guided brain tumor biopsies. However, its use was stopped because of specific safety issues. Three years later, using the same machine at the Imperial College in England, a transurethral resection of the prostate was performed [9]. This system was called the PROBOT and became the first self-navigated, robotic-based surgical procedure. The navigational plan consisted of a three-dimensional model of the prostate, and the determination of the resection area by the surgeon. Using this plan, the calculation of the cutting trajectories and execution of the procedure was carried out by the robot. A few years later in 1992, the ROBODOC was developed by International Business Machines (IBM, New York, USA) Corporation and associates to help surgeons to mill out precision prosthetic fittings in the femur for total hip replacement [10]. This became the first robot approved by the Food and Drug Administration (FDA) for medical use. Simultaneously, robotic telepresence or telesurgery technology was developed at the Stanford Research Institute (SRI), National Aeronautics and Space Administration (NASA), and the Department of Defense (DOD) [11]. These efforts developed the technologies for surgeons to remotely perform procedures at a distance from the operating room, with target applications such as immediate operative care in the battlefield. The commercialization of immersive telepresence for robotic medical laparoscopy (where a surgeon can operate across the room from a patient by directing robotic arms via controls and a video display) was achieved with the da Vinci Surgical System (Intuitive Surgical Inc., Sunnyvale, CA), [12]. It received FDA approval in 2000 as the first comprehensive robotic system for laparoscopic surgery. Aside from a vision console, this robotic system consists of a surgeon-side console (master), controlled by a surgeon, and a patient-side console (slave), a robotic module consisting of three or four arms, one for holding the laparoscope and rest of the arms for surgical instruments. These instruments are inserted into the patient through ports similar to those used for laparoscopic/endoscopic surgery. The arms of the slave console follow the commands received from input manipulators on the surgeon-side console (Fig. 17.1 from [13]).

Using this system, tremor filtering, movement scaling, increased range of motion, and improved ergonomics could be achieved. The input manipulators allow for seven DOFs, i.e., the surgeon

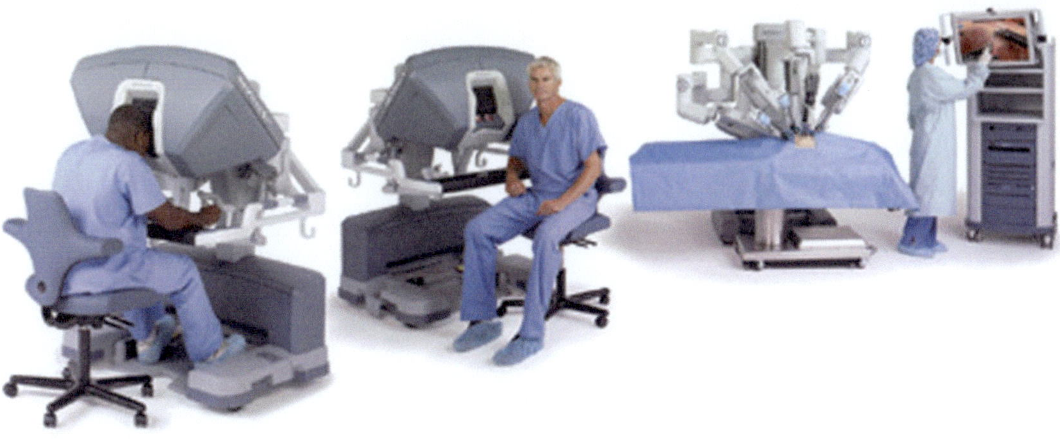

Fig. 17.1 Da Vinci Surgical System 2010 Intuitive Surgical, Inc. (With permission) [13]

can roll; pitch; yaw; move in x, y, z direction; and grip using the laparoscopic tools. The imaging system provides the surgeon with a high-definition, 3D magnified image of the operative field with the use of two independent cameras in the dual-channel endoscopes [6].

Around the same time of the introduction of the da Vinci robot, Computer Motion (merged with Intuitive Surgical Inc. in 2003) revealed the AESOP (Automated Endoscopic System for Optimal Positioning) as the first laparoscopic camera holder, while voice activation was added later [12]. After that, Computer Motion produced an integrated robotic system termed the ZEUS surgical system [11, 12]. ZEUS has three robotic arms that are mounted on the operating table [14]. One robotic arm is AESOP, which helps the surgeon with a better vision from inside the patient's body. The other two arms of ZEUS are the extension of the left and right arms of the surgeon to support precise incisions and extractions. Similar to the da Vinci system, surgeons sit at a console and wear special glasses to see a three-dimensional image. However, ZEUS differs from the da Vinci system because its AESOP part can respond to voice commands. The FDA cleared AESOP and ZEUS in 1994 and 2001, respectively.

Historically, robotic have contributed to and impacted surgery areas such as neurosurgery, orthopedics, maxillofacial, ophthalmology, urology, gastrointestinal surgery, and cardiac surgery [12]. The da Vinci robot has been used in many different procedures such as cardiothoracic surgery, general surgery, gynecology, and urology [15]. For example, in glottis cancer, the adaptation of laser cutters to the suite of da Vinci robotic instruments has made a robotic approach practical [16]. What's more, the design of flexible robots advances robotic surgery further by addressing the limitations related to rigid endoscopy [16]. Recently, intraoperative image-based techniques have also been shown to help surgeons to more accurately localize and to reach desired structures without violating neighboring critical structures [17–19].

17.4 Advantages and Disadvantages of Robotics in the Medical Field

Compared to conventional open surgery, robots have been purported to provide many advantages. A list of these advantages, paramount in otologic surgery, is summarized below [6]:

1. Increased accuracy and surgical precision
2. Improved three-dimensional visualization and magnification relative to binocular microscopy
3. Less invasive access with the potential for minimizing recovery time and downstream surgical costs
4. Improved stability through scaling of surgical maneuvers
5. Improved ergonomics for the surgeon
6. Better access due to afforded higher degree of freedom
7. Articulation beyond normal manipulation
8. Ability to perform operations from a distance (telesurgery)

In spite of the main advantages acquired by a surgical robot, some limitations have been reported as well [6]:

1. High initial and subsequent maintenance costs
2. Need to train surgeon and staffs
3. Prolonged learning curve
4. Lack of haptic feedback to the operator
5. Need to get FDA approval, which is expensive and time consuming

17.5 Robotics in Otologic Surgery

Robotic systems in otologic surgery can be categorized in three classes: (1) telerobotic, (2) cooperative, and (3) autonomous robotic system. Each category is described below.

Previous efforts incorporating robotics into otologic surgery are summarized in Table 17.1 and will be further discussed below.

17.5.1 Telerobotic Systems

This type of robotic system consists of a master and a slave component with a surgeon included in the control loop. In other words, the surgeon uses a master robot or a joystick to send commands to the slave robot to perform a task on a patient. Telerobotic systems consist of two different types: (1) unilateral telerobotic system and (2) bilateral telerobotic systems. Unilateral telerobotic system does not provide force feedback on the master side, while bilateral telerobotic systems provide force feedback on the master side. For example, the da Vinci robot is a unilateral telerobotic system. Otologic surgery is exceedingly delicate as Nguyen et al. [20] showed that a 5 μm positional resolution and an angular resolution of 0.3° are required. This degree of accuracy is quite difficult to achieve for even the most skilled surgeon. However, a telerobotic system which supports position scaling could possibly make this level of accuracy more universally attainable. Improved visualization within the middle ear could also be achieved by powerful high-definition endoscopic systems, held distally in the surgical field, thus preserving the field of vision.

Table 17.1 Summary of reported robotic system studies in otologic surgery

Author name and year of publication	Type of robot	Study type	Clinical application	Figure number
Nguyen et al. [20] (2011)	Telerobotic system 6 DOF	Phantom	Stapedectomy	2
Liu et al. [21] (2014)	Telerobotic system 7 DOF	Cadaveric (*$N = 1$)	Cochlear implant	3
ROTHBAUM et al. [23] (2002)	Cooperative robotic system 6 DOF	Phantom	Stapedectomy	4
Majdani et al. [27] (2009)	Autonomous robotic system	Phantom	Cochlear implant electrode insertion	5
Schurzig et al. [26] (2010)	1 DOF			
Bell et al. [17] (2012)	Autonomous robotic system 5 DOF	Cadaveric ($N = 15$)	Cochlear electrode insertion	6
Dillon et al. [18] (2014)	Autonomous robotic system 4 DOF	Phantom	Temporal bone milling	7
Danilchenko et al. [19] (2011)	Autonomous robotic system 6 DOF	Cadaveric ($N = 3$)	Mastoidectomy	8

*N Number of studies

17.5.1.1 Examples in Otologic Surgery

- *RobOtol* [20]: Nguyen et al. developed a telerobotic system including a master robot and a slave robot. The slave robot's kinematic chain was composed of three perpendicular linear links at the base and three rotary links at the distal part of the arm, as shown in Fig. 17.2. During otologic surgery, the field of view is quite limited. The vision axis and the approach are almost collinear. The tools have to be very thin and are held far from the tip to avoid blocking of the target. To reduce the visual impairment, a cable transmission mechanism was used to allow for the placement of the two last actuators at the base of the robot arm. The master robot consists of the surgeon controlling the arm remotely using by a pen-like interface with six degrees of freedom (Phantom Omni, Sensable Technologies, Inc., Woburn, MA). Otosclerosis surgery was considered as a model to define the specifications of this robot for a tele-operated otologic surgery. The prototype was tested in human temporal bone specimens by otologists. Duration of procedure, distance covered by the tool, and the number of times the emergency button was pressed were three measures that were considered during the evaluation of the system performance in both position mode and velocity control mode. The operator was able to reach all four target points on the tympanic membrane, the stapes footplate, and the round window in all three temporal bones in velocity command mode. Incus-stapes disjunction and stapes removal were performed successfully under the microscope and with the endoscope in two temporal bones. All participants were able to complete placement of the piston prosthesis in the stapedotomy in both velocity-to-position and position-to-position command modes.
- *Modified tool for the da Vinci robot* [21]: Liu et al. reported on a cadaveric feasibility study of usage of the da Vinci system for cochlear implantation. For this purpose, the group developed an attachment which allowed for a pneumatic-powered drill to be coupled to one of the working arms of the da Vinci robot, as shown in Fig. 17.3. For this study, integration of augmented reality through segmentation of

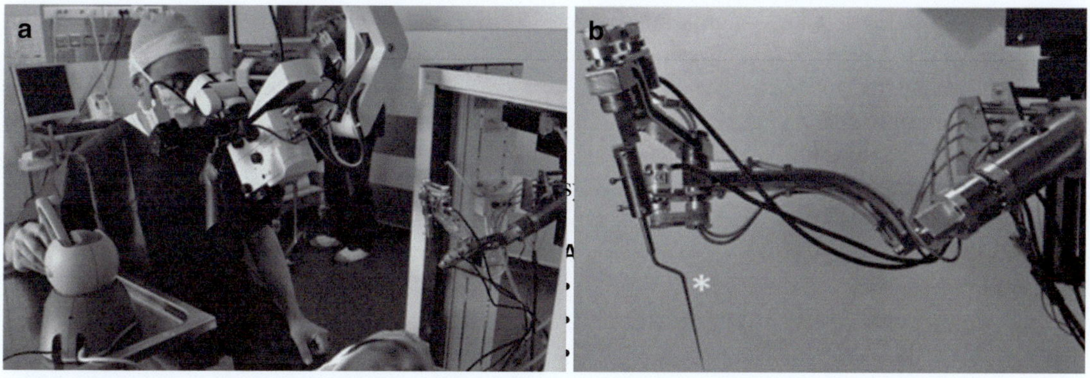

Fig. 17.2 Telerobotic system. (**a**) Phantom Omni interface (Master robot), (**b**) the RobOtol prototype (Slave robot) [20]

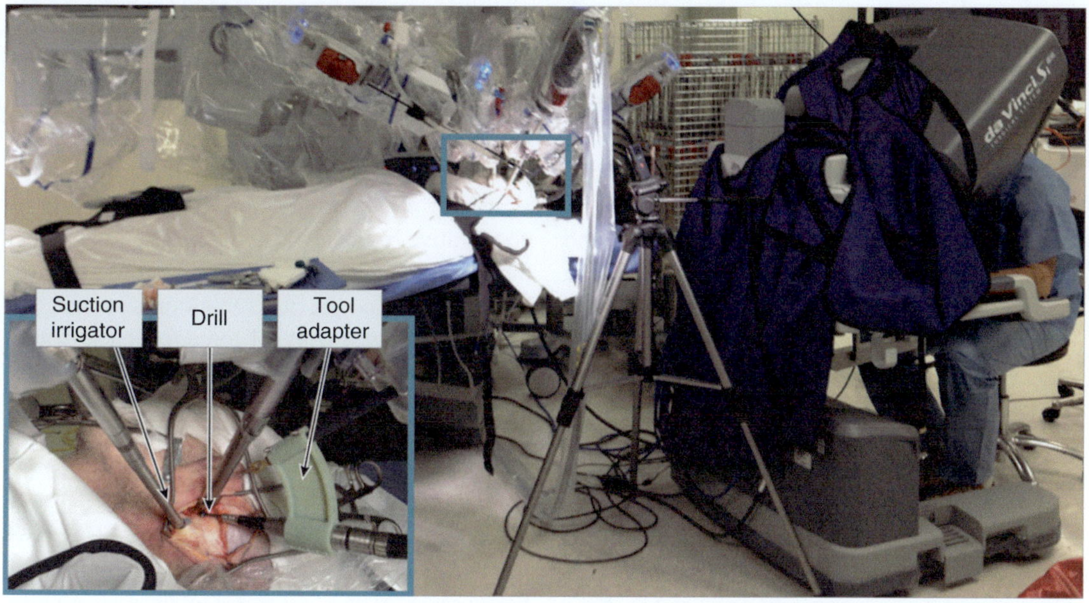

Fig. 17.3 Operating room with the da Vinci Si for otologic surgery. *Inset* is a close-up of the initial position of the endoscope, suction/irrigator, and drill attached with the custom tool adapter (With permission) [21]

implementation. First, the magnification of the robotic 3D endoscope for improved visualization through the posterior tympanostomy was felt to be noticeably inferior. Second, the study reported that the existing robotic arm surgical tools, such as the suction irrigator, were found to be too large for dissection through the posterior tympanostomy approach to the cochlea. However, though the lack of haptic feedback is an undesired effect, it was

- Comfortable pose for surgeon
- Safety enforcement using forbidden zone concept (virtual fixture)
- Improved dexterity in limited space because of small slave robots
- Better line of sight

Disadvantages

- Limited perception of contact by surgeon for unilateral telerobotic system

- Possibility of instability highlighting the requirement for more robust control system for bilateral telerobotic system
- Lack of haptic feedback in currently available commercial systems such as the da Vinci.
- Longer procedure time with currently available systems

17.5.2 Cooperative Robotic System

Cooperative robotic system are designed to extend human performance to permit fine manipulation tasks that are normally considered difficult or impossible and allow for even less experienced surgeons achieve higher performance outcomes. In this type of robotic system, the surgeon and the robot cooperate to perform a task. Robotics are therefore incorporated to allow surgeons to overcome to human natural physical limitations in both dexterity (tremor, jerk, drift, and overshoot) and tactile sensitivity [22, 23].

According to the Committee on Hearing and Equilibrium, primary stapedotomy has a reported success rate of approximately 70 %. Complications associated with stapedotomy typically result from either cochlear or labyrinthine trauma. As manifested by decreases in pure tone thresholds and speech discrimination scores, cochlear trauma leads to sensorineural hearing loss in 5–15 % of patients. Vertigo occurs in approximately 2 % of patients. For stapedotomy, surgical skill is among the most important variables predicting outcome. In fact, it has been postulated that given a wide large learning curve for this surgical procedure, only surgeons with significant experience should perform the operation [24, 25].

17.5.2.1 Examples in Otologic Surgery

- *Steady-hand (SH) robot* [23]: In the SH robotic system, the operator shares the control of surgical tool with a robot arm, as illustrated in Fig. 17.4. The surgeon and robot comanipulate the surgical tool. The robot senses the forces exerted by the surgeon on the handle as well as the tool-tip forces and synthesizes this information to provide tremor-free positional control. The SH robot dampens high-frequency movement (i.e., tremor) like a viscous system. While using the SH robot, the surgeon has reported to feel like he/she is manipulating the surgical tool in a "viscous fluid." For certain tasks, the SH robot has been shown to enhance dexterity.

Rothbaum et al. performed experimental studies using SH robot and a surgical model of stapedotomy based on a human temporal bone, to show the effect of force feedback provided by cooperative robots on five fenestrations under three different experimental conditions: (1) free hand (FH), that is, no robotic assistance, (2) robotic assistance with 1:1 force feedback (force-feedback mode), and (3) robotic assistance with 2:1 force scaling (force-scaling mode). For evaluating the efficacy of SH robot, stapedotomy performance was investigated and compared for (1) manual and (2) with robotic assistance. Furthermore, to evaluate subspecialty expert/novice differences, the performance of micropick fenestration of the stapes footplate was studied. The SH robot significantly (approximately 58 %) reduced the cumulative force applied to the stapes footplate in the force-feedback mode. Cumulative force was not significantly affected by surgeon experience. Neither surgeon experience nor SH robotic assistance affected maximum force or fenestration targeting (displacement) in force-feedback mode. Both cumulative force and duration of fenestration were significantly reduced by SH

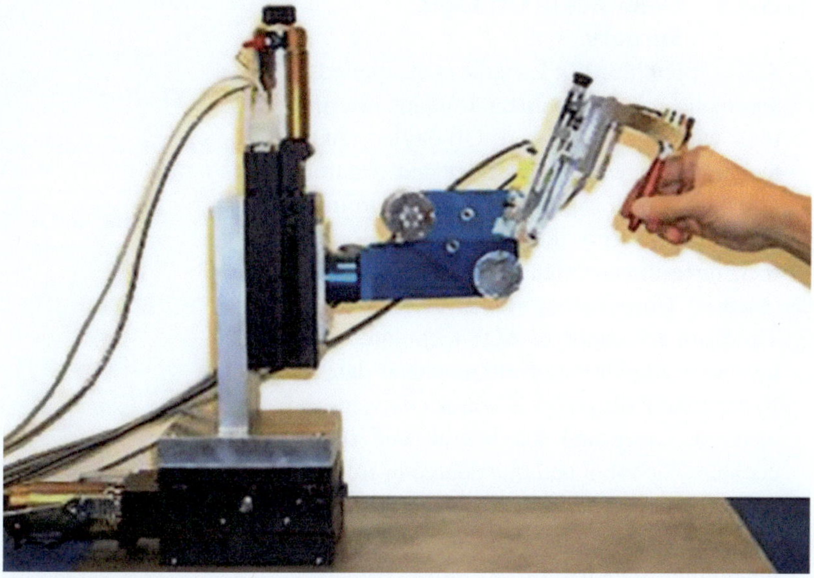

Fig. 17.4 The Johns Hopkins University steady-hand robot for cooperative human-machine microsurgical manipulation [22]

robot assistance in force feedback. Tremor reduction significantly affected two performance variables: (1) cumulative force applied to the stapes footplate and (2) fenestration targeting. The reductions in the duration of fenestration caused reduction in cumulative force. According to Rothman et al., the mechanism by which tremor reduction decreases duration of fenestration is uncertain; perhaps the steadying nature of the system could make operators more confident in the precise movements of fenestration.

Advantages and disadvantages of cooperative robotic system for ear surgery are listed next.

Advantages

- Surgeon's hand tremor elimination.
- Safety enforcement using forbidden zone concept (virtual fixture).
- More precise motions.
- Force feedback and force-scaling may be integrated.

Disadvantages

- May limit dexterity of the surgeon.
- Robot may obstruct the surgeon's line of sight and requires that the surgeon modify the angle of approach to the footplate.
- Longer procedure time.

17.5.3 Autonomous Robotic System

In an autonomous robotic system, the robot itself can perform part of or the entire task. In ear surgery, this kind of robot usually requires preoperative imaging, such as MRI or CT data, to perform path planning. In the field of otology, a main task of otological cases is the mastoidectomy, in which bone is milled away while exposing but not damaging vital anatomy. Mastoidectomy could be a good fit for an autonomous robotic approach since: (a) the tissue to be resected is encased in rigid bone, and (b) critical anatomical features remain hidden until they are revealed by ablation. The first of these two reasons makes surgery with the autonomous robot feasible; the second makes it useful since less intracochlear trauma would occur especially considering that the rupture force of the basilar member in a human cadaver is 0.029–0.039 N [26]. The robot, guided by images that see beneath the surface, can safely ablate bone to which the human operator would be blind.

The rigidity of bone is essential because it ensures that the three-dimensional structure of the target anatomy remains the same during preoperative imaging/planning and during subsequent intervention.

17.5.3.1 Examples in Otologic Surgery

- *A.K. A robot* [26, 27]: Labadie et al. applied an automatic robotic cochlear implant insertion tool with the Advanced Off-Stylet (AOS) technique, in which the stylet and electrode array are withdrawn simultaneously, to insert the electrode array into an anatomically correct, three-dimensional scala tympani model (Med-el Corporation; Innsbruck, Austria). The main advantage of AOS technique is the decreased likelihood of intracochlear damage by restricting the physical contact between the electrode array and the lateral wall of the cochlea. The robot had one degree of freedom and used two independent piezoelectric step motors with positional accuracy of 1 μm and maximum velocity of 5 mm/s (SmarAct GmbH; Oldenburg, Germany). The electrode array was grasped by a modified surgical alligator forceps, and stylet was held via a stainless steel hooked wire. During the insertion, the force resulting from the contact between the electrode array and scala tympani model was measured by four semiconductor strain gauges (model SS-060-033-1000 PB; Micron Instruments, Inc.; Simi Valley, CA) coupled to the insertion tool. In Fig. 17.5, the experimental setup using a scala tympani model is shown. The insertion force generated by this technique was compared with the human operators and the robotic insertion tool via the traditional technique, in which the stylet is removed after complete insertion of the electrode, respectively in [26, 27]. Compared to human operators, the robot achieved more repeatable results, fewer relative force peaks, and slightly higher average force values, may not be clinically significant. Additionally, beyond 7 mm insertion depth, cochlear implant electrode insertion via AOS could reach to a significant reduction in both average and maximal force in comparison with the traditional insertion technique.
- *Bone-attached robotic system* [17, 18]: The robotic system developed in [17], shown in Fig. 17.6, was specifically designed for lateral skull-based surgery. It consists of a table-mounted robotic arm (Fisso, Baitella AG, Switzerland), a force-torque sensor (Mini40, ATI, USA) for moving the tool tip to any desired position by a surgeon, an optical tracking system for verifying the tool position, an image-guidance system for preoperative and postoperative analysis, head fixation system (FixIT, Medicon Medical Instruments, Germany), and a touch screen interface for controlling the robot actions and status. Compared to the existing approaches based on industrial robots, this robot showed equal or better accuracy levels with a better compatibility with a clinical environment because of its overall weight (5.5 kg) and size (total arm length = 65 cm). However, this design was dependent on a tracking system and the error related to the monitoring and alignment of the patient with the robot. To eliminate the mentioned limitation, Dillon et al. proposed a compact and bone-attached robot with a preoperative CT scan-based plan for temporal bone milling [18]. The robot in discussion, illustrated in Fig. 17.7, a four-axis milling

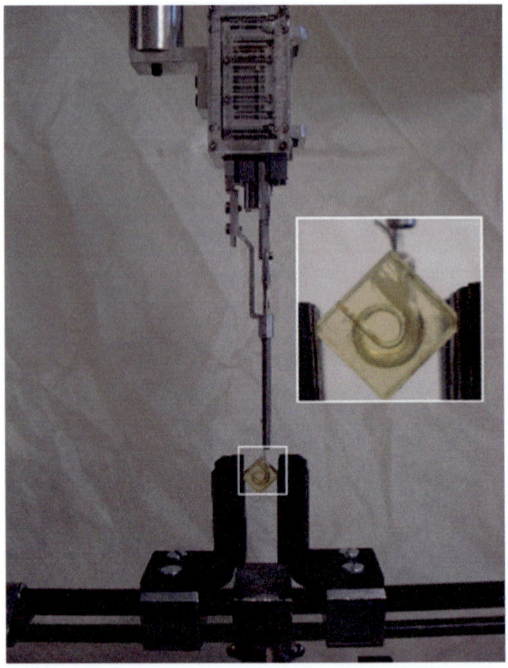

Fig. 17.5 Experimental setup of electrode insertion above the scala tympani model [26]

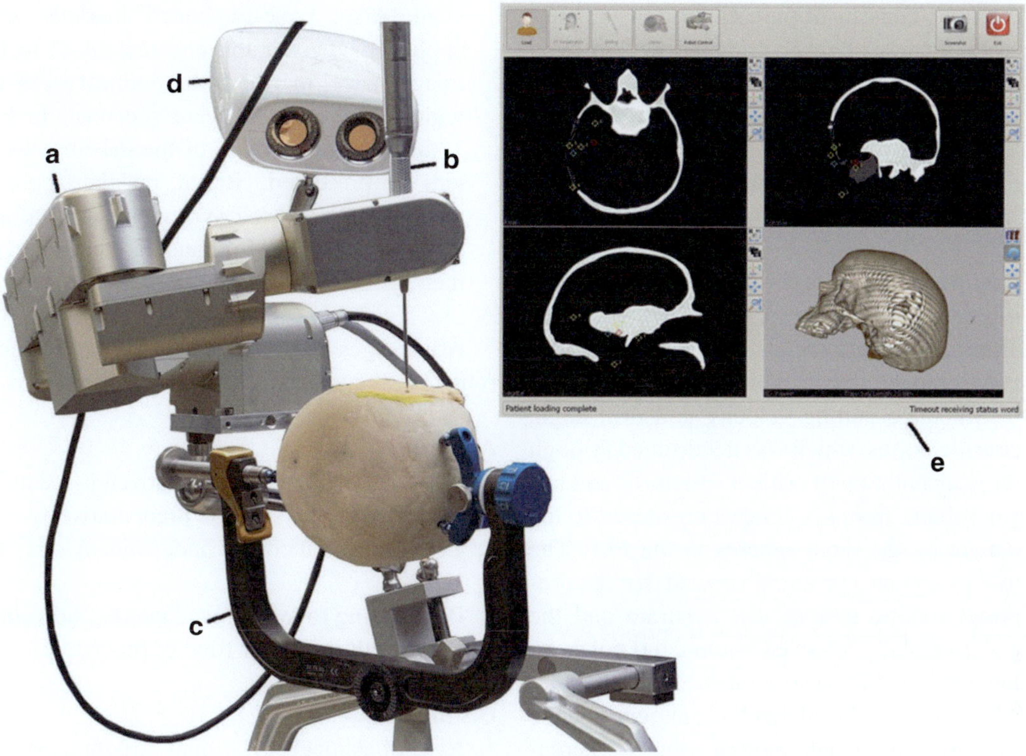

Fig. 17.6 Overview of the robot navigation system. (**a**) The mounted robot to the OR table, (**b**) a conventional surgical drill, (**c**) a head clamp, (**d**) an optical tracking system, and (**e**) a touch screen interface [17]

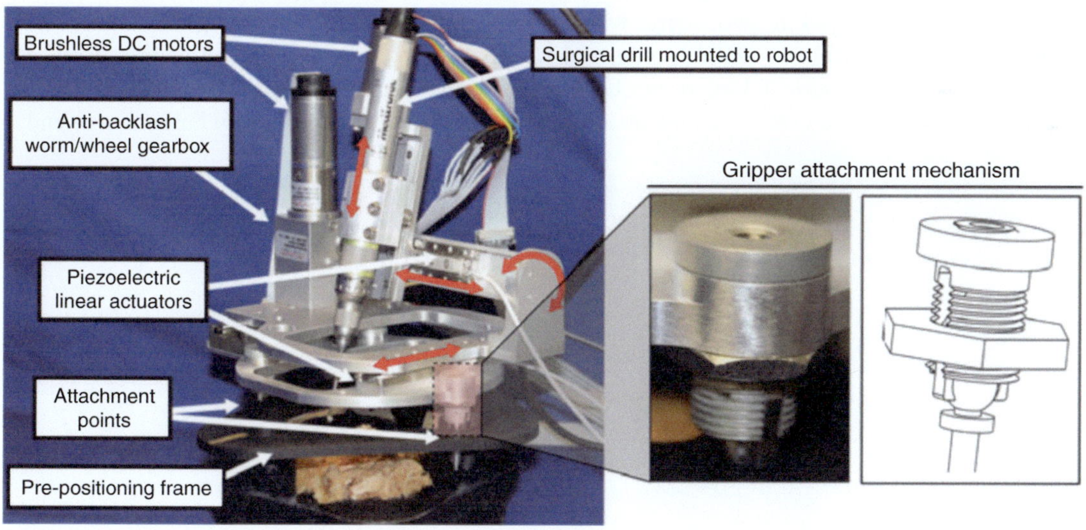

Fig. 17.7 Compact and bone-attached robot with test sample attached the prepositioning frame (PPF) using spherical gripper mechanisms [18]

machine, consists of piezoelectric linear actuators (SmarAct GmbH, Oldenburg, Germany) for moving along the x- and y-directions, a brushless DC motor (Maxon Precision Motor, Inc., Fall River, MA, USA) with a lead screw for moving along the z-direction, and a brushless DC motor and anti-backlash worm-wheel gearbox (Gysin AG, Itingen, Switzerland) for rotating about the x-direction. Moreover, the robot was attached to the patient via three titanium spheres on a prepositioning frame (PPF). Preoperative planning for the robot trajectory incorporated cutting velocity and drill angle considerations, which was determined through the segmentation of critical structures and target volume from CT images registered to the patient by the three spheres in the PPF. The trial results on a phantom showed that the proposed robotic system was accurate and the experimentally removed volume did not overlap with the critical structures.

- *OTOBOT* [19]: Danilchenko et al. reported the first usage of an autonomous robot for percutaneous placement of a cochlear implant in a cadaveric model using infrared tracking to monitor the motion of both the specimen and the robot. In their work, a developed version of the OTOBOT system was used, which incorporates a Mitsubishi RV-3S industrial robot (Mitsubishi Electric & Electronics USA, Inc., Cyprus, CA) controlled by custom software. Also, bone-implanted markers were applied to register the physical space to CT image space, in which the boundaries of the regions to be milled were specified. In Fig. 17.8, the configuration of the developed system is presented. Based on the acquired results, the proposed system is accurate and reliable, but its performance is dependent on the registration accuracy level.

Advantages and disadvantages of autonomous robotic systems for ear surgery are listed next.

Advantages

- The target volume to be removed is manually identified by the surgeon preoperatively.
- Consistent outcome independent of the surgeon.
- Preplanning to avoid facial nerves and veins.
- May result in shorter time of procedure.

Disadvantages

- Risk of damage to critical structures if preplanning is not accurate enough.
- Setup time may prolong the procedure time.
- Possible requirement for multiple CT scans with attendant radiation exposure, i.e., both the preoperative and intraoperative CT scan.
- Necessity for surgeons and patients to take a "leap of faith" in terms of allowing a robot to complete the surgery from beginning to end.

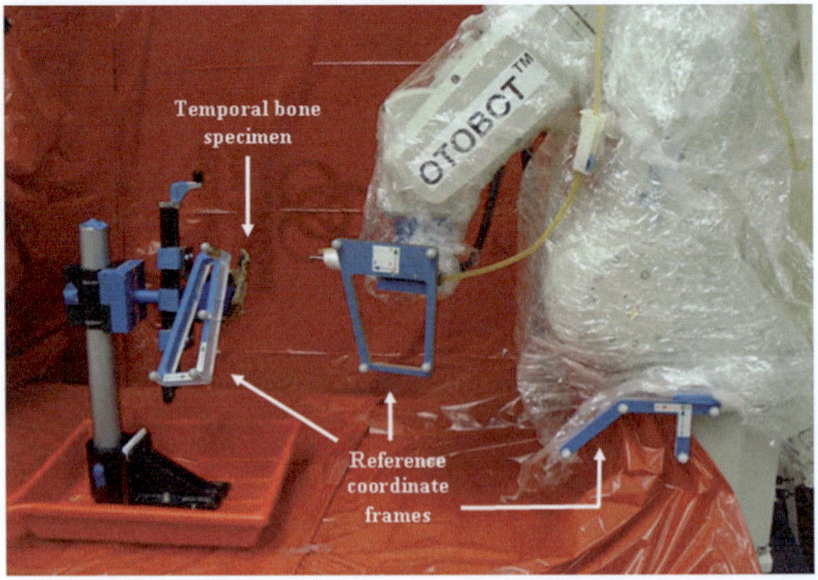

Fig. 17.8 Setup of the OTOBOT robotic system to perform mastoidectomy on patient [19]

Conclusion

Otologic surgery combines difficulties of microsurgery and endoscopic surgery. This surgery is performed on fragile millimetric structures. Therefore, precise control of movement and forces under microscopic magnification (up to 40 times) is a necessity. In addition, many tasks are performed through a keyhole approach represented by the external auditory canal. Thus, to maximize the field of vision, appropriate instruments should be thin and long. Therefore, endoscopes are less likely to be employed in ear surgery due to their large diameters and the risk of trauma to the ossicular chain during placement in the tympanic cavity. While several characteristics of the da Vinci Surgical System (e.g., remote center of motion, near-field 3D vision) may be important in the otologic surgery, the current overall dimensions of the da Vinci robot, especially the distal diameter of its tools (5 mm), seem to be too large for otologic surgery.

The researched robotic systems in otologic surgery could be categorized in three classes, including (1) telerobotic system, (2) cooperative robotic system, and (3) autonomous robotic system. As described in the previous subsections, each of these categorized robotic systems has distinct advantages and disadvantages. Since there are complex anatomy and presence of many critical structures embedded within the bone area, we believe that the latter approach, i.e., image-guided autonomous robotic intervention, is well suited for inner ear surgery compared to the others. While some phantom and cadaveric studies have been reported in the literature of this field, based on the information summarized in Table 17.1, and to the best of our knowledge, there is no reported clinical study using autonomous robotic systems in otologic surgery so far.

As a future work, in order to make the robotic-assisted otologic surgery clinically practical, the following issues should be addressed.

1. Reduction in the robotic instrument size
2. Improving the path planning and trajectory planning
3. Improving patient safety features
4. Improving the tactile and haptic perception during surgery
5. Minimal change in the surgical workflow in order to switch ability to the manual procedures in the case of complication

References

1. Mudry A. The history of the microscope for use in ear surgery. Am J Otolaryngol. 2000;21:877–86. Nguyen
2. Pothier DD. Introducing endoscopic ear surgery into practice. Otolaryngol Clin N Am. 2013;46:245–55.
3. Marchioni D, Alicandri-Ciufelli M, Pothier DD, Rubini A, Presutti L. The round window region and contiguous areas: endoscopic anatomy and surgical implications. Eur Arch Otorhinolaryngol. 2015;272(5):1103–12.
4. Adunka OF, Buchman CA. Scala tympani cochleostomy I: results of a survey. Laryngoscope. 2007;117: 2187–94.
5. Adunka OF, Radeloff A, Gstoettner WK, Pillsbury HC, Buchman CA. Scala tympani cochleostomy II: topography and histology. Laryngoscope. 2007;117:2195–200.
6. Maan ZN, Gibbins N, Al-Jabri T, D'Souza AR. The use of robotics in otolaryngology-head and neck surgery: a systematic review. Am J Otolaryngol. 2012;33:137–46.
7. Spong MW, Hutchinson S, Vidyasagar M. Robot modeling and control. 1st ed. Hoboken, NJ: Johne Wiley and Sons; 1989.
8. Kwoh YS, Hou J, Jonckheere EA, Hayati S. A robot with improved absolute positioning accuracy for CT guided stereotactic brain surgery. IEEE Trans Biomed Eng. 1988;35:153–60.
9. Davies BL, Hibberd RD, Coptcoat MJ, Wickham JEA. A surgeon robot prostatectomy – a laboratory evaluation. J Med Eng Technol. 1989;13:273–7.
10. Bauer A, Borner M, Lahmer A. Clinical experience with a medical robotic system for total hip replacement. In: Nolte LP, Ganz R, editors. Computer assisted orthopedic surgery. Bern: Hogrefe & Huber; 1999. p. 128–33.
11. Satava RM. Robotic surgery: from past to future – a personal journey. Surg Clin N Am. 2003;83:1–6.
12. Dharia SP, Falcone T. Robotics in reproductive medicine. Fertil Steril. 2005;84:1–11.
13. Intuitive Surgical. Da Vinci surgical system. 2005. http://www.intuitivesurgical.com.
14. ZEUS robotic surgical system, the official medical robotics news center sponsored by; AVRA medical robotics Inc. http://allaboutroboticsurgery.com/zeus-robot.html.
15. Patel VR, Chammas Jr MF, Shah S. Robotic Assisted laparoscopic radical prostatectomy: a review of the current state of affairs. Int J Clin Pract. 2007;61:309–14.

16. Byrd JK, Duvvuri U. Current trends in robotic surgery for otolaryngology. Curr Otorhinolaryngol Rep. 2013;1:153–7.
17. Bell B, Stieger C, Gerber N, Arnold A, Nauer C, Hamacher V, Kompis M, Nolte L, Caversaccio M, Weber S. A self-developed and constructed robot for minimally invasive cochlear implantation. Acta Otolaryngol. 2012;132:355–60.
18. Dillon NP, Balachandranb R, dit Falissec AM, Wannab GB, Labadieb RF, Withrowa TJ, Fitzpatrickd JM, Webster RJ. Preliminary testing of a compact, bone-attached robot for otologic surgery. Proc SPIE Int Soc Opt Eng. 2014;9036:1–17.
19. Danilchenko A, Balachandran R, Toennies JL, Baron S, Munske B, Fitzpatrick JM, Withrow TJ, Webster 3rd RJ, Labadie RF. Robotic mastoidectomy. Otol Neurotol. 2011;32:11–6.
20. Nguyen Y, Miroir M, Kazmitcheff G, Ferrary E, Sterkers O, Grayeli AB. From conception to application of a tele-operated assistance robot for middle ear surgery. Surg Innov. 2012;19:241–51.
21. Liu WP, Azizian M, Sorger J, Taylor RH, Reilly BK, Cleary K, Preciado D. Cadaveric feasibility study of da vinci si–assisted cochlear implant with augmented visual navigation for otologic surgery. JAMA Otolaryngol Head Neck Surg. 2014;140:208–14.
22. Taylor R, Jensen P, Whitcomb L, Barnes A, Kumar R, Stoianovici D, Gupta P, Wang Z, deJuan E, Kavoussi L. A steady-hand robotic system for microsurgical augmentation. Int J Robot Res. 1999;18: 1201–10.
23. Rothbaum DL, Roy J, Stoianovici D, Berkelman P, Hager GD, Taylor RH, Whitcomb LL, Francis HW, Niparko JK. Robot-assisted stapedotomy: micropick fenestration of the stapes footplate. Otolaryngol Head Neck Surg. 2002;127:417–26.
24. Watson GJ, Byth K, da Cruz M. Outcomes in stapedotomy surgery: the learning curve redefined. Otol Neurotol. 2015;36:1601–3.
25. Lial PI, Soares VY, Viana LM, Sampaio AL, Oliveira CA, Bahmad Jr F. Stapedotomy in a residency training program. Int Tinnitus J. 2013;18:163–7.
26. Schurzig D, Webster RJ, Dietrich MS, Labadie RF. Force of cochlear implant electrode insertion performed by a robotic insertion tool: comparison of traditional versus Advance Off-Stylet techniques. Otol Neurotol. 2010;31:1207–10.
27. Majdani O, Schurzig D, Hussong A, Rau T, Wittkopf J, Lenarz T, Labadie RF. Force measurement of insertion of cochlear implants in vitro: comparison of surgeon and automated insertion tool. Acta Otolaryngol. 2009;29:1–6.

18 Complications and Postoperative Care

Eugene L. Son and Neil D. Gross

18.1 Introduction

No matter what measures are taken, doctors will sometimes falter, and it isn't reasonable to ask that we achieve perfection. What is reasonable is to ask that we never cease to aim for it [1]. The da Vinci Surgical System (Intuitive Surgical, Inc., Sunnyvale, CA) was approved by the US Food and Drug Administration (USFDA) in 2009 for transoral robotic surgery (TORS) of the upper aerodigestive tract. Since approval, TORS has been described for the treatment of benign and malignant neoplasms of the upper aerodigestive tract. Interest in TORS has increased because of its minimally invasive nature when compared to traditional open approaches that require mandibulotomy for access to the oropharynx. This technology has also been applied to surgical procedures for benign indications such as obstructive sleep apnea (OSA) including lingual tonsillectomy [2]. TORS using the da Vinci Surgical System provides high-resolution three-dimensional visualization and increased magnification with angled scopes [3]. Another system, the Flex Robotic System (Medrobotics Corp., Raynham, MA), has been developed and was approved for transoral surgery by the USFDA in July 2015.

Although TORS has proven to be a less morbid approach compared to traditional open surgery, it has predictable sequelae and risks of complications. Sequela can be defined as an expected event following surgery. TORS produces the well-recognized sequelae of throat pain, odynophagia, and dysphagia. When these sequelae are poorly managed, complications can develop including dehydration, weight loss, and aspiration pneumonia. Life-threatening complications can result as well. In addition, there is a very serious risk of bleeding after TORS with the possibility of airway compromise and death. Self-reported complication rates following TORS have been relatively low. Proper training, careful technique, and appropriate management of the sequelae of TORS can lead to a decreased rate of complications. In this chapter, the incidence and management of sequela and complications will be explored.

18.2 Sequelae

Swallowing is a complex function with multiple coordinated voluntary and involuntary actions of the surrounding muscles. There are four stages which include the oral preparatory stage, the oral stage, the pharyngeal stage, and the esophageal

E.L. Son
Department of Otolaryngology – Head and Neck Surgery, The University of Texas Medical Branch, 301 University Boulevard, Galveston, TX 77555-0521, USA
e-mail: elson@utmb.edu

N.D. Gross (✉)
Department of Head and Neck Surgery, Unit 1445, Division of Surgery, The University of MD Anderson Cancer Center, 1400 Pressler Street, Houston, TX 77030, USA
e-mail: ngross@mdanderson.org

Z. Gil et al. (eds.), *Atlas of Head and Neck Robotic Surgery*, DOI 10.1007/978-3-319-49578-1_18

stage [4]. TORS can affect one or multiple sites of the upper aerodigestive tract (UADT) causing dysfunctional swallowing. When mucosa and muscle are violated in the pharynx, the result is pain and dysfunction of specific muscles. After TORS in the oropharynx, all patients are expected to experience odynophagia and dysphagia.

18.2.1 Odynophagia

Odynophagia is derived from the Greek roots odyno meaning pain and phagia meaning to eat. The UADT from the oral cavity to the larynx is innervated by branches of cranial nerves V, VII, IX, and X. Postoperative pain is expected after surgery in the upper aerodigestive tract. There are no guidelines nor studies performed regarding optimal postoperative pain management following TORS. Opioids are commonly administered intravenously in the immediate postoperative period. Patient-controlled anesthesia (PCA) can be employed for the acute demands expected immediately postoperatively, but is not commonly used at our institution. The cumulative amount of opioid administered within a 24 h period can be collected and then converted to a scheduled per os (PO) dose with allowance of breakthrough doses for outpatient pain management. Other classes of pain medication including acetaminophen, nonsteroidal anti-inflammatory drugs (NSAID), and neurotransmitter modulators such as gabapentin may aid as an adjunct but have not been well studied for pain control in this population. A Cochrane review found perioperative local anesthesia such as lidocaine injection in the oropharynx does not reduce postoperative pain and does not decrease the need for analgesics following routine tonsillectomy [5].

Patients have different thresholds of pain which merit individualized titration of medication. In general, we start postoperative pain management with 5–10 milligrams (mg) of oxycodone oral solution every 3–4 h. The liquid form provides an easy transition from enteral to oral administration. Hydrocodone and codeine elixirs contain acetaminophen, which limits the ceiling dose of these opioids. Oxycodone is available as a single drug, preventing potential toxicity with acetaminophen. Intravenous (IV) opioids including morphine (2.5–5 mg every 3–4 h) and fentanyl (25–30 micrograms (mcg) every 1–3 h) are placed as standing orders as needed for breakthrough pain. In addition to this, acetaminophen and tramadol are provided as a third line for breakthrough pain. All of these medicines are available in liquid form making an easy transition for outpatients after discharge from the hospital. At about 1 week when patients have been discharged, patients are called to monitor pain control and can be instructed to start ibuprofen if the current regiment is not adequate. Currently, there is no evidence on the effect of NSAID use on postoperative bleeding. Consultation with a pain specialist may be beneficial in patients with a history of chronic pain and opioid dependence. It must be stressed that pain regiments should be tailored to individual patients.

Administration of steroids after tonsillectomy has been shown to decrease throat pain, decrease time to resume oral intake, and decrease postoperative nausea and vomiting [5]. Until recently, there has not been any studies on the effect of steroids in the perioperative period specifically for patients following TORS. However, the results of an important randomized, double-blinded, placebo-controlled trial of extended (up to 4 days after surgery) administration of dexamethasone versus placebo after TORS for oropharyngeal squamous cell carcinoma (OPSCC) are expected imminently (unpublished data). In the meantime, the best available evidence would support a single intraoperative dose of steroids such as 8–10 mg of dexamethasone.

18.2.2 Dysphagia

Dysphagia can lead to aspiration or inefficient swallowing causing pneumonia, malnutrition, dehydration, and weight loss [4]. Any significant surgical intervention in the oropharynx will result in dysphagia. Less extensive procedures (e.g., resection of lingual tonsil tissue versus resection of tongue musculature) are generally expected to result in less dysphagia. Many patients undergoing TORS tolerate early initiation of an oral diet and have a short hospital length of stay. Vicini et al. reviewed complications after 243 TORS procedures for sleep-related disorders and reported patients returning to mechanical soft diets on an average of 1.15 days, ranging from 1 to 4 days [6]. Hoff et al. reviewed complications after TORS for benign disease in 293 procedures with the average hospital stay of 1.8 days [7]. Easa et al. evaluated swallowing outcomes for 78 patients that underwent TORS for OSA [8]. Although they performed tracheostomy in 82% of patients, who were all decannulated on postoperative day 4, the average timing to start PO feeding was 1.05±0.25 days, and no patients required feeding tubes. Richmon et al. reviewed outcomes after TORS in 91 patients treated mostly for OPSCC (86.8%) [9]. The mean time to initiation of oral diet was 1.26 days with the average length of hospital stay of 1.5 days. Early initiation of oral intake was not associated with an increase in postoperative complications.

Patients with malignancy undergoing larger resections may have longer average hospital stays due to the expected increase in severity of dysphagia. Moore et al. reported 45 patients undergoing TORS for OPSCC with an average hospital stay of 3.8 days (range 1–10 days) [10]. Weinstein et al. reported the result of TORS for malignancy in 177 patients, who had average hospital stays of 4.2 ± 2.7 days [11]. The presence of tracheostomy, free flap transfers, and previous therapies for malignancy can impact length of stay.

The use of a temporary feeding tube after TORS varies depending upon the extent of resection. We place nasogastric feeding tubes intraoperatively in all patients undergoing TORS for malignancy. These are removed when the patient demonstrates adequate oral intake which is usually around postoperative day 3–5. Glazer et al. reviewed 166 patients following TORS for OSA and reported only 1 patient who required a gastrostomy tube, which was removed after 4 months [12]. Hoff et al. reviewed complications after TORS for benign disease in 293 procedures and only placed feeding tubes in 2 patients intraoperatively, both of which were removed on postoperative day 1 [7]. In the setting of resections for malignancy, studies show an increased use of feeding tubes. Moore et al. reviewed 45 patients who underwent TORS for OPSCC with 48.9% of these patients having a nasogastric feeding tube for an average of 12.5 days (range 2–41 days) [10]. Weinstein et al. reviewed 177 patients who underwent TORS for malignancy and had 6.7% of patients relying on a gastrostomy tube for nutrition at 12-month follow-up [11]. Twenty-five percent of these patients had previous radiation therapy. Patients without previous radiation had a 5.0% gastrostomy tube dependency rate. Although feeding tube placement is not routine after TORS for benign indications, temporary feeding tubes are often required after TORS for malignancy with a low rate of long-term dependence depending upon baseline swallowing function and the extent of adjuvant therapies applied.

Chia et al. performed a voluntary survey study of TORS surgeons in the United States. Their results provided normative data after TORS for malignancy (88.8%) [13]. 62.2% of the respondents initiated oral diet on postoperative day 0–1 with a minority of 6.7% respondents delaying oral intake until 1 week after surgery. In that study, the majority of respondents (71.1%) routinely placed a nasogastric feeding tube at the time of TORS. Patients with a history of prior radiation therapy had a higher rate of prolonged gastrostomy tube dependency at 6.5% compared to those without one at 0.3% ($p < 0.0001$). The presence of previous radiation therapy should merit consideration of prophylactic placement of a gastrostomy tube.

Preoperative swallow studies are predictive of posttreatment swallow function in the setting of head and neck cancer. All patients undergoing TORS should have a preoperative swallow assessment to stratify those patients who may potentially have severe dysphagia postoperatively [9]. Thus, consultation with a speech and language pathologist should be completed routinely prior to TORS. A modified barium swallow study is beneficial prior to TORS in patients with substantial baseline dysphagia. The speech and language pathologist is also critical for advising the safer resumption of oral intake after surgery.

The tumor (T) classification OPSCC has been shown to correlate with swallowing outcomes following TORS for malignancy. Hutcheson et al. performed a systemic review of functional outcomes after TORS for oropharyngeal cancer [14]. Time to oral intake varied by group of T classification studied. Studies excluding T4 tumors had earlier time to oral diet than ones that included T4 tumors.

A study that included only T1 and T2 OPSCC had 96% of patients beginning oral intake by postoperative day 1. Studies that included all T classes of OPSCC had only 51% of patients beginning oral intake by postoperative day 1. Therefore, a prophylactic gastrostomy tube should be considered in patients undergoing TORS with bulky (T3, T4), endophytic cancers.

18.3 Complications

Avoidable and unavoidable complications can occur after TORS. Exploring the factors that contribute to complications can minimize the frequency and severity of injury. There are a number of complications that can be expected after TORS with postoperative bleeding being the most deadly. Chia et al. conducted a multi-institutional survey with TORS-trained surgeons (45 surgeons responded) performing a combined 2015 procedures [13]. There was an overall major complication rate of 10.1%. Postoperative bleeding was the most common complication at 3.1% (Table 18.1).

An increased risk of complications may be seen in OSA patients. Richmon et al. reported 43% of OSA patients undergoing TORS experienced at least one complication compared to 10% of non-OSA patients ($p = 0.04$). The authors attributed the increased risk of complications in the OSA patient population to an increased number of comorbidities including obesity [9]. Glazer et al. reviewed postoperative complications in 166 patients following TORS for OSA and concluded that the number of specific OSA procedures performed and preoperative ASA (American Society of Anesthesiologists) score were both independent predictors of having a complication [12].

Table 18.1 Postoperative complications [15]

Complication	% cases
Hemorrhage	3.10
Tooth injury	1.40
Dehydration requiring admission	1.30
Aspiration pneumonia	1.10
Temporary (<2 months) hypoglossal nerve injury	0.90

18.3.1 Postoperative Bleeding

Richmon et al. assessed the factors that contributed to length of stay after TORS in 91 patients [9]. Twelve percent of patients in their cohort experienced a complication. Postoperative bleeding occurred in 7% of patients with two patients having recurrent postoperative bleeding. Nearly all (94%) of the complications occurred in the first postoperative week with 38% of the complications occurring within 24 h of surgery. Asher et al. examined factors that contributed to bleeding after TORS in 147 patients [16]. They reported 11 (7.5%) patients with postoperative bleeding at a mean occurrence of 11.1 ± 9.2 days after surgery. The majority (82%) of these bleeds required management in the operating room. Another large study of 293 TORS procedures reported an average time to onset of bleeding being 7.3 days postoperatively (range 0–18 days) [7]. Glazer et al. reported all major postoperative bleeding occurred within 10 days [12]. Pollei et al. concluded that the greatest bleeding risk is present from postoperative day 7 to 14 [17]. The mean postoperative day for bleeding was day 10 with 83.6% of those bleeds occurring within 2 weeks of surgery. Thus, there seems to be a bimodal distribution of bleeding similar to what is observed in patients after tonsillectomy (Fig. 18.1). Patients should be educated about the risk of bleeding with TORS as well as the most likely times for bleeding.

Although there is a wide range of complication rates between studies, the rate of postoperative bleeding appears greater in patients undergoing TORS for malignancy compared to patients undergoing TORS for benign indications (Tables 18.2 and 18.3).

In the USFDA indication trial for TORS with the da Vinci Surgical System, the postoperative bleeding rate was 7.3% (2.8% requiring return to operating room) among 177 patient treated at 3 institutions [11]. Vergez et al. reviewed 130 patients undergoing TORS with 93% having a diagnosis of malignancy. The postoperative bleeding rate was 11.5% with 93% of patients treated in the operating room [20]. In comparison, a cohort of 243 patients undergoing TORS for sleep-related breathing disorders experienced a postoperative

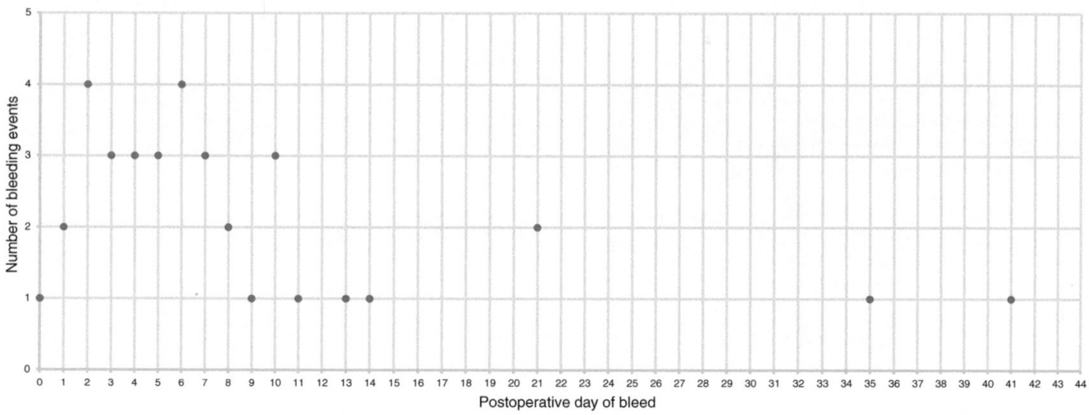

Fig. 18.1 Timing to postoperative bleed (33 events). Combined data from Asher et al. [16] and Mandel et al. [18]

Table 18.2 Incidence of complications after TORS for malignancy

Authors	Institution(s)	# patients	# malignancy (%)	# OP cases (%)	# complications (%)	# POB (%)	# OP bleeds (%)
Aubry et al. [15]	TORS's French Group (9 centers)	178	178 (100%)	51 (28.7%)	73 (41%)	33 (18.5%)	10 (30.3%)
Asher et al. [16]	University of Alabama at Birmingham (UAB)	147	136 (92.5%)[a]	102 (69.4%)[a]	N/A	11 (7.5%)	10 (90.9%)
Cognetti et al. [19]	Thomas Jefferson University	61	53 (87%)	46 (82%)	5 (8.2%)	2 (3.3%)	2 (100%)
Mandal et al. [18]	University of Pittsburgh Medical Center	224	185 (82.6%)	N/A	N/A	22 (9.8%)	11 (50%)
Pollei et al. [17]	Mayo Clinic (3 centers)	269	269 (100%)	269 (100%)	N/A	16 (5.9%)	16 (5.9%)
Richmon et al. [9]	Johns Hopkins University	91	79 (91%)	91 (100%)	11 (12.1%)	8 (8.8%)	8 (8.8%)
Weinstein et al. [11]	Multi-institutional (Univ. of Pennsylvania, UAB, Mayo Clinic)	177	177 (100%)	139 (78.5%)	29 (16%)	13 (7.3%)	N/A

Abbreviations: *OP* oropharyngeal, *POB* postoperative bleeds
[a]At least this number; more may be present but not specified

bleeding rate of 5% with only 34% managed in the operating room [6]. A study of 293 TORS procedures performed for benign disease experienced a postoperative bleeding rate of 4.1% [7]. A cohort of 166 patients who underwent TORS for OSA had a postoperative bleeding rate of 7.2% with 58% going to the operating room for cauterization; all but one patient had bleeding that originated from the tonsillar fossa [12]. Aubry et al. reported the highest rate of postoperative bleeding at 18.5% in 178 patients [15]. Interestingly, this group had a very high proportion of laryngeal and hypopharyngeal tumors (71%) suggesting that the decreased working space and more limited expo-

Table 18.3 Incidence of complications after TORS for benign indications

Authors	Institution(s)	# patients	# OP cases (%)	# complications (%)	# POB (%)	# OP bleeds (%)
Hoff et al. [7]	Multi-institutional (University of Michigan, University of Pennsylvania, Middlesex Hospital)	285	285 (100%)	59 (20.7%)	12 (4.1%)	N/A
Vicini et al. [6]	Multi-institutional (Morgagni-Pierantoni Hospital, University of Michigan, University of Pennsylvania, Columbia University, Clinica Universidad de Navarra, Louvain University Hospital of Mont Godinne, University of Pavia)	243	243 (100%)	50 (20.5%)	11 (4.6%)	N/A

Abbreviations: *OP* oropharyngeal, *POB* postoperative bleeds

sure of the larynx and hypopharynx can contribute to poorer hemostatic control.

Anticoagulation and antiplatelet therapy can affect postoperative bleeding rates and are usually withheld and/or bridged during the perioperative period. A review of 147 patients undergoing TORS revealed that 72% of the patients who had postoperative bleeding were on an antithrombotic medication for other comorbidities [16]. The postoperative bleeding rate in patients taking antithrombotic medication was significantly higher at 17% versus 3% ($p = 0.02$). They also noted that postoperative bleeding risk was greatest on postoperative days 7–14. A French review found that anticoagulation and/or antiplatelet therapy was a significant risk factor for postoperative bleeding ($p < 0.05$) [15]. Richmon et al. reported similar trends stating 50% of the patients who had postoperative bleeding were found to be on anticoagulation therapy [9]. Hoff et al. reported a postoperative bleeding rate of 4.1% and contributed two late postoperative bleeding episodes after re-initiation of clopidogrel or warfarin [7]. Patients who had anticoagulation at the time of surgery had higher rates of postoperative bleeding compared to patients not anticoagulated (13.5% vs. 8.1%) although this did not reach statistical significance ($p = 0.2785$) [7]. The authors in this study were so convinced of the association between bleeding after TORS and perioperative anticoagulation that they recommended withholding anticoagulation for 4 weeks postoperatively. However, at this time it remains unclear the optimal duration of time to withhold or bridge anticoagulation in patients treated using TORS.

18.3.2 Transcervical Ligation

The majority of bleeding after TORS is venous and self-limiting. However, potentially catastrophic arterial bleeding can occur after TORS. The incidence of life-threatening bleeding after TORS is unknown. No deaths from bleeding after TORS were reported in the USFDA indication trial [11]. However, by 2013, there were seven deaths from bleeding after TORS self-reported in a voluntary survey of TORS surgeons in the USA [13]. This is likely a gross underestimation, underscored by the fact that the response rate for the study was low and that the respondents were heavily weighted to high volume TORS surgeons. A variety of surgical techniques have been developed to minimize the risk of catastrophic bleeding after TORS, and some authors have advocated for routine transcervical ligation of feeding vessels to minimize or eliminate the risk of arterial bleeding after TORS.

Pollei et al. reviewed factors affecting bleeding rates in patients undergoing transoral oropharyngectomy by different approaches which included TORS, transoral laser microsurgery (TLM) and handheld cautery in 906 patients [17]. Of the 5.4% of patients with postoperative bleeding, 67% required operative intervention. In that retrospective study, prophylactic transcervical ligation of the external carotid system was performed during the primary surgery in 15.6% of patients. They reported no overall difference in bleeding rate after ligation compared to those patients who were not ligated ($p = 0.21$). Severe postoperative bleeding, defined as bleeding resulting in hypoxia/airway compromise requiring tracheostomy, cardiopulmonary arrest, or hemodynamic instability requiring of a blood transfusion, occurred less frequently in patients who had concurrent transcervical vessel ligation at 11.1% versus 25.8%. The difference was clinically meaningful but not statistically significant ($p = 0.66$). Vessel ligation was performed more frequently in patients with higher T classification ($p = 0.002$) since these patients were most likely to develop bleeding after TORS. So the authors recommended that patients with higher T classification should be considered for prophylactic transcervical ligation to decrease the rate and severity of bleeding after TORS.

More recently, Mandal et al. reviewed factors for postoperative bleeding after TORS in 224 patients with 185 cases performed for malignancy and 39 performed for benign indications [18]. 9.82% of these patients had varying degrees of bleeding after TORS. Prophylactic transcervical arterial ligation (9.1%) did not decrease overall postoperative bleeding rates when compared to the non-prophylactically ligated group (9.9%) ($p = 1.00$). There was a decreasing trend in frequency of severe bleeding after TORS, but this did not reach statistical significance ($p = 0.70$). Prior radiation therapy or chemoradiation therapy increased postoperative bleeding rates but not significantly ($p = 0.09$). Many experienced TORS surgeons routinely ligate branches of the ipsilateral external carotid system despite the paucity of data to date to support the effectiveness of the procedure. This is likely because the consequences of arterial bleeding after TORS can be dire and, although rare, may be preventable with a simple maneuver. A better understanding of the incidence and pathogenesis of catastrophic bleeding after TORS is needed to more clearly define the optimal strategies for prevention.

18.3.3 Neurologic Injury

There are multiple cranial nerves that can be encountered performing TORS, especially for malignancy. The severity of injury can include neuropraxia, axonotmesis, and neurotmesis. In cases that involve malignancy, important nerves may be intentionally sacrificed for adequate resection. The glossopharyngeal, hypoglossal, and lingual nerves are all at risk during TORS. Every effort should be made to preserve these nerves as they are collectively instrumental in the function of swallowing. It is also important to remember that neurologic injuries can be either direct or indirect. Direct nerve injury (e.g., cutting the nerve) is far less common than indirect injury (e.g., nerve compression).

The glossopharyngeal nerve serves as the main afferent innervation for the tonsillar fossa and oropharynx. It descends from the jugular foramen and courses with the stylopharyngeus through the superior and middle constrictor muscles. The nerve can be visualized anterior and medial to these muscles [21]. A branch of this nerve is frequently encountered during TORS for tonsillar malignancy as it courses between the stylopharyngeus and styloglossus muscles (Fig. 18.2). Sacrifice of this branch is often necessary to ensure an oncologic resection of cancers involving the inferior tonsil and or glossopharyngeal sulcus. The functional impact of sacrifice of a branch of the glossopharyngeal nerve during TORS has not been formally described but appears inconsequential in the context of soft tissue and mucosa loss.

In contrast, injury to the hypoglossal nerve during TORS can be functionally devastating. In well-selected TORS cases, the hypoglossal nerve is typically not at risk. However, an increased risk of injury is observed in patients with recurrent disease, a history of radiation treatment, and/or bulky primary tumors. Muscle movement of the ipsilateral tongue during electrocautery dissection can be an important, albeit traumatizing, signal of proximity to the nerve. It is also important to recognize that hypoglossal nerve injury can occur during placement of surgical clips to control or prevent bleeding. The lingual nerve is also at risk during TORS. Risk of direct injury to the lingual nerve is particularly relevant for cancers that extend anteriorly toward the floor of the mouth.

A critical understanding of the anatomy of the submandibular triangle from an "inside-out" perspective is paramount to avoiding injury to the hypoglossal and lingual nerves. Early recognition of the submandibular gland and posterior belly of the digastric muscle during TORS for cancers involving the glossopharyngeal sulcus can help avoid direct nerve injury. The hypoglossal nerve is at most risk during TORS as it passes over the hyoglossus and runs along the superior border of the hyoid bone, deep to the digastric and mylohyoid muscles [21]. The lingual nerve which gives afferent and taste sensation to the anterior two-thirds of the tongue can be found on the lateral surface of the styloglossus muscle [22].

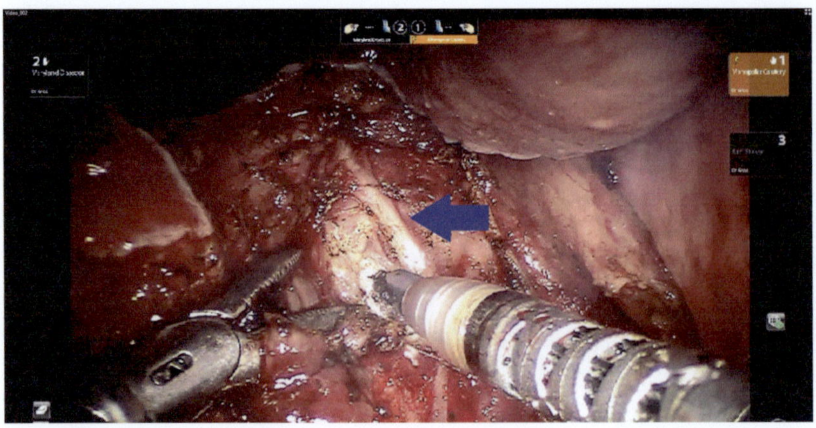

Fig. 18.2 Right glossopharyngeal nerve (*blue arrow*) exposed and preserved during TORS for tonsil cancer

Finally, the internal branch of the superior laryngeal nerve is at risk during TORS for supraglottic cancers. After piercing the thyrohyoid membrane, the internal branch of the superior laryngeal nerve provides afferent innervation for the supraglottic laryngeal mucosa [23]. It is involved with the cough reflex and aspiration prevention. This nerve travels in close proximity to the superior laryngeal artery which requires deliberate ligation during TORS of the larynx.

The incidence of significant neurologic injury after TORS is reportedly low. In a large survey study, temporary (<2 month) hypoglossal nerve injury occurred in 0.9% out of 2015 patients undergoing TORS, prolonged (>2 month) hypoglossal nerve injury occurred in 0.1%, and inadvertent lingual nerve injury occurred in 0.6% of cases [13]. Richmon et al. reported there were no hypoglossal nor lingual nerve palsies in 91 consecutive patients [9]. Weinstein et al. reported only 1 patient with tongue numbness out of 192 patients undergoing TORS for malignancy [11]. Many large retrospective studies have not reported nerve injuries. In contrast, Vicini et al. reported a hypogeusia rate of 14.2% in 243 TORS procedures for sleep-related disorders with all resolving within 8 months [6]. This likely represents indirect compression injury to the lingual nerve which may be underreported in other TORS series for malignancy. The risk of compression injury to the lingual nerve would seem proportional to the size of the tongue, duration and extent of retraction, as well as the surgical defect. Anecdotally, many patients undergoing TORS will have some extent of temporary sensation or taste change of their tongue. As with all risks, this should be communicated with patients preoperatively.

18.3.4 Aspiration and Pneumonia

With swallowing being compromised from odynophagia and dysphagia, the risk of aspiration and subsequent pneumonia is increased after TORS. Easa et al. evaluated swallowing outcomes for 78 patients that underwent TORS for OSA [8]. Gastrografin fluoroscopy was performed in the first postoperative week with only 6% having signs of significant aspiration. These patients all were without any swallowing complaints within 3 months and had no resulting significant weight loss. There was also no significant correlation between the volumes of tissue removed and the incidence of aspiration. A large review of TORS for benign indications reported pneumonia occurring six times in a cohort of 285 patients [7].

The risk of aspiration and pneumonia is likely greatest after TORS for malignancy, although there is a wide range in the incidence reported. In the USFDA indication trial for TORS, there was a 2.8% rate of pneumonia with two out of these five patients developing life-threatening complications of acute respiratory distress syndrome and pneumothorax [11]. Chia et al. noted 1.1% rate of aspiration pneumonia out of survey study of 2015 patients [13]. In a systemic review, Hutcheson et al. reported an incidence of postoperative pneumonia ranging from 0% to 7% in patients following TORS for oropharyngeal malignancy [14]. Recently, Aubry et al. reported an aspiration pneumonia rate of 15.5% and found that higher T-stage (T3, T4) and laryngeal location of the primary tumor were significant risk factors ($p < 0.05$) [15]. These authors attributed the high rate of aspiration pneumonia to the high percentage of patients with laryngeal tumors (47.2%). The reporting of aspiration after TORS is likely linked to the extent and timing of investigation as some degree of laryngeal penetration is common on early swallowing studies after TORS. Aggressive management of pain with early and frequent speech and language pathology coaching are critical to preventing aspiration and pneumonia.

18.3.5 Dehydration

Dehydration is a well-known complication from inadequate oral intake when odynophagia is not well controlled. Decreased urine output, tachycardia, and hypotension are some of the signs and symptoms of dehydration that will need to be treated with intravenous fluid hydration. Reported rates of dehydration following TORS ranges from 1.3% to 9.6% [7, 9, 11–13]. Dehydration is also relatively uncommon after TORS for benign indications. Richmon et al. reported dehydration to occur more frequently in OSA patients ($p < 0.001$) [9]. Educating patients on the importance of adequate oral intake and signs of dehydration can reduce emergency room visits and readmissions. Many TORS surgeons will place a nasogastric feeding tube during surgery. Some patients will require continued use of the feeding tube at home to avoid dehydration. Careful assessment of realistic oral intake prior to removal of the feeding tube and discharge is important to minimize the risk of dehydration.

18.3.6 Airway Compromise

Surgery in the upper airway always carries the risk of obstructive postoperative edema. Extended (e.g., overnight) intubation or prophylactic tracheostomy should always be considered when there are concerns of potential airway obstruction. The use of prophylactic tracheostomy was increased in early TORS series, likely reflecting the learning curve of TORS surgeons. In 130 patients treated with TORS primarily for malignancy (95%), Vergez et al. reported planned tracheostomy in 17 patients and emergent tracheostomy in 2 patients for postoperative edema [20]. In contrast, Hoff et al. reviewed complications after TORS for benign disease in 293 procedures with only 1 patient undergoing planned tracheostomy and 2 patients undergoing reintubation [7]. Oral tongue edema secondary to compression from the retractor and reperfusion is the most common cause of obstruction. For resections of oropharyngeal neoplasms, the amount of tissue excised can help offset resulting airway edema allowing for immediate postoperative extubation. Sleep apnea patients often have known difficult airways and could be at risk for obstructive postoperative edema. Perioperative steroids should be given routinely to decrease expected oropharyngeal edema after TORS. Extended intubation may be prudent in TORS cases where significant tongue swelling is observed during surgery.

Differing philosophies exist regarding concomitant tracheostomy with TORS as some surgeons perform tracheostomies routinely. Vicini et al. reported 110 tracheostomies performed after 243 TORS procedures for sleep-related disorders [6]. Two of seven institutions in this study routinely performed tracheostomy concomitantly with TORS. Patients with tracheostomy were capped after 3.85 ± 1.57 days and decannulated after 5.83 ± 1.96 days. Easa et al. performed tracheostomy in 82% of patients, which were all removed by postoperative day 4 [8].

In general, the need for tracheostomy after TORS is low. In a review involving 11 studies, Hutcheson et al. reported tracheostomy rates ranging from 0% to 31% [14]. A total of 411 patients were included, and only two had permanent tracheostomy dependence with a mean tracheostomy dependence ranging from 7 to 8 days. Chia et al. reported 2.8% of 2015 patients undergoing TORS required tracheostomy [13]. Patients undergoing salvage surgery for recurrent disease, with a history of radiation, or having bulky primary tumors are at greatest risk of needing a tracheostomy. Therefore, the indication for tracheostomy with TORS is essentially no different than that for open procedures of the oral tongue. In the setting of transoral bleeding, the airway may need to be secured with emergent tracheostomy. In a large survey study including 2015 patients, five patients had emergent tracheostomy performed in the setting of acute bleeding [13]. Prophylactic tracheostomy should be considered in any TORS procedure where the risk of postoperative bleeding is increased [18].

Postoperative airway management is similar as in traditional head and neck surgery. For example, placement of an oral airway or nasal trumpet will be based on factors such as short thyromental distance or an enlarged tongue. Anesthesiologists can also make decisions about placement of these airway tools at the time of extubation. Routine tracheostomy is not performed at our institution. Patients are also not routinely kept intubated unless intraoperative findings reveal significant tongue edema. Properly selected patients such as those with non-bulky primary tumors will not need to be intubated for an extended period. Intensive care unit (ICU) placement is usually needed only when extended (>4 hrs) intubation will be needed.

18.3.7 Death

Reported mortality rates following TORS are low with most cases attributed to postoperative bleeding. Chia et al. reported an overall 0.3% mortality rate with four reported causes of death due to hemorrhage [13]. Seven of the 62 patients (11.3%) who experienced a postoperative bleeding died. Vergez et al. reported 3 of 130 patients died from complications including one due to pulmonary embolism and two due to postoperative bleeding [20]. Mandal et al. reported a mortality rate of 0.9% with two patients who experienced severe bleeding [18]. Pollei et al. had an overall postoperative bleeding rate of 5.4% with a 1.1% severe or life-threatening postoperative bleeding rate [17]. One patient who developed anoxic brain injury and died 8 months postoperatively. Multiple large retrospective studies reported no TORS-related mortalities [6, 7, 11, 12, 19, 24]. Of course, given that most patients considered for TORS have an excellent prognosis, any mortality after TORS is tragic. Every effort should be made to minimize the risk of death after TORS. This is best achieved by minimizing the risk of severe bleeding after TORS.

18.3.8 Other Complications

Additional minor complications have been reported inconsistently after TORS. Dental complications occur at 1.4% [13]. Lip burns can occur up to 1.2% [12]. Local bacterial infections are very uncommon in the immediate postoperative course. Best evidence would suggest a single dose of IV antibiotics given preoperatively. Oral thrush has been known to occur with a reported incidence of 2% [9]. This can be treated with swish and spit nystatin solution. Better reporting these types of complications in the future may increase the rate of total complications but can help surgeons and patient understand the frequency of these risks.

18.4 Avoiding Complications

18.4.1 Training

The learning curve for surgeons performing TORS is now well known. Chia et al. studied the effects of case numbers and complications in TORS surgeons. Complication rates significantly decreased when surgeons performed more than 50 cases at 6.1% compared to those performing less than 50% ($p < 0.0001$) [13]. Surgeons performing fewer than 25 cases had a postoperative bleeding rate of 4.5%, those performing 26–50 cases had a rate of 2.5%, and those performing more than 50 cases had a rate of 2.8%. Vergez et al. had six cases where TORS was converted to an open procedure due to lack of exposure and noted that all of these came in the first half of their review hinting that experience increased ability for exposure [20]. White et al. reviewed a 4-year period of 168 patients undergoing TORS divided into 4 groups of 42 patients by time and compared outcomes [25]. There was a significant decrease in total operative time ($p < 0.001$), decrease in total intubation time ($p < 0.001$), and decrease in length of hospital stay ($p < 0.001$). There was a 47% decrease in operative time and 87% decrease in total intubation time from the first to the last group. There was a decrease in complications including postoperative bleeding and airway edema, but these were not significant. The first group had seven patients with postoperative bleeding and six patients with airway edema, whereas group 4 had 1 and 1, respectively. Although outcomes of operative time and intubation time may not reflect the surgeon's skill level independently, experience of a hospital and its staff may also contribute to better outcomes when performing TORS.

Training is paramount to summiting the learning curve with TORS. In other specialties, there are established guidelines for surgeons to become trained and credentialed robotic surgery. Requirements typically include formal training through a residency and/or fellowship program or an independent structured training curriculum [26]. Consensus guidelines were recently established for TORS as well [27]. These guidelines are meant to provide guidance to aspiring TORS surgeons and to hospitals charged with credentialing. Historically, most TORS surgeons were trained after residency or fellowship. A survey of 45 TORS surgeons showed 86.7% of respondents were trained through industry-sponsored training and 15.6% were trained through fellowship experience [13]. Yet, there is a clear difference in the quality of training afforded during residency or fellowship (graduate) compared to postgraduate training. Residency programs have reported development of curriculums to increase safety and efficiency [28]. During periods of inactivity, biweekly practice of 1 h has been shown to retain robotic surgical skills [29]. There are increasing efforts to provide TORS training free from industry influence. However, to date, no national organization has taken the lead in the oversight of training and credentialing of TORS.

18.4.2 Tumor Selection

Proper patient selection is paramount to successful outcomes with TORS. Patient and tumor factors impact patient selection; experience is needed to recognize these factors which can be subtle. Exposure of the target tissue is imperative to precise surgery and avoidance of complications. A good clinical exam in the office and under anesthesia can help determine the likelihood of good exposure intraoperatively (Fig. 18.3). Trismus and obstructive dentition can be rate-limiting factors as is the opportunity for neck extension. Medical conditions including kyphosis and previous cervical spine surgery can negatively impact the exposure for TORS. For malignancy, tumor factors will also heavily influence the decision for TORS. TORS is best suited for small primary (T1–T2) OPSCC. For larger primary tumors, the value of TORS may be diminished by the larger expected surgical defect and incumbent increased morbidity. One exception is bulky, pedunculated primary tumors where the surgical defect would be expected to be no larger than that for a smaller primary (Fig. 18.4). In these cases, a primary surgical approach using TORS may be most beneficial in allowing for a more focused delivery of adjuvant radiation (e.g., unilateral versus bilateral).

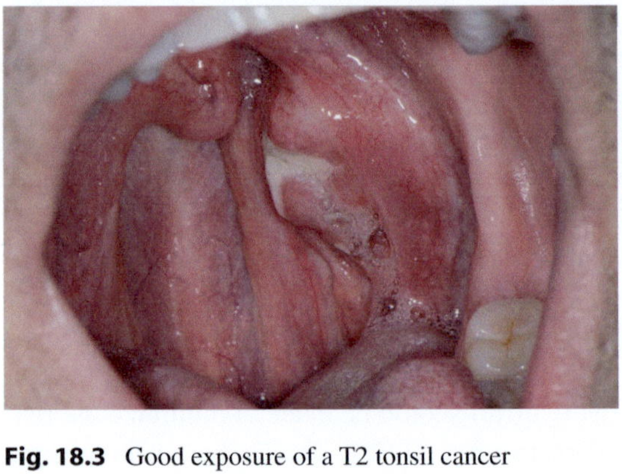

Fig. 18.3 Good exposure of a T2 tonsil cancer

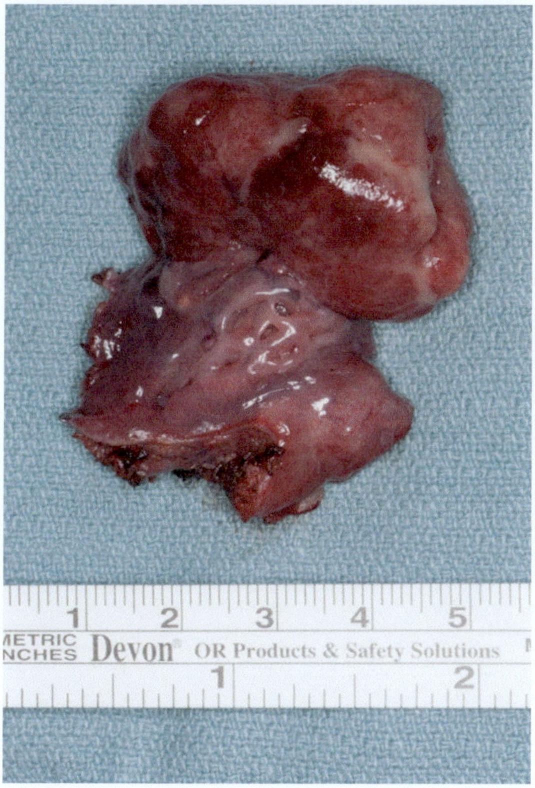

Fig. 18.4 Specimen after TORS of a pedunculated T3 tonsil cancer

18.4.3 Tools

The correct use of available tools can minimize complications. The oral cavity, eyes, and face are vulnerable to collateral damage during TORS. Application of eye protection (e.g., eye shields) is important for TORS cases. Tooth guards can be helpful in protecting the maxillary dentition from damage as well as protecting the tongue from being lacerated by the lower incisor teeth during suspension laryngoscopy (Fig. 18.5). Keeping the lips moist and protected can prevent from desiccation and trauma during TORS as well.

There are many retractors that can be used during TORS including a Crow-Davis mouth gag and a Dingman mouth gag. The only retractors specifically designed for TORS are the Feyh-Kastenbauer (F-K) retractor (Olympus, Barlett, TN) and the Flex retractor (Medrobotics, Raynham, MA). Multiple blades have been developed for use with the TORS retractor to access specific parts of the upper aerodigestive tract.

When encountering vessels, especially named vessels, application of surgical clips are necessary to prevent postoperative bleeding. In a survey taken by 45 surgeons, exposed arterial vessels in the oropharynx are most commonly managed intraoperatively with surgical clips (93.3%) and electrocautery (55.6%) [13].

The use of different forms of energy for cutting and ablating tissue is usually dependent on the surgeon and institution. Hoffman et al. studied the use of four different resection methods on porcine tongues including CO_2 laser, Tm:YAG laser, monopolar blade, and radiofrequency needle [30]. The radiofrequency needle had the most favorable cutting width and smaller coagulation defects in that study. Still, the monopolar blade is the most widely used tools for dissection during TORS.

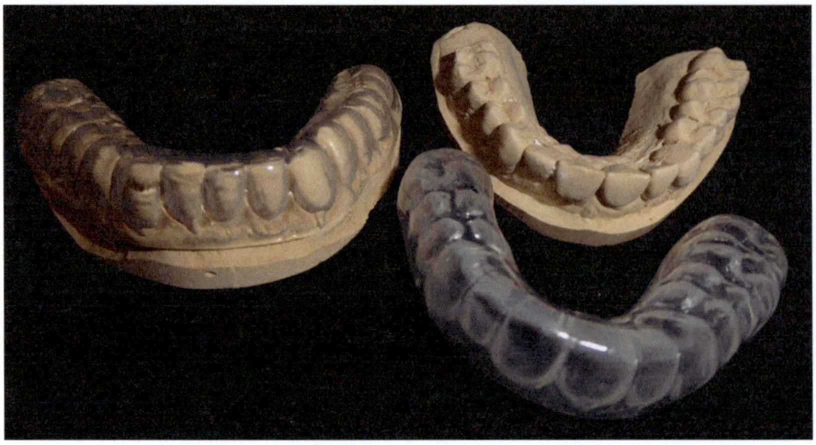

Fig. 18.5 Teeth guards

18.4.4 Technique

18.4.4.1 General

Meticulous surgical technique is crucial for all head and neck surgery. For TORS, this may be more difficult to achieve given the lack of haptic feedback with current technology. Most importantly, with TORS there is an increased reliance of visual cues, and any bleeding during TORS can obscure visualization of the anatomy. So the importance of careful, layer-by-layer dissection with careful hemostasis during TORS cannot be overstated. Coordination between the console surgeon and bedside assistant is very important in this regard.

18.4.4.2 Management of Blood Vessels and Intraoperative Bleeding

During TORS, there are named arteries that may need to be identified and ligated, especially for malignancy. Branches of the facial, lingual, and ascending pharyngeal artery supply the pharynx. Cautery can control mucosal and muscle bleeding as well as small unnamed vessels. However, larger vessels such as the dorsal lingual artery require vascular clip application. During TORS of the supraglottis, the superior laryngeal artery should always be identified and ligated [23]. Pollei et al. recommends using hemoclips on all arteries 2 mm or larger and suture ligation on arteries larger than 4 mm [17]. Brickman et al. recommended that any vessel larger than 1 mm should be meticulously clipped and divided [31]. Regardless of vessel size, the liberal use of surgical clips is advised by more experienced TORS surgeons (Fig. 18.6). Any exposed artery should be clipped and/or covered with adjacent soft tissue when possible. This is particularly important in the setting of previous radiation therapy.

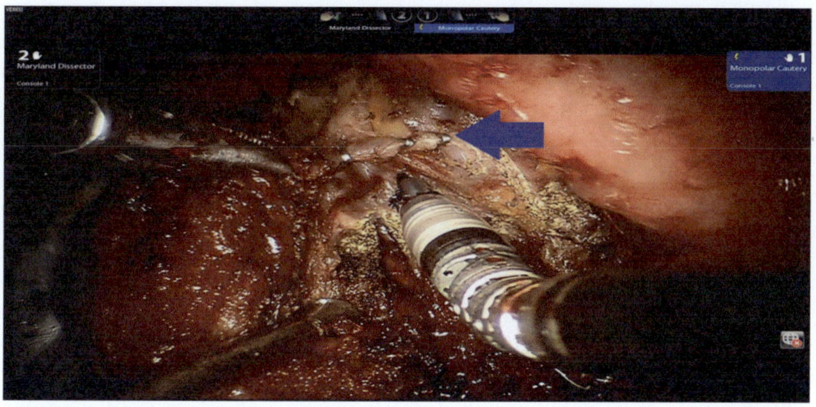

Fig. 18.6 Multiple surgical clips applied to ascending pharyngeal artery (*blue arrow*) during TORS for right tonsil cancer

18.4.4.3 Management of the Neck

Currently, there is no consensus on the ideal timing of neck dissection in patients with malignancy undergoing TORS. Benefits from concomitant TORS and neck dissection include a single anesthetic exposure, convenience, decreased length of treatment, concurrent vessel ligation, and decreased cost. Staged neck dissections have the benefit of potentially decreasing postoperative fistula formation and decreasing postoperative upper aerodigestive tract edema since ipsilateral lymphatics are undisturbed. Additionally, if margins were positive on initial tumor resection, then re-resection can be performed concurrently with a staged neck dissection. Staged neck dissection before TORS has the advantage of ligating named arteries to decrease bleeding risk during and after TORS.

The extent of neck dissection influences the risk of pharyngocutaneous fistula after TORS. Resection of the submandibular gland significantly increases the risk of fistula. Moore et al. reviewed 148 patients who underwent concurrent TORS and neck dissection for oropharyngeal cancer [32]. Twenty-nine percent of these patients were identified to have a communication between the oropharynx and neck during surgery. All patients had level I–IV neck dissections with removal of the submandibular gland. All had a combination of primary closure, local advancement flap, fibrin glue application (Tisseel), and cervical drain placement. 14.3% of these patients developed postoperative pharyngocutaneous fistulae which required incision and drainage with daily packing. All other fistulae resolved with clinical therapy and without return to the operating room. All patients with fistula formation had tonsillar fossa or lateral pharyngeal involvement; no patients with purely base of tongue involvement developed fistulae. None of the patients without intraoperative communication developed fistulae.

In contrast, Kucur et al. reviewed the safety of concurrent neck dissection with TORS in 113 patients with OPSCC where the submandibular gland was persevered in all cases except 2. Six intraoperative communications were found and repaired with either primary repair or muscle advancement flap reconstruction resulting in no postoperative fistulae [33]. The techniques included primary closure, primary closure with acellular dermal matrix reinforcement, submandibular gland transposition, anterior belly of digastric muscle rotational flap, posterior belly of digastric muscle rotational flap, and omohyoid muscular pedicled rotational flap.

Mockelmann et al. compared 21 patients who underwent concurrent TORS and neck dissection and 20 patients who underwent staged neck dissection on average 8.4 days (3–28 days) after TORS [34]. The group with concurrent surgery had a 9.5% rate of intraoperative communication that developed no postoperative fistulae after primary repair. These were repaired with primary closure and a pedicled muscle flap. However, there was no significant difference observed between the two groups for rates of fistula formation, postoperative bleeding, hematoma, and seroma. The group with concurrent surgery had a median hospital stay of 8 days (5–9 days), and the staged group had a median stay of 15 days (11–35 days). The average delay in surgery accounted for the difference in length of stay. Howard et al. compared 96 patients who underwent ipsilateral submandibular gland (SMG) preservation and 157 who underwent SMG resection during concomitant TORS and neck dissection [35]. The incidence of intraoperative communication was significantly lower in cases with SMG preservation compared to those with SMG removal, 2.1% vs. 14.1% ($p = 0.0017$). All postoperative fistulae occurred in those patients who underwent SMG removal (7.6%) compared to 0% in the SMG preservation group. Tonsil location of the primary tumor had a significant effect on fistula formation ($p = 0.0039$). T-stage was associated with intraoperative communication formation ($p = 0.0048$) but not for postoperative fistula formation ($p = 0.3410$). There was no significant difference in disease-free survival, disease-specific survival, disease-specific survival, nor overall survival at 5 years.

Overall, preservation of the submandibular gland has been reported to decrease the rate of postoperative pharyngocutaneous fistula formation after concurrent TORS and neck dissection.

Preservation of the submandibular gland has also shown to be oncologically safe [36]. Rotational muscle flaps can decrease the frequency of fistula formation by increased vascularized bulk and allowing for a robust partition between the oropharynx and neck. These techniques may be utilized to decrease the rate of postoperative pharyngocutaneous fistula formation after concurrent TORS and neck dissection.

Conclusion

TORS has proven to be a safe procedure with a low overall complication rate. As the volume of TORS increases, further analysis can be performed to identify factors that contribute to the frequency and severity of complications. Swallowing function is impacted by TORS and, in most cases, the sequelae of dysphagia and odynophagia is short-lived. Judicial use of prophylactic feeding tubes and tracheostomy placement may further decrease complication rates. Postoperative bleeding continues to be an infrequent but potentially lethal complication. Transcervical ligation does not affect overall postoperative bleeding rates but may decrease the risk of catastrophic arterial bleeding after TORS. Neck dissection concomitant with TORS is safe with an acceptably low pharyngocutaneous fistula rate.

References

1. Gawande A. Complications: a surgeon's notes on an imperfect science. New York: Picador; 2002.
2. Crawford JA, Montevecchi F, Vicini C, Magnuson JS. Transoral robotic sleep surgery: the obstructive sleep apnea-hypopnea syndrome. Otolaryngol Clin North Am. 2014;47(3):397–406. doi:10.1016/j.otc.2014.03.004.
3. O'Mallet Jr BW, Weinstein GS. Robotic skull base surgery: preclinical investigations to human clinical application. Arch Otolaryngol Head Neck Surg. 2007;133(12):1215–9.
4. Logemann JA. Mechanisms of normal and abnormal swallowing. In: Cummings CW, Flint PW, editors. Cummings otolaryngology head & neck surgery. 5th ed. Philadelphia: Mosby/Elsevier; 2010. p. 1215–21.
5. Baugh RF, Archer SM, Mitchell RB, et al. Clinical practice guideline: tonsillectomy in children. Otolaryngol Head Neck Surg. 2011;144(1 Supple): S1–30. doi:10.1177/0194599810389949.
6. Vicini C, Montevecchi F, Campanini A, et al. Clinical outcomes and complications associated with TORS and OSAHS: a benchmark for evaluating an emerging surgical technology in a targeted application for benign disease. ORL J Otorhinolaryngol Relat Spec. 2014;76(2):63–9. doi:10.1159/000360768.
7. Hoff PT, D'Agnostino MA, Thaler ER. Transoral robotic surgery in benign diseases including obstructive sleep apnea: safety and feasibility. Laryngoscope. 2015;125(5):1249–53. doi:10.1002/lary.25026.
8. Eesa M, Montevecchi F, Hendawy E, et al. Swallowing outcome after TORS for sleep apnea: short- and long-term evaluation. Eur Arch Otorhinolaryngol. 2015;272(6):1537–41. doi:10.1007/s00405-014-3480-x.
9. Richmon JD, Feng AL, Yang W, et al. Feasibility of rapid discharge after transoral robotic surgery of the oropharynx. Laryngoscope. 2014;124(11):2518–25. doi:10.1002/lary.24748.
10. Moore EJ, Olsen KD, Kasperbauer JL. Transoral robotic surgery for oropharyngeal squamous cell carcinoma: a prospective study of feasibility and functional outcomes. Laryngoscope. 2009;119(11):2156–64. doi:10.1002/lary.20647.
11. Weinstein GS, O'Malley Jr BW, Magnuson JS, et al. Transoral robotic surgery: a multicenter study to assess feasibility, safety, and surgical margins. Laryngoscope. 2012;122(8):1701–7. doi:10.1002/lary.23294.
12. Glazer TA, Hoff PT, Spector ME. Transoral robotic surgery for obstructive sleep apnea: perioperative management and postoperative complications. JAMA Otolaryngol Head Neck Surg. 2014;140(12):1207–12. doi:10.1001/jamaoto.2014.2299.
13. Chia SH, Gross ND, Richmon JD. Surgeon experience and complications with Transoral Robotic Surgery (TORS). Otolaryngol Head Neck Surg. 2013;149(6):885–92. doi:10.1177/0194599813503446.
14. Hutcheson KA, Holsinger FC, Kupferman ME, Lewin JS. Functional outcomes after TORS for oropharyngeal cancer: a systemic review. Eur Arch Otorhinolaryngol. 2015;272(2):463–71. doi:10.1007/s00405-014-2985-7.
15. Aubry K, Vergez S, de Mones E, et al. Morbidity and mortality revue of the French group of transoral robotic surgery: a multicentric study. J Robot Surg. 2015;11 [Epub ahead of print]
16. Asher SA, White HN, Kejner AE, et al. Hemorrhage after transoral robotic-assisted surgery. Otolaryngol Head Neck Surg. 2013;149(1):112–7. doi:10.1177/0194599813486254.
17. Pollei TR, Hinni ML, Moore EJ, et al. Analysis of postoperative bleeding and risk factors in transoral surgery of the oropharynx. JAMA Otolaryngol Head Neck Surg. 2013;139(11):1212–8. doi:10.1001/jamaoto.2013.5097.
18. Mandal R, Duvvuri U, Ferris RL, et al. Analysis of post-transoral robotic-assisted surgery hemorrhage: frequency, outcomes, and prevention. Head Neck. 2015; doi:10.1002/hed.24101.

19. Cognetti DM, Luginbuhl AJ, Nguyen AL, Curry JM. Early adoption of transoral robotic surgical program: preliminary outcomes. Otolaryngol Head Neck Surg. 2012;147(3):482–8. doi:10.1177/0194599812443353.
20. Vergez S, Lallemant B, Ceruse P, et al. Initial multi-institutional experience with transoral robotic surgery. Otolaryngol Head Neck Surg. 2012;147(3):475–81. doi:10.1177/0194599812443221.
21. Moore EJ, Janus J, Kasperbauer J. Transoral robotic surgery of the oropharynx: clinical and anatomic considerations. Clin Anat. 2012;25(1):135–41. doi:10.1002/ca.22008.
22. Dallan I, Seccia V, Faggiono L, et al. Anatomical landmarks for transoral robotic tongue base surgery: comparison between endoscopic, external and radiological perspectives. Surg Radiol Anat. 2013;35(1):3–10. doi:10.1007/s00276-012-0983-2.
23. Gun R, Ozer E. Surgical anatomy of oropharynx and supraglottic larynx for transoral robotic surgery. J Surg Oncol. 2015;112:690–6. doi:10.1002/jso.24020.
24. Blanco RG, Fakhry C, Ha PK, et al. Transoral robotic surgery experience in 44 cases. J Laparoendosc Adv Surg Tech A. 2013;23(11):900–7. doi:10.1089/lap.2013.0261.
25. White HN, Frederick J, Zimmerman T, et al. Learning curve for transoral robotic surgery: a 4-year analysis. JAMA Otolaryngol Head Neck Surg. 2013;139(6):564–7. doi:10.1001/jamaoto.2013.3007.
26. Herron DM, Marohn M, SAGES-MIRA Robotic Surgery Consensus Group. A consensus document on robotic surgery: prepared by the SAGES-MIRA robotic surgery consensus group. Surg Endosc. 2008;22(2):313–25. discussion 311-2
27. Gross ND, Holsinger FC, Magnuson JS, et al. Robotics in otolaryngology and head and neck surgery: recommendations for training and credentialing. Head Neck. 2016; doi:10.1002/hed.24207. [Epub ahead of print]
28. Curry M, Malpani A, Li R, et al. Objective assessment in residency-based training for transoral robotic surgery. Laryngoscope. 2012;122(10):2184–92. doi:10.1002/lary.23369.
29. Guseila LM, Saranathan A, Jenison EL, et al. Training to maintain surgical skills during periods of robotic surgery inactivity. Int J Med Robot. 2014;10(2):237–43. doi:10.1002/rcs.1562.
30. Hoffman TK, Schuler PJ, Bankfalvi A, et al. Comparative analysis of resection tools suited for transoral robot-assisted surgery. Eur Arch Otorhinolaryngol. 2014;271(5):1207–13. doi:10.1007/s00405-013-2615-9.
31. Brickman D, Gross ND. Robotic approaches to the pharynx: tonsil cancer. Otolaryngol Clin North Am. 2014;47(3):359–72. doi:10.1016/j.otc.2014.03.002.
32. Moore EJ, Olsen KD, Martin EJ. Concurrent neck dissection and transoral robotic surgery. Laryngoscope. 2011;121(3):541–4. doi:10.1002/lary.21435.
33. Kucur C, Durmus K, Gun R, et al. Safety and efficacy of concurrent neck dissection and transoral robotic surgery. Head Neck. 2015; doi:10.1002/hed.24033.
34. Mockelmann N, Busch CJ, Münscher A, et al. Timing of neck dissection in patients undergoing transoral robotic surgery for head and neck cancer. Eur J Surg Oncol. 2015;41(6):773–8. doi:10.1016/j.ejso.2015.02.002.
35. Howard BE, Hinni ML, Nagel TH, et al. Submandibular gland preservation during concurrent neck dissection and transoral surgery for oropharyngeal squamous cell carcinoma. Otolaryngol Head Neck Surg. 2014;150(4):587–93. doi:10.1177/0194599813519041.
36. Takes RP, Robbins KT, Woolgar JA, et al. Questionable necessity to remove the submandibular gland in neck dissection. Head Neck. 2011;33(5):743–5. doi:10.1002/hed.21451.

19 TORS with the Flex® Robotic System

David Goldenberg and Michael D.F. Goldenberg

19.1 Background and Current Technology

Robot-assisted surgery has become a popular alternative to many open traditional surgical procedures. While modern robotic surgical techniques have been described since the late 1980s, telesurgery (i.e., surgery done at a distance from the patient) was first successfully performed in 2001, when physicians situated in New York removed the gallbladder of a 62-year-old patient in Strasbourg, France [1]. Since then, technology has improved and remote robotic surgery has become quite prevalent and sophisticated. Used primarily in urology and gynecology at its inception, transoral robotic surgery (TORS) was eventually developed for use in head and neck procedures. The da Vinci system® (Intuitive Surgical Inc., Sunnyvale, CA, USA) is one such advanced robot, studied extensively at the University of Pennsylvania for its application in TORS in order to perfect and standardize its use [1, 2]. The da Vinci was the only tool available to perform TORS on the head and neck, yet has its own limitations. The newest iteration of robotic surgical equipment is the Flex® Robotic System (Medrobotics, Raynham, MA, USA), which improves upon some of the shortcomings of its predecessors. This chapter will focus on the present state of TORS of the head and neck and the future possibilities which improved technology can provide.

19.2 Linear Systems

Until now, Intuitive Surgical's da Vinci system® has been the most commonly used robotic system for TORS. This linear system is composed of several components: a visualization cart which holds the lighting and cameras, the surgeon console which allows the surgeon to remotely control the robotic arms, and the patient cart which holds the various robotic tools [1]. The system's arms and wristed instruments essentially act as an extension of the surgeon's hands, allowing for a smaller initial opening and more movement within a limited size surgical cavity [2].

Two providers, at a minimum, are required to perform TORS with the da Vinci system® [2]. The first is the console surgeon, who performs the surgery at the robot console removed from the operating table [2]. The second is the bedside assistant, charged with a number of tasks, including additional retraction, smoke evacuation, preventing clashing of the right and left arms,

D. Goldenberg, MD, FACS (✉)
M.D.F. Goldenberg, BA, MA
Penn State University College of Medicine and Penn State Hershey Medical Center, Division of Otolaryngology — Head and Neck Surgery, Hershey, PA, USA
e-mail: dgoldenberg@pennstatehealth.psu.edu

Z. Gil et al. (eds.), *Atlas of Head and Neck Robotic Surgery*, DOI 10.1007/978-3-319-49578-1_19

and protection of the patient from unwanted movements of the robotic arms [2].

The orientation of the operating room (OR) may be different than more traditional surgery. The patient cart must approach the operating table at an angle of ~30° [2], and, as such, other carts that would normally be situated in its way must be placed elsewhere. The anesthesia cart is moved away from the head of the patient bed and instead placed at its foot, to ensure there is no interference with the robot console, the robot arms, or the bedside assistant [2]. This is achieved by placing the patient's head at the foot of the table and then spinning it 180° [2]. This may cause instability in larger patients and may be corrected by placing stabilizing furniture (i.e., adjustable stool or OR platforms) under the foot of the bed where the patient's head is now positioned [2]. Instead of the anesthesia cart, the bedside assistant is placed at the patient's head to ensure proper manipulation of the robotic instruments and patient safety [2].

There should be at least three people maneuvering the patient cart: one pushing the cart to approach the operating table at 30°, the second holding the robotic arms in place to avoid damage to them, the patient, or other OR equipment, and the third ensuring that the cart does not collide with anything in the room [2]. It should be noted that, in setting up the operating theater, certain stabilization equipment (e.g., Mayo stands) cannot be used as they potentially interfere with the robot arms [2].

19.3 Limitations of Current Technology

Despite its advantages, there have been noted difficulties with current robot technology in TORS [3, 4]. Its large size is one principal inconvenience, as it limits the space available in the OR [1]. Another is the interconnected nature of the machines across the operating room, which may lead to accidents involving the patient or providers and/or damage to the robotic components themselves [1]. Certain cases may also require multiple changes of robotic instruments, which in effect stop the surgical procedure, increasing the amount of time the case requires and prolonging anesthesia time [1]. For instance, a change from a 0° to a 30° camera may be necessary every time the surgeon wishes to change a viewing angle in the vicinity of the oropharynx or larynx. The da Vinci does not have its own suction unit or smoke evacuation and must rely on a bedside assistant for these tasks [5].

Robot setup times of up to an hour have been reported, with a mean of ~25 min [1, 3]. Specific to TORS, we must recall that the da Vinci was not designed for head and neck use, and, as such, its size and the size of its instruments do not always lend themselves to such surgeries [1, 3]. Clashing of the right and left arms is a common problem and often results in pausing the surgery multiple times in order to reposition the robotic arms. This is necessary to avoid harming the patient or damaging the robot and may significantly lengthen surgery time.

19.4 The Flex® Robotic System

The Flex® Robotic System is specifically designed and FDA cleared for TORS [6]. Unlike previous robotic surgical instruments before it, which were linear and dependent on different angled cameras (0 and 30°) in order to change viewing direction, the Flex® Robotic System is based on a flexible robotic scope and flexible instrumentation [6]. In addition to the ability to maneuver the surgical tools in three dimensions, the surgeon has the option to change the shape and position of the scope itself, changing the viewing angle and position of the camera at will. The robotic scope alternates between semirigid and completely rigid states, allowing the surgeon the ability to advance and position the scope as needed, yet maintain a stable surgical platform for the procedure [6].

The system itself is composed of two carts. One cart houses a stand, the attached Flex® Base and the working end of the robot. A second cart is called the Flex® Console. The Flex® Console is placed directly at the operating table so that the surgeon can easily access it (Fig. 19.1) [6]. This console, on which a monitor is mounted, also houses the control unit through which the surgeon manipulates the robotic scope (Fig. 19.2) [6]. From here, the surgeon may maneuver the scope with either gross or fine movements in order to ensure the correct position of all instrumentation. The second unit, called the Flex® Cart, is placed at the side of the operating table and connects to the reusable Flex® Base and can be positioned via various lockable joints. The Flex® Base is the portion of the robot to which the single-use Flex® Drive and reusable scope are attached (Fig. 19.3) [6]. The system is aligned

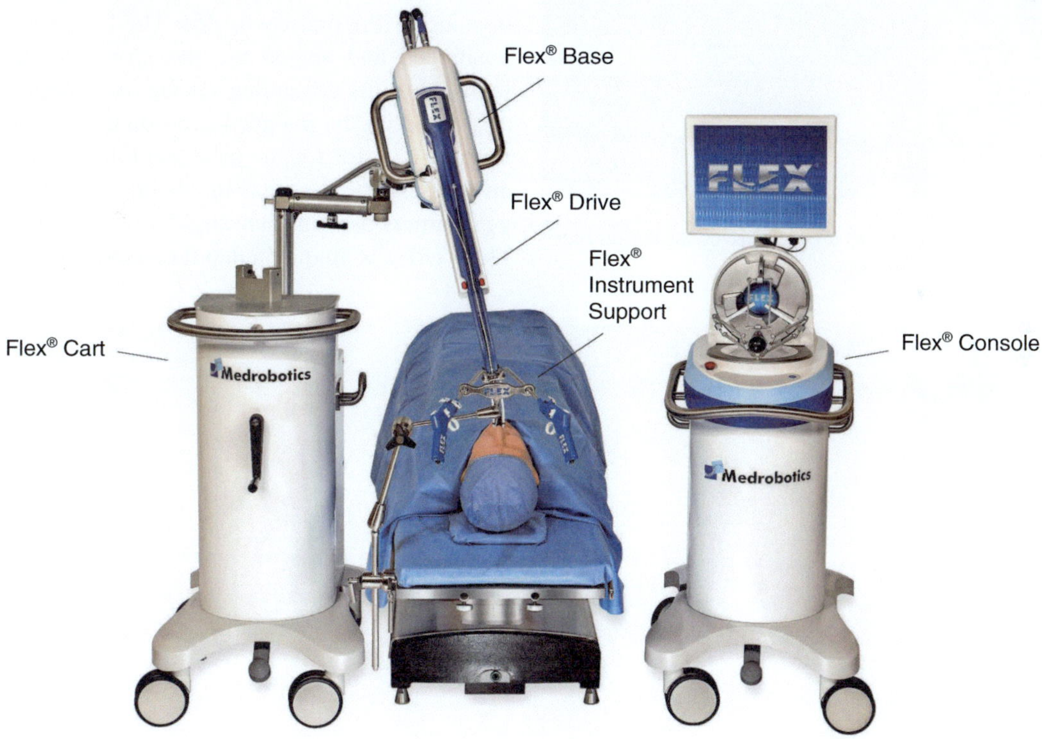

Fig. 19.1 Components of the Flex® Robotic System

at the distal part of the operating table to be positioned appropriately to reach the oral cavity.

The robotic scope is comprised of two mechanisms, an inner and outer, which are arranged in a concentric mechanical assembly. The distal segment, which is controlled by the surgeon using a 3D joystick-like controller, embodies a digital camera providing HD vision, LED lamps, a lens washer, and two external accessory channels. The scope is equipped with two external accessory channels for introducing 3.5 mm flexible instruments. The surgeon moves the scope under visual control on a monitor on the Flex® Console or an external monitor. The Medrobotics® Flex® Robotic System consists of four primary components: (A) the Flex® Console which houses the physician control handle, a touch screen visual display, and the touch screen monitor; (B) the Flex® Base, a reusable assembly that transfers electronic signals from the console into mechanical motions; (C) the Flex® Drive, a sterile, single-use component that mounts on the Flex® Base and houses the flexible portion of the robot and components to move it as well as the Flex® Camera; and the (D) Flex® Cart and Stand as support for the Flex® Base and Flex® Drive.

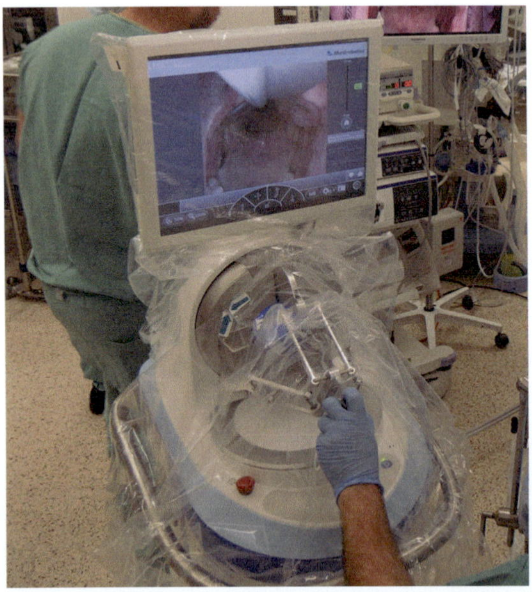

Fig. 19.2 Surgeon uses joystick-like controller on Flex® Console to position scope

Setup time for the entire system is reported at less than 10 min [6]. In preparation for surgery, the Flex® Base is placed midline on the patient, and the Flex® Drive is positioned directly at the opening of the oral cavity [6]. The base can be positioned and angled via the aforementioned lockable joints depending on the view required and based on the intended procedure being performed, e.g., for tongue base and tonsil surgery, an obtuse angle is used (Fig. 19.3a), while laryngeal surgery uses an acute angle (Fig. 19.3b). The Flex® Drive is unique in that it can move in three

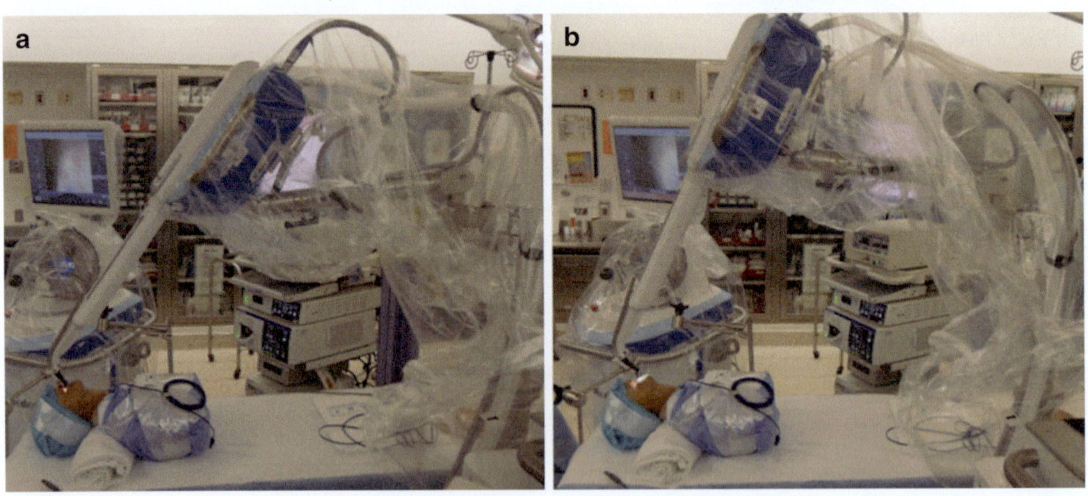

Fig. 19.3 The base can be angled via the lockable joints on the stand to position the Flex® Drive based on the intended procedure being performed: for oropharyngeal surgery, a more obtuse angle is used (**a**), while laryngeal surgery uses a more acute angle (**b**)

dimensions without the requirement of external support and then made rigid once in the desired location—again, in either gross or fine motions [6]. When the scope requires removal, the "Home" button on the Flex® Console may be pressed to cause the scope to retract out of the oropharynx, hypopharynx, or larynx and return to its default starting position. This "homing" may also be also be used to "guide" removal of the excised mass, with the surgeon gripping it with forceps or clamps and pulling back slowly as the scope returns to its home position. To either side of the scope, there are small channels that follow its contour and allow various compatible flexible tools to reach the operation site without additional maneuvering (Figs. 19.4 and 19.5). In this system, there are no external arms. Instead, the flexible instruments act as an extension of the surgeon's hands, allowing for a smaller initial opening and more movement within a limited size surgical cavity. The small size, flexibility, and easy maneuverability of the instruments allow for a rapid exchange of surgical instruments or their handedness by the surgeon himself, with no need for assistance (Fig. 19.6). This, in turn, greatly enhances the procedure's pace and flow when compared to halting the procedure to reposition outer components.

The technological advancements address some of the limitations described with performing TORS with older linear systems. The size of the Flex® Robotic System is markedly smaller than previous surgical robots, allowing for more room within the operating theater and for greater unit portability [6]. This, along with the bedside nature of the consoles, may reduce the amount of potential accidents cited above caused by the spread out nature of the da Vinci and similar systems. The smaller size, mobility, and simpler layout also result in shorter setup time, as is mentioned above. Finally, the acquisition cost is roughly half that of the da Vinci robot, potentially allowing for more widespread adoption of TORS [6].

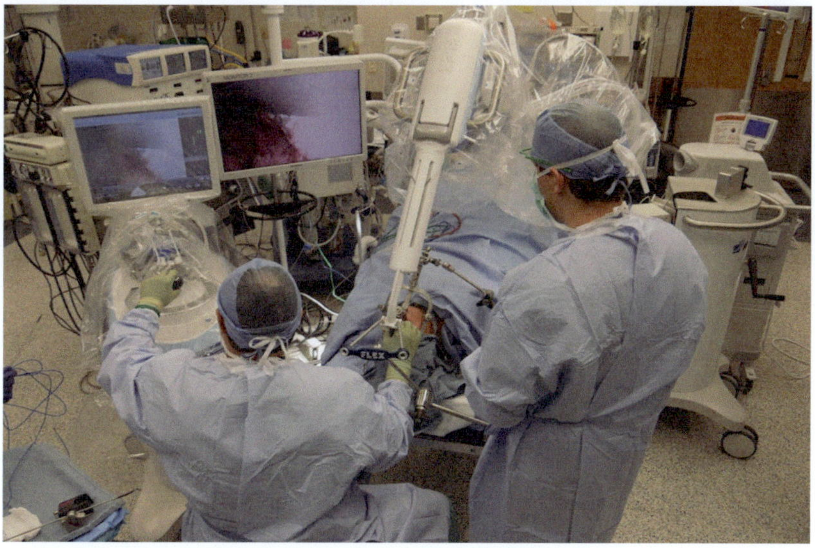

Fig. 19.4 Surgeon driving the Flex® Drive into position

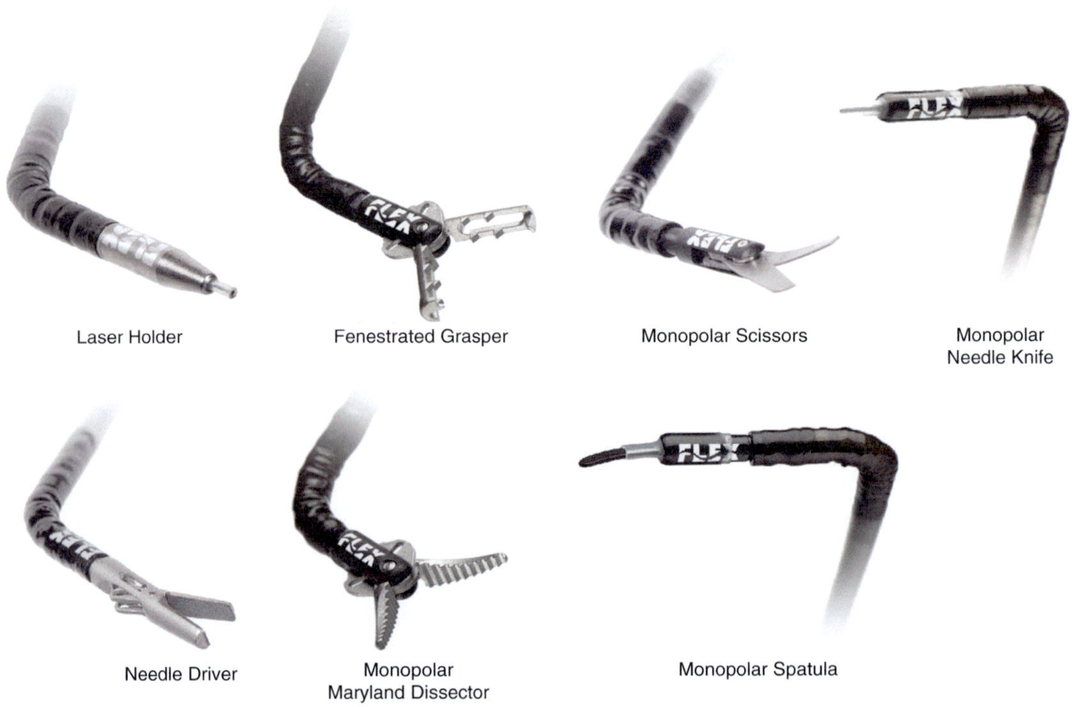

Fig. 19.5 Instruments currently available for use with the Flex® Robotic System

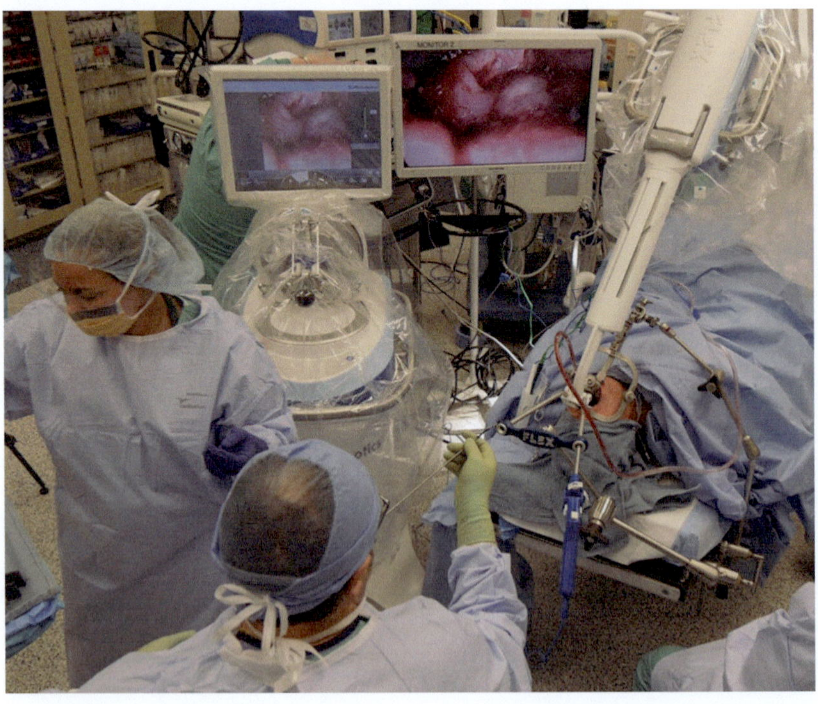

Fig. 19.6 Surgeon placing compatible Flex® Instruments into side channels of positioned flexible robotic scope

19.5 Available Instruments and Tools

While the flexible robotic scope of the Flex® Robotic System is its major component, the procedures themselves are performed by those instruments that are placed in the two working channels. As mentioned above, these channels match the contour of the camera and allow a variety of compatible third-party instruments to be used. Figure 19.7 shows an assortment of available Flex® Instruments at the time of writing, including a laser holder, fenestrated grasper, monopolar Maryland dissector, monopolar scissors, needle driver, monopolar spatula, and monopolar needle knife [Flex® instrument IFUs].

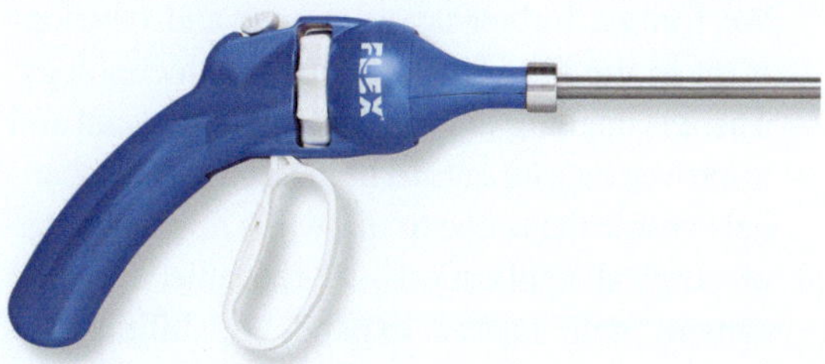

Fig. 19.7 Handle for the interchangeable instruments of the Flex® Robotic System

Conclusions

The Medrobotics Flex® Robotic System represents the natural progression and new generation of robotic technology for transoral surgery. It combines a highly flexible robotic scope with a variety of flexible instruments that reach the operative site quickly and efficiently. This system has a small footprint that easily fits in most ORs, is lean and mobile for efficient scheduling, and has a quick setup time for fast room turns. We foresee further advancement and development in the next few years of this technology. There is ongoing development of additional and improved instruments to fit in the two side channels beside the scope to allow for a wider range of surgical applications. A reusable, 3D HD camera will further expand capabilities for visualization.

References

1. Valero R, Ko YH, Chauhan S, et al. Cirugía robótica: Historia e impacto en la enseñanza. Actas Urol Esp. 2011;35(9):540–5. doi:10.4321/S0210-48062011000900006.
2. Weinstein GS, O'Malley BW. Transoral robotic surgery. 1st ed. San Diego: Plural Publishing; 2011.
3. Chauvet D, Missistrano A, Hivelin M, Carpentier A, Cornu P, Hans S. Transoral robotic-assisted skull base surgery to approach the sella turcica: cadaveric study. Neurosurg Rev. 2014;37(4):609–17. doi:10.1007/s10143-014-0553-7.
4. Weinstein GS, O'Malley BW, Desai SC, Quon H. Transoral robotic surgery: does the ends justify the means? Curr Opin Otolaryngol Head Neck Surg. 2009;17(2):126–31. doi:10.1097/MOO.0b013e32832924f5.
5. Esteban F, Menoyo A, Abrante A. Critical analysis of robotic surgery for laryngeal tumours. Acta Otorrinolaringol Engl Ed. 2014;65(6):365–72.
6. Medrobotics Corporation. Flex scope instructions for use (IFU). March 2014.

Intraoperative Imaging and Navigation in Robotic Surgery

20

Wen P. Liu

20.1 Introduction

A clinician performing head and neck robotic surgery currently relies on volumetric preoperative and diagnostic images (e.g., computed tomography (CT) and/or magnetic resonance images (MRI)) to develop a surgical plan. However, intraoperative imaging provides in situ information about the presence of pathology and its anatomic relationship to vital structures in real time, potentially allowing for more targeted, safer, and less morbid surgery. Literature on intraoperative imaging for robotics in otolaryngology (e.g., irradiative modality, cone beam computed tomography (CBCT); and non-irradiative modalities, ultrasound (US), narrow band imaging (NBI), or near-infrared fluorescence) shows researchers adapting traditionally diagnostic imaging techniques for intraoperative needs. Surgical objectives include planning traversals for target resection, margin delineation, and reconstruction while controlling or preserving critical functional structures. Intraoperative imaging has been explored not only to visualize this workspace but also to provide an anchoring modality for registering higher-resolution preoperative images and plans. This requires establishing the correspondence of image coordinates in preoperative to intraoperative space and to the surgical scene by using registration algorithms. Rigid registration is an arguably solved issue with a mainstay of commercially available systems used in standard surgical procedures. However, nonrigid registration in real time, involving reliably modeling intraoperative deformations from setup and intervention, continues to be a challenge. In addition to high fidelity registration, effective navigation and visualization in robotic surgery in otolaryngology are also very active areas of research. In this chapter, we survey how research and development in various modalities of intraoperative imaging have addressed these technical challenges in state-of-the art navigation for robotic surgery in otolaryngology.

20.2 Background

20.2.1 Intraoperative Imaging Modalities

20.2.1.1 C-arm and Flat-Panel Cone Beam Computed Tomography (CBCT)

For 2D intraoperative imaging, X-ray has long been established as a cost-effective, real-time modality. Fluoroscopy was used by Goding et al. to observe hypoglossal nerve stimulation and to evaluate airway changes for otolaryngology [5]. However, 3D imaging better informs the surgeon about the precise extent for dissection and can be

W.P. Liu
Intuitive Surgical, Sunnyvale, CA, USA
e-mail: wen.p.liu@gmail.com

Z. Gil et al. (eds.), *Atlas of Head and Neck Robotic Surgery*, DOI 10.1007/978-3-319-49578-1_20

used to update intraoperative stereotactic navigation. The emergence of intraoperative CBCT has proved useful in complex skull base and endoscopic surgery, especially in cases in which the extent of bony resection is critical to the successful outcome of the operation [6]. Unlike anterior skull base surgery, the use of intraoperative image guidance has only recently gained popularity in the field of lateral skull base surgery. While conventional multi-detector computed tomography (MDCT) is able to better resolve soft tissue, flat-panel CBCT scanners generally deliver less radiation to the patient and have less metal artifact effects. In a retrospective case review of 12 patients, Conley et al. [6] compared a conventional CT system (NeuroLogica CereTom® (NeuroLogica Corporation, Danvers, MA)) to two 2D flat-panel CBCT systems (O-ARM® (Medtronic Inc., Minneapolis, MN), and Xoran xCAT® (Xoran Technologies Inc., Ann Arbor, MI)), evaluating the ease of use, image characteristics, and integration with image guidance for skull base and endoscopic sinus surgery. In their study, all three scanners provided good quality images, but more significantly their results showed that intraoperative CBCT was not only technically feasible but was also useful for surgical decision-making in three out of four of their cases. For example, the intraoperative scan was used to facilitate a novel approach (retrolabyrinthine) to acoustic tumor removal by precisely delineating the extent of bony removal vis-à-vis the needed exposure. This would have been less certain, by standard means of caliper estimation. In one of these cases, the use of the O-arm was impossible secondary to morbid obesity, which precluded safe positioning of the patient for image acquisition. Other limitations noted include restrictions on the type of head reference array that can be used in lateral approaches and the lack of integration of the navigation systems and the operating microscope.

20.2.1.2 Ultrasound Imaging

The advent of minimally invasive approaches has further integrated ultrasound devices for otolaryngology in both diagnostics and intervention. In diagnostic techniques for otolaryngology, ultrasound has become an extended component of the physical examination in head and neck patients, particularly those with diseases of the thyroid, salivary gland, lymph node, and tongue [7–9]. For surgery in otolaryngology, the risk of inadvertent tissue injury requires in situ imaging techniques that can be used to visualize the operative field dynamically and beyond the visible surface. In Doppler mode, US provides temporal 4D data to assess vascular flow in the oral and maxillofacial regions [10] and is an efficient modality to image the morphology of soft tissue in 3D, allowing for applying differential pressure on retropharyngeal metastases to determine their spatial mobility relative to the carotid artery. Transoral ultrasound has been shown to be a cost-effective modality for evaluating the retropharyngeal space [11–13]. In base of tongue cancer, clinicians have successfully used ultrasound to guide core biopsies [12, 14, 15], interstitial photodiagnosis, and photodynamic therapy [16]. Furthermore, registration of ultrasonography to CT has demonstrated advantages in staging and surgical planning for papillary thyroid carcinoma (PTC). In a tertiary center prospective study, Lesnik et al. [17] measured sensitivity, specificity, and positive/negative predictive value of nodal diagnostics in central/lateral cervical compartments in 162 PTC patients undergoing preoperative lymph node evaluation by PE, US, and CT. The gold standard for diagnostic accuracy is surgical pathology. In patients undergoing primary (Group I)/revision (Group II) surgical treatment for PTC, the cases that used US registered to CT yielded significantly higher sensitivity for macroscopic lymph node detection in both lateral and central neck, most marked in Group I central compartment.

20.2.1.3 Optical Imaging

In endoscopic surgery, the unique advantage of optical imaging techniques, such as autofluorescence and narrow band imaging, over all other modalities discussed in this chapter, is the direct coregistration of white light and augmented information in the primary visual field. If the photons required for optical imaging can be gathered from the same endoscope/laryngoscope used to guide the robotic surgery, the nontrivial issue of organ deformation is intrinsically addressed [18]. In fact, near-infrared visualization of fluorescence tracers (e.g., indocyanine green (ICG)) have shown promise in identifying and guiding tumor resection because of their favorable characteristics, such as minimal scattering, enhanced tissue penetration depth, and high-quality contrast [18]. Currently in robotics, the da Vinci® Surgical System (Intuitive Surgical Inc., Sunnyvale, CA) supports integrated near-infrared imaging to visualize fluorescence. Fluorescence in robotic surgery has been used successfully in urologic and general laparoscopic surgery [19–21]. The potential of their application in head and neck oncology can be seen in the study by Rosenthal et al. [22] which assessed the safety and tumor specificity of a fluorescently labeled epidermal growth factor receptor (EGFR)-targeted agent. A 30-day dose escalation study of the EGFR was performed with 12 patients undergoing surgical resection of squamous cell carcinoma. Multi-instrument fluorescence imaging was performed in the operating room and in surgical pathology. Fluorescence levels positively correlated with EGFR levels, and results showed that fluorescence imaging with an intraoperative, wide-field device can successfully differentiate tumor from normal tissue during resection (average tumor-to-background ratio of 5.2 in the highest dose range). This study is the first to demonstrate that commercially available antibodies can be fluorescently labeled and safely administered to humans to identify cancer with submillimeter resolution, which has the potential to improve outcomes in clinical oncology.

Narrow band imaging is another type of optical imaging technology, typically integrated in an endoscopy system that can display the mucosal surface layer in high contrast, especially hemoglobin-rich areas such as blood vessels and microvascular patterns. Magnifying endoscopy (ME) enhances the capabilities of standard video endoscopy with higher resolution and higher contrast, compared to endoscopes with NBI used in otolaryngology, such as ENF-VQ and ENF-VH (Olympus Medical Systems, Tokyo, Japan) [23]. Researchers have shown that ME-NBI enables detection of early superficial laryngopharyngeal cancers, which are difficult to detect by standard endoscopy or nonmagnifying endoscopy with NBI [24]. For transoral robotic surgery (TORS), Tateya et al. report two advantages of using ME-NBI [25]. One is that the combination facilitates early diagnosis of pharyngeal cancers, and the detection of superficial lesions is expected to increase with the advent of ME-NBI. The second advantage is associated with improved resection of invasive cancer lesions. ME-NBI provides improved lesion boundary visualization, which will be beneficial in avoiding excessive resection. This is especially helpful for the superficial part of the invasive cancer, thus resulting in better functional outcomes, such as swallowing and voice function. The limitation of ME-NBI is that it is not useful for examining deeper tissue beneath the epithelium. Thus pathological diagnosis via biopsy is therefore still necessary for checking the vertical margin.

20.2.2 Intraoperative Navigation Through Registration and Visualization

20.2.2.1 Registration

A common form of navigation in surgery for head and neck registers preoperative image data (i.e., diagnostic CT, MRI) using either optical or electromagnetic (EM) technology. In this context, registration is the spatial alignment of a medical image data set to the coordinate system of the patient and/or operating room. Commercially available optical and EM systems have had the most success in workspaces with rigid structures, such as skull base surgery, craniomaxillofacial surgery, and neurosurgery [26, 27]. Intraoperatively, these guidance systems provide real-time tracking of a pointer or other tools with respect to the registered image data. The accuracy attainable with optical systems in clinic has been reported to be approximately 2 mm in target registration error [28]; however studies using EM tracking in clinical settings have noted higher errors [29]. Optical systems generally provide better spatial uniformity with a larger field of view than EM solutions, which are subject to interference from magnetic objects and stray electromagnetic fields [30]. The major disadvantage of an optical system is the requirement of line of sight between the camera and the tracked markers. Although each of these conventional platforms has individual trade-offs and potential deficiencies, they have been readily applied in image-guided surgical interventions [31].

For example, in 2008, Desai et al. [32] presented a series of three case studies using EM-based tracking to guide transoral resection of oropharyngeal and pharyngeal space lesions. Using the Brainlab EM-tracking system (Munich, Germany), preoperative CT was registered to the patient through identification of bony landmarks. This allowed surgeons to localize an intraoperative pointer with respect to the preoperative CT throughout the procedure. The study showed that the provided guidance was especially helpful in assessing the anatomy during the dissection, particularly in the deep lateral parapharyngeal space close to the carotid artery and lateral pharyngeal wall. The limitation, other than the technical disadvantages of EM tracking as discussed above, is the reliance on preoperative data, which does not account for intraoperative deformations. Additionally, the guidance provided is viewed separately from the primary visual field and must be mentally correlated.

While rigid registration is arguably solved with optical and EM systems, deformable workspaces, where nonrigid changes necessitate an update to the preoperative surgical plan, continue to challenge researchers. For example, in transoral base of tongue surgery, deformations begin with setup: the patient's neck is flexed, with the mouth open and tongue retracted. To capture these setup deformations for TORS, Liu et al. [33, 34] experimented with the alignment of preoperative CT to presurgical CBCT. Reaungamornrat et al. [35] developed a four-step nonrigid transformation, where a volume of interest (e.g., tongue and hyoid bone) is segmented in both the moving image (i.e., CT) and the fixed image (i.e., CBCT). These segmentation "masks" provide surface meshes from which two point clouds are defined. First, a Gaussian mixture (GM) [36] registration is used to compute a rigid initial global alignment of the two point clouds. Second, a GM nonrigid registration uses a thin-plate spline approach to perform deformable alignment of the point clouds. For both the moving and fixed mask, a distance transform [37] (DT) consisting of the distance of each voxel to the surface mesh is computed in step three. Lastly, in the fourth step, a fast-symmetric-force variant of the Demons algorithm [38] is applied to register the two DTs. Operating on distance transforms allows the combined registration module to be intensity-invariant and thereby supports registration of surgical CAD/CAM derived from other modalities, such as MRI, in addition to CT. Aside from this hybrid approach, many other deformable registration methods exist and substantiate further investigation for otolaryngology, but are beyond the scope of this chapter.

20.2.2.2 Visualization

Viewing navigational data in interventional suites can be accomplished through a variety of mediums. Traditional imaging systems present their images on a 2D computer monitor, which requires the clinician to mentally register the given information with the operative scene. However, navigational information can be absorbed through audio, visual, and haptic means with obvious advantages through fusion of multiple sources of information. For example, we can overlay live fluoroscopy onto 3D volumes from CBCT angiographies. However, in endoscopic head and neck interventions, direct overlay of navigational information onto video images [26] provides a more natural integration with the primary visual displays. Video augmentation has been shown to be advantageous in monocular endoscopic skull base procedures [39], while stereoscopic augmented reality has been realized in operating microscopes and robotic surgical case studies [40]. With the advent of 3D visualization in consumer products (e.g., Google glass, Microsoft HoloLens, Magic Leap, etc.), the millennial generation of surgeons and patients can expect visualization to advance in these directions.

For robotic surgery in otolaryngology, similar methods of navigation through video augmentation have been explored for cochlear implant [41], TORS studies using ex vivo animal and cadaveric models [33, 34], and clinical TORS with retrospective analysis [40]. In 2012, in a single clinical case study for TORS, Pratt et al. [40] augmented the da Vinci stereoscopic view by manually aligning models of segmented anatomy derived from preoperative plans. Their retrospective analysis of procedure footage noted beneficial opportunities for guidance in TORS along with observations that the degree of tongue muscle deformation induced by gag placement is significant. The need to bridge the gap between preoperative images and intraoperative setup was further emphasized with ex vivo studies by Liu et al. [33, 34]. Using porcine tongue phantoms, they tasked a TORS surgeon with placing pins into embedded targets in order to evaluate target localization using varied methods of image guidance: (1) Simulated current practice with preoperative images on a computer monitor. (2) Intraoperative images on a computer monitor. (3) Video augmentation with intraoperative images. Experiments not only showed a statistically significant improvement in target localization error when comparing (1) to (3) (4.9 ± 4.6 mm to 1.7 ± 1.8 mm, respectively, when measured from the edge of the target), but improvements from (1) to (2) also showed the value of navigating with intraoperative imaging, as compared to relying on preoperative data.

The experiments from Liu et al. [34] further highlight one of the main challenges in augmented reality, namely, stereopsis, or depth perception. Incorrect stereopsis has been a topic of discussion since the 1990s, as researchers noted natural spatial errors affecting virtual reality when systems portrayed 3D space using a 2D display [42]. Poor calibration or registration amplifies stereopsis incorrectly, and the user will empirically observe that virtual anatomy appears to be detached and floating in front of the real scene. To counter such effects, Bichlmeier et al. [43] adjusted the transparency according to the position and line of sight of the observer, creating a significantly improved fusion of virtual objects to a realistic viewpoint in the scene. To directly address ambiguity in stereopsis for TORS, Liu et al. [44] extended their video augmentation guidance system with tool localization. Using the joint values of the robotic arm, their system tracked the primary surgical tool and communicating explicit depth information, with respective to tool localization, through dynamic color changes of virtual anatomical models. Further details of their experiment are discussed below in 20.3.

20.3 Preclinical Studies of Intraoperative Imaging and Navigation in Robotic Surgery

20.3.1 C-arm and Flat-Panel Cone Beam Computed Tomography (CBCT)

Continued advancements in imaging and robotics have led to the development of hybrid operating rooms with integrated intraoperative imaging systems (e.g., ultrasound, fluoroscopy, and cone beam computed tomography) with minimally invasive surgical systems (e.g., robotics, laparoscopy, and endoscopy) [18]. The design of these advanced ORs must consider functional needs in order to accommodate different perioperative setups and workflows [45]. The workspace for C-arms may range from mobile bases to ceiling- or floor-mounted systems. Image quality and resolution differ widely, with older technology using image intensifiers to newer technology using motor-actuated flat-panel detectors that are synchronized with an X-ray source. Thus, the imaging capabilities of intraoperative C-arms can vary from single 2D planar X-rays images to 3D reconstructed volumes (e.g., CBCT [33, 34, 41, 46]).

Room setup and surgical workflow are even more complex in cases that involve both CBCT and robotic assistance. In designing a hybrid operating room, the "free" or available workspace, after surgical setup, shared between an imaging system and a surgical robotic system, must be evaluated. For otolaryngology, workspace ergonomics were explored in a 2015 preclinical study of the Artis zeego (Siemens AG, Berlin, Germany) and a da Vinci Si (Intuitive Surgical Inc., Sunnyvale, CA) as an extension of experiments conducted by Liu et al. [44] in 2015. Their experimental setup (Fig. 20.1a) showed that a full CBCT can be acquired with the base of the da Vinci® patient-side cart (PSC) positioned for intervention, however, with all robotic arms retracted. The ability to acquire a full CBCT image without repositioning the PSC (with robotic arms retracted) was also confirmed in an investigation for intraoperative CBCT guidance for a cadaveric cochlear implant [41] (Fig. 20.1d). Therefore, their work showed that the free workspace for these two procedures supports intraoperative CBCT acquisition.

In the TORS experiments, Liu et al. [44] injected two synthetic tumors into the base of tongue of in vivo porcine models and ex vivo porcine tongue models. Using the da Vinci® and zeego setup above, they obtained a presurgical CBCT angiography, which allowed them to derive models of segmented critical anatomy after surgical positioning. Segmentations included the lingual arteries, synthetic tongue resection targets (centroid and boundary), registration fiducials, oral tongue, and tongue base volume. A head and neck surgeon, proficient in TORS, performed mock tumor resections (with and without video augmentation as guidance) with the goal of achieving a 10 mm margin while controlling the lingual artery. Similar to Pratt et al. [40], in experiments with video guidance, the models of critical anatomy were directly displayed as a transparent overlay in the stereoscopic viewport. However, in contrast to the preoperative data and manual updates used by Pratt et al., these images captured surgical setup and were automatically updated by using the joint values of the robotic camera arm.

In addition to the overlay of critical anatomy, the guidance system also tracked the primary surgical tool (5 mm monopolar cautery) and rendered a virtual transparent sphere at an offset to the tip. The color of the sphere changed from green, to yellow, to red, when the estimated distance from tracked sphere was <=2 mm outside of the margin, inside the margin by 2 mm, and inside the margin by 4 mm, respectively (Fig. 20.2, center target sphere is green, indicating a desired distance <=2 mm outside of the margin). In addition, a quantitative depth gauge was shown on the tool calipers, displaying the estimated relative distance to the target (Fig. 20.2, white numeric label on end effector). To further disambiguate depth, not just for the tool tip, they implemented a novel supplemental view of tracked tools. This auxiliary camera perspective, rendered picture-in-picture, could be changed dynamically but was observed to be most useful when displaying the lateral left-to-right sagittal plane, orthogonal to the camera plane (Fig. 20.2, lower left-hand corner). Results from ex vivo and in vivo porcine models measuring resection ratios showed improved resection efficiency, when comparing current practice to their proposed dynamic visual navigation with explicit stereoscopic depth information. Compared to previous literature, these studies uniquely integrate continuous augmented visual guidance in 3D in the primary visual field for robotics in otolaryngology.

The limitation from this experiment is the lack of continuous imaging updates to capture deformation from resection as the intervention progressed. However, in this setup (similar for da Vinci®-assisted cochlear implantation [41]), with the robotic arms positioned for intervention, they verified that the zeego C-arm can still achieve a scan range of ~40°. Thus, in these surgical scenarios, live dual 2D X-ray fluoroscopy images have the potential to apply and provide not only real-time planar projection of the resection throughout the procedure but also stereotactic triangulation, which is useful for tool localization [44]. More confidence can be achieved by visualization of the workspace throughout intervention than by factoring in the known error of registration to pre-resection scans. In a follow-up study, workspace ergonomics of the single-port da Vinci® Sp and the zeego were investigated further using a configuration for transoral intervention (Fig. 20.3). In these experiments, a cadaveric model was injected with synthetic tumors, and presurgical CBCT angiography (CBCTA) images were obtained. From these images, the carotid arteries were identified (Fig. 20.3d), and experienced TORS surgeons were able to successfully remove the tumor with and without guidance (live fluoroscopic overlay onto CBCTA (Fig. 20.3c)).

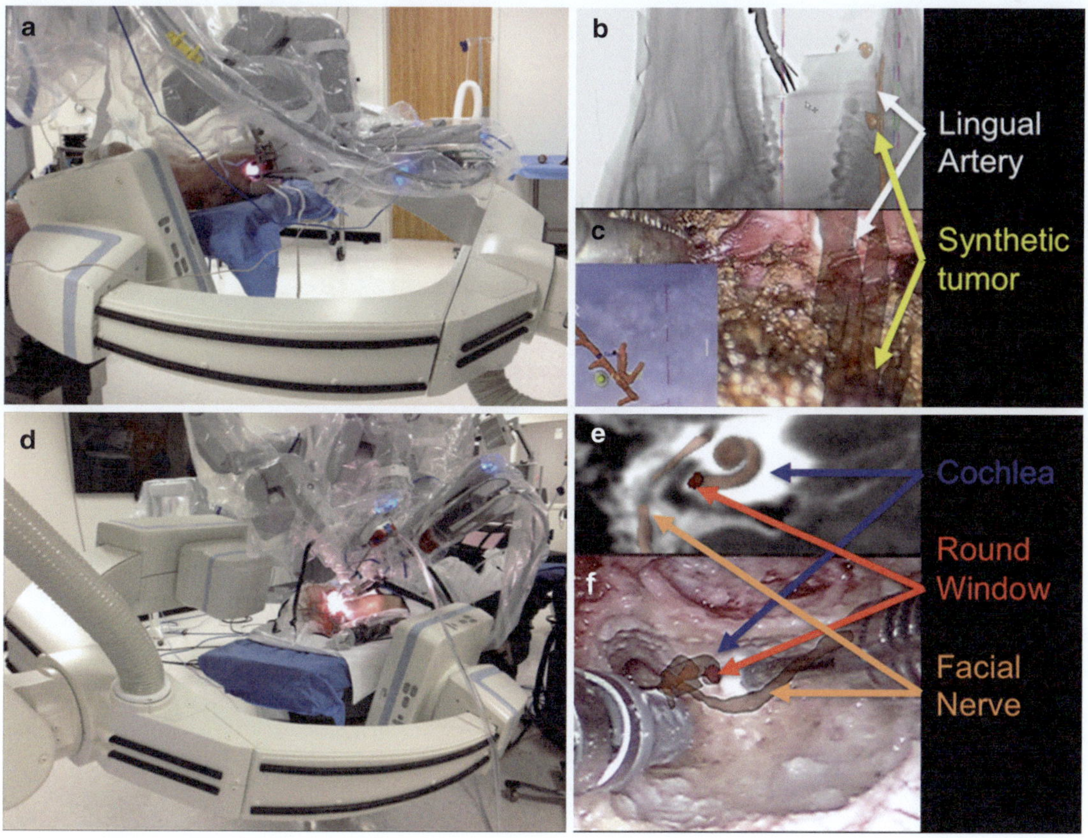

Fig. 20.1 Photographs of the da Vinci Si-zeego workspace. (**a**) Configuration for transoral robotic surgery using an in vivo porcine phantom with (**b**) fluoroscopy and (**c**) video augmentation. (**d**) Configuration for cochlear implant using a cadaveric phantom with (**e**) segmented critical structures from CBCT and (**f**) video augmentation

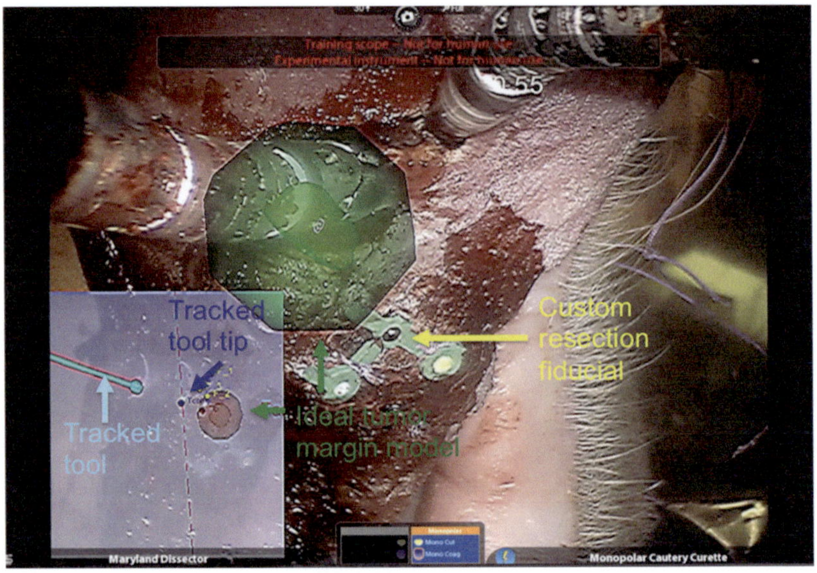

Fig. 20.2 Screen capture of an ex vivo phantom experiment using video augmentation of margins and tool tracking in a novel view (*lower left picture-in-picture*) for image guidance. The spherical representation of an ideal margin is green since tool tip is within +2 mm proximity (Initially published in IJORS 2015)

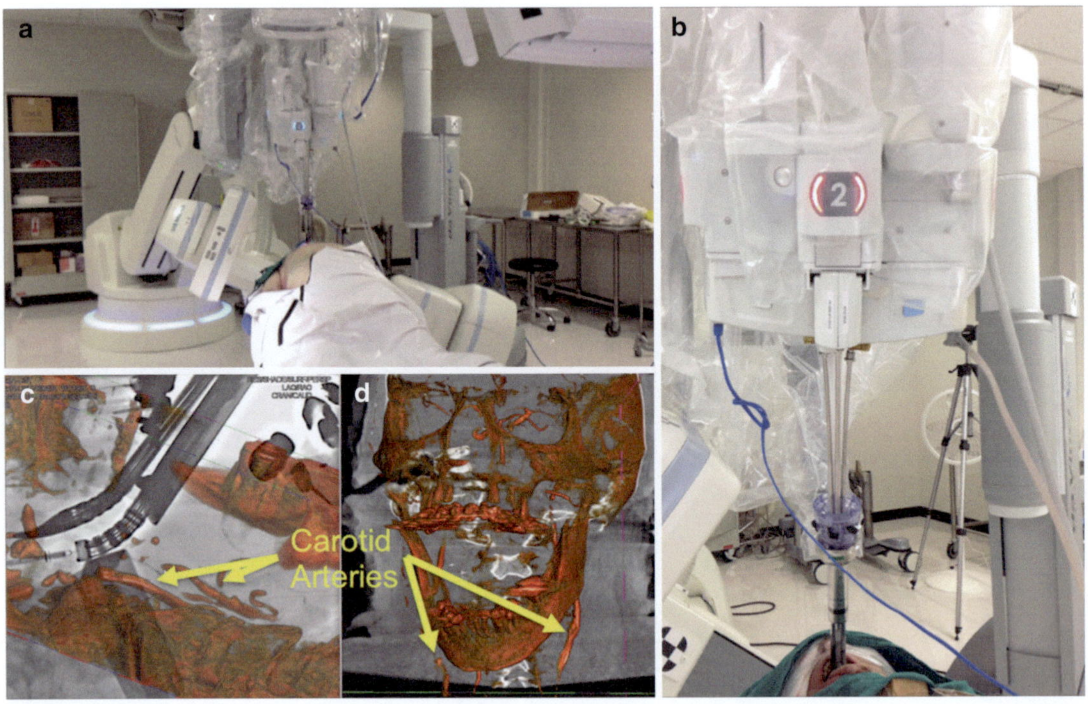

Fig. 20.3 (**a**, **b**) Photographs of the da Vinci Sp-zeego workspace configuration for transoral robotic surgery using a cadaveric phantom. (**c**) Fluoroscopy overlay on CBCTA. (**d**) Single sagittal slice viewed with intraoperative CBCTA reconstruction

20.4 Clinical Studies of Intraoperative Imaging and Navigation in Robotic Surgery

20.4.1 Ultrasound

Adaptation of commercial ultrasound systems for intraoperative imaging in head and neck surgery has been demonstrated in robotic case studies. In 2015, Goepfert et al. [47] used an endocavity transducer for intraoperative imaging in a single complex reoperative TORS case study. Their patient, previously treated with total thyroidectomy, with left central and lateral neck dissection, was found to have an isolated 2.6 cm left retropharyngeal nodal metastasis on MRI (confirmed to be papillary thyroid carcinoma on fine needle aspiration biopsy). After intubation and prior to the incision, the ultrasound guidance assisted in localizing the node in its location lateral to the superior constrictor muscle and medial to the internal carotid artery and jugular vein and aided in the placement of the mucosal incision and planning of the subsequent dissection with the da Vinci® system.

In comparison, Clayburgh et al. [48] used the Aloka Alpha 7 ultrasound system (Hitachi Aloka Medical, Ltd., Wallingford, CT) with various ultrasound probes to guide six da Vinci-assisted TORS cases. For applications in the posterior and lateral oropharynx (e.g., tonsillar fossa, parapharyngeal space), a neuro-spine straight ultrasound probe was used. In order to image the lateral and posterior pharyngeal walls, the robotic arms were removed from the patient's mouth while the camera was left in position, and the ultrasound probe was inserted alongside the camera. For the base of tongue, a liver ultrasound probe was used instead. This probe is aligned at a 90° angle and has a small tab on its backside that could be grasped with the Maryland dissector on the robotic arm. Thus, while imaging the tongue base with this probe, at least one and potentially both robotic arms could remain in place. US images, displayed in the TilePro™ screen of the surgeon side console, were primarily used to identify vascular anatomy. For example, in a case involving a 78-year-old female presenting with a superficially invasive squamous cell carcinoma of the left tonsil and lateral pharyngeal wall with extension to the tongue base, surgeons visualized the pulsation of the carotid system as well as other vessels near the lesion. These studies noted that real-time US images were particularly helpful in identifying larger-caliber blood vessels within the operative field prior to encountering them visually and in delineation of margin in deep tumor resections. The primary limitation of these experiments is the visualization gap between imaging and endoscope.

20.4.2 Optical Imaging

In 2014, Tateya et al. [24] reported the first clinical study combining ME-NBI with TORS in a treatment of squamous cell carcinoma on the base of tongue. A superficial cancer lesion, about 1.5 cm in diameter, was identified in the left side of the tongue base with an otolaryngological videoendoscope with NBI (ENF-type VQ). NBI clearly visualized the lesion as a brownish area, whereas the lesion was hardly recognizable under white light. For this patient, the cancer lesion was not recognizable by computed tomography, magnetic resonance imaging, or positron emission tomography (PET). Neither neck lymph node metastasis nor distant metastasis was found on CT, MRI, or PET. The lesion was clinically diagnosed as T1N0M0.

Prior to surgery, ME-NBI visualized the flat lesion as a brownish area with scattered dots of abnormal vessels, which were invisible in white light. The boundary of the tumor was easily traceable with ME-NBI. The extent of the lesion was confirmed by iodine staining. Boundary markings of the lesion and an incision line at the lower boundary of the lesion were made with the electric needle knife, and the procedure was switched to TORS using the da Vinci® Surgical System. Successful tongue base resection, with a depth and safety margin of 5 mm (confirmed by a negative margin in the frozen sections), was conducted by two cooperating gastroenterologists using the 8 mm Maryland dissector and 8 mm monopolar cautery. No neck dissection was performed. In this case, combining ME-NBI with TORS made it possible to estimate the horizontal extent of the superficial lesion precisely, which was beneficial in determining the extent of resection.

20.5 Related Clinical Research

20.5.1 Ultrasound

Studies at Johns Hopkins Hospital have evaluated the feasibility of using intraoperative, transcervical ultrasound concurrently with TORS at the base of tongue. Blanco et al. [49] hypothesized that transcervical ultrasound could provide clinically relevant characteristics that may not otherwise be appreciable. In their study of 22 patients with suspected BOT tumors in comparison to 18 controls, 100 % of BOT tumors were visualized with US. Using a transcervical probe, 90.9 % and 95.5 % of the BOT tumors were found to be hypoechoic and exhibiting irregular margins, respectively. Their results show that ultrasound could be used to characterize adjacent site involvement, midline, and endophytic extent, in addition to visualizing the lingual artery.

20.5.2 Optical Imaging

In optical imaging for otolaryngology, researchers have shown extensive interest in the application of ICG for interventional imaging. In parapharyngeal space tumor resections, Yokoyama et al. [50] observed fluorescent images of ICG injected via the cephalic vein using the HyperEye Medical System (MIZUHO Corporation Tokyo, Japan). At 10–30 min after injection, they confirmed the visibility of bright fluorescence emission with all tumors, including those behind the carotid artery, lower cranial nerves, and submucosal tumors hidden under fascia. Nakamura et al. [51] compared cervical sentinel node biopsies using the standard technique (blue dye and a gamma probe) in 20 basins of 18 patients (group A) and using fluorescence navigation along with the standard technique in 12 basins of 16 patients (group B). The detection rate of sentinel nodes was 83 % (29/35 in group A) and 95 % (36/38 in group B), while the false-negative rate was 6 % (1/18 patients in group A) and 0 % (in group B). In another study, Betz et al. [52] recruited 11 patients with free flap reconstructions of the upper aerodigestive tract to undergo ICG fluorescence angiography. Results showed feasibility of providing guidance with real-time information about the perfusion state of the tissue without greater patient discomfort or risk of side effect.

ICG characterization of tissue perfusion has also been applied to guide intraoperative decision-making in complicated reconstructions in otolaryngology. Lee et al. [53] conducted a pilot study using intraoperative laser-assisted ICG imaging measurements and fluorescence videos to objectively measure the benefit of vascular delay procedures in patients with head and neck defects and wound healing risk factors requiring locoregional flap reconstruction. Two patients were identified based on comorbid conditions that resulted in a higher risk of flap failure, as well as the need for a locoregional flap for reconstruction. At the initial elevation of the flap, quantitative results from flap imaging demonstrated low perfusion numbers and minimal fluorescence, suggesting poor tissue perfusion and increased likelihood of postoperative flap compromise or failure. Following a vascular delay of 3 weeks, repeat measurements were substantially improved.

These studies not only show the potential of ICG but also active clinical interest for its usage for interventional purposes in otolaryngology. Historically, obtaining Food and Drug Administration (FDA) approval for routine clinical use of such promising agents has been difficult to achieve [18]. For example, although ICG's natural excretion path is through the hepatobiliary system, Intuitive Surgical had to run a new clinical trial to receive approval to use its Firefly Fluorescence system for cholangiography [54]. Furthermore, clinicians routinely use ICG for lymph node detection in a variety of anatomic locations, as recommended in the National Comprehensive Cancer Network guidelines; however, no organization has sought FDA approval due to the high cost of trials. Another fluorescence agent, methylene blue, visualized with white light, has consistently shown added value for localization during neck dissection [55], but is not currently FDA approved for any use. These clinical use scenarios, along with the applications of ICG discussed above, are considered to be off-label by US regulatory agencies. More sufficient and consistent evidence showing the impacts of these methods is necessary in order to justify their use in routine clinical practice.

Conclusion

Head and neck surgery has seen tremendous technical advances over the last decade in minimally invasive approaches to the upper aerodigestive track and neck as well as the introduction and widespread adoption of robotic platforms. Literature reviewed in this chapter has highlighted how intraoperative imaging can identify and preserve adjacent neurovascular structures of the retropharyngeal and parapharyngeal spaces while maximizing and the adequacy of resection. Certainly, as technology continues to evolve, the ability to treat pathology with greater precision and less morbidity will follow. Nonetheless, various challenges remain, including the use of very large robotic systems without haptic feedback while operating in the narrow, deep confines of the head and neck, which can be disorienting. Image-guided navigation offers a promising tool to overcome these limitations by providing the surgeon with augmented visual information regarding the surgical environment. Clearly, researchers are pushing to adapt and evaluate diagnostic and preoperative techniques for navigation in robotic surgery for otolaryngology. Exciting but limited preclinical studies and clinical case studies demonstrate the potential utility of these systems. The widespread application and cost-effectiveness of such technology remain to be seen.

References

1. Abdullah A, Mahmud MR, Maimunah A, Zulfiqar MA, Saim L, Mazlan R. Preoperative high resolution CT and MR imaging in cochlear implantation. Ann Acad Med Singap. 2003;32:442–5.
2. Sahani D, Mehta A, Blake M, Prasad S, Harris G, Saini S. Preoperative hepatic vascular evaluation with CT and MR angiography: implications for surgery. Radiographics. 2004;24:1367–80.
3. Ozsarlak O, Tjalma W, Schepens E, Corthouts B, Op de Beeck B, Van Marck E, Parizel PM, De Schepper AM. The correlation of preoperative CT, MR imaging, and clinical staging (FIGO) with histopathology findings in primary cervical carcinoma. Eur Radiol. 2003;13:2338–45.
4. Cheng L, Cao R, Meng G, Huang Q, Hou D, Hu L. Application of computer assisted navigation system in endoscopic sinus and skull base surgery. Lin Chung Er Bi Yan Hou Tou Jing Wai Ke Za Zhi. 2012;26:796–8.
5. Goding Jr GS, Tesfayesus W, Kezirian EJ. Hypoglossal nerve stimulation and airway changes under fluoroscopy. Otolaryngol Head Neck Surg. 2012;146:1017–22.
6. Conley DB, Tan B, Bendok BR, Batjer HH, Chandra R, Sidle D, Rahme RJ, Adel JG, Fishman AJ. Comparison of intraoperative portable CT scanners in skull base and endoscopic sinus surgery: single center case series. Skull Base: Off J North Am Skull Base Soc [et al]. 2011;21:261–70.
7. Pfeiffer J, Kayser G, Ridder GJ. Sonography-assisted cutting needle biopsy in the head and neck for the diagnosis of lymphoma: can it replace lymph node extirpation? Laryngoscope. 2009;119:689–95.
8. Helbig M, Krysztoforski K, Krowicki P, Helbig S, Gstoettner W, Kozak J. Development of prototype for navigated real-time sonography for the head and neck region. Head Neck. 2008;30:215–21.
9. Wakasugi-Sato N, Kodama M, Matsuo K, Yamamoto N, Oda M, Ishikawa A, Tanaka T, Seta Y, Habu M, Kokuryo S, Ichimiya H, Miyamoto I, Kito S, Matsumoto-Takeda S, Wakasugi T, Yamashita Y, Yoshioka I, Takahashi T, Tominaga K, Morimoto Y. Advanced clinical usefulness of ultrasonography for diseases in oral and maxillofacial regions. Int J Dent. 2010;2010:639382.
10. Eida S, Sumi M, Yonetsu K, Kimura Y, Nakamura T. Combination of helical CT and Doppler sonography in the follow-up of patients with clinical N0 stage neck disease and oral cancer. AJNR Am J Neuroradiol. 2003;24:312–8.
11. Miyashita T, Tateno A, Ablimit I, Nakamizo M, Kumazaki T, Yagi T. Ultrasonographic demonstration of retropharyngeal lymph nodes: preliminary report. Ultrasound Med Biol. 2003;29:633–6.
12. Fornage BD, Edeiken BS, Clayman GL. Use of transoral sonography with an endocavitary transducer in diagnosis, fine-needle aspiration biopsy, and

intraoperative localization of retropharyngeal masses. AJR Am J Roentgenol. 2014;202:W481–6.
13. Isa K, Yasaka M, Kimura K, Nagatsuka K, Minematsu K. Transoral carotid ultrasonography for evaluating internal carotid artery occlusion. Intern Med. 2005;44:567–71.
14. Chen CN, Lin CY, Ko JY, Lou PJ, Wang CP, Chen TC, Hsiao TY, Yang TL. Application of ultrasound-guided core biopsy as a novel diagnostic tool for base of tongue cancer: our experiences with ten patients. Clin Otolaryngol: Off J ENT-UK; Off J Netherlands Soc Oto-Rhino-Laryngol Cervico-Facial Surg. 2015;34:1537–46.
15. Meacham RK, Boughter Jr JD, Sebelik ME. Ultrasound-guided fine-needle aspiration of the tongue base: a cadaver feasibility study. Otolaryngol Head Neck Surg. 2012;147:864–9.
16. Osher J, Jerjes W, Upile T, Hamdoon Z, Morley S, Hopper C. Adenoid cystic carcinoma of the tongue base treated with ultrasound-guided interstitial photodynamic therapy: a case study. Photodiagn Photodyn Ther. 2011;8:68–71.
17. Lesnik D, Cunnane ME, Zurakowski D, Acar GO, Ecevit C, Mace A, Kamani D, Randolph GW. Papillary thyroid carcinoma nodal surgery directed by a preoperative radiographic map utilizing CT scan and ultrasound in all primary and reoperative patients. Head Neck. 2014;36:191–202.
18. Fong Y, Giulianotti PC, Lewis J, Koerkamp BG, Reiner T. Imaging and visualization in the modern operating room. New York: Springer.
19. Daskalaki D, Aguilera F, Patton K, Giulianotti PC. Fluorescence in robotic surgery. J Surg Oncol. 2015;112:250–6.
20. Autorino R, Zargar H, White WM, Novara G, Annino F, Perdona S, De Angelis M, Mottrie A, Porpiglia F, Kaouk JH. Current applications of near-infrared fluorescence imaging in robotic urologic surgery: a systematic review and critical analysis of the literature. Urology. 2014;84:751–9.
21. Bjurlin MA, Gan M, McClintock TR, Volpe A, Borofsky MS, Mottrie A, Stifelman MD. Near-infrared fluorescence imaging: emerging applications in robotic upper urinary tract surgery. Eur Urol. 2014;65:793–801.
22. Rosenthal EL, Warram JM, de Boer E, Chung TK, Korb ML, Brandwein-Gensler M, Strong TV, Schmalbach CE, Morlandt AB, Agarwal G, Hartman YE, Carroll WR, Richman JS, Clemons LK, Nabell LM, Zinn KR. Safety and tumor specificity of cetuximab-IRDye800 for surgical navigation in head and neck cancer. Clin Cancer Res. 2015;21:3658–66.
23. Muto M, Nakane M, Katada C, Sano Y, Ohtsu A, Esumi H, Ebihara S, Yoshida S. Squamous cell carcinoma in situ at oropharyngeal and hypopharyngeal mucosal sites. Cancer. 2004;101:1375–81.
24. Tateya I, Ishikawa S, Morita S, Ito H, Sakamoto T, Murayama T, Kishimoto Y, Hayashi T, Funakoshi M, Hirano S, Kitamura M, Morita M, Muto M, Ito J. Magnifying endoscopy with narrow band imaging to determine the extent of resection in transoral robotic surgery of oropharyngeal cancer. Case Rep Otolaryngol. 2014;2014:604737.
25. Tateya I, Morita S, Muto M, Miyamoto S, Hayashi T, Funakoshi M, Aoyama I, Hirano S, Kitamura M, Ishikawa S, Kishimoto Y, Morita M, Mahattanasakul P, Morita S, Ito J. Magnifying endoscope with NBI to predict the depth of invasion in laryngo-pharyngeal cancer. Laryngoscope. 2015;125:1124–9.
26. Varma TR, Eldridge P. Use of the NeuroMate stereotactic robot in a frameless mode for functional neurosurgery. Int J Med Robot Comp Assist Surg: MRCAS. 2006;2:107–13.
27. Ecke U, Luebben B, Maurer J, Boor S, Mann WJ. Comparison of different computer-aided surgery systems in skull base surgery. Skull Base: Off J North Am Skull Base Soc ... [et al.]. 2003;13:43–50.
28. Yaniv Z, Wilson E, Lindisch D, Cleary K. Electromagnetic tracking in the clinical environment. Med Phys. 2009;36:876–92.
29. Hauser R, Westermann B. Optical tracking of a microscope for image-guided intranasal sinus surgery. Ann Otol Rhinol Laryngol. 1999;108:54–62.
30. Glossop ND. Advantages of optical compared with electromagnetic tracking. J Bone Joint Surg Am. 2009;91(Suppl 1):23–8.
31. Cleary K, Peters TM. Image-guided interventions: technology review and clinical applications. Annu Rev Biomed Eng. 2010;12:119–42.
32. Desai SC, Sung CK, Genden EM. Transoral robotic surgery using an image guidance system. Laryngoscope. 2008;118:2003–5.
33. Liu WP, Reaugamornrat S, Deguet A, Sorger JM, Siewerdsen JH, Richmon J, Taylor RH. Toward intraoperative image-guided transoral robotic surgery. J Robot Surg. 2013;7:217–25.
34. Liu WP, Reaugamornrat S, Sorger JM, Siewerdsen JH, Taylor RH, Richmon JD. Intraoperative image-guided transoral robotic surgery: pre-clinical studies. Int J Med Robot Comp Assist Surg: MRCAS. 2014;11:256–67.
35. Reaungamornrat S, Liu WP, Wang AS, Otake Y, Nithiananthan S, Uneri A, Schafer S, Tryggestad E, Richmon J, Sorger JM, Siewerdsen JH, Taylor RH. Deformable image registration for cone-beam CT guided transoral robotic base-of-tongue surgery. Phys Med Biol. 2013;58:4951–79.
36. Jian B, Vemuri BC. Robust point set registration using gaussian mixture models. IEEE pattern analysis and machine. Intelligence. 2011;33:1633–45.
37. Maurer Jr CR, Rensheng Q, Raghavan V. A linear time algorithm for computing exact Euclidean distance transforms of binary images in arbitrary dimensions. IEEE Pattern Analysis and Machine. Intelligence. 2003;25:265–70.
38. Vercauteren T, Pennec X, Malis E, Perchant A, Ayache N. Insight into efficient image registration techniques and the demons algorithm. Proc Inf Process Med Imaging. 2007;4584:495–506.
39. Balicki M, Xia T, Jung MY, Deguet A, Vagvolgyi B, Kazanzides P, Taylor, R. "Prototyping a hybrid

cooperative and tele-robotic surgical system for retinal microsurgery", in MICCAI workshop on systems and architectures for computer assisted interventions, Toronto, Sept. 18, 2011. p. Available online in Insight (Online Journal) [http://www.midasjournal.org/browse/publication/815]. PMCID: PMC3880681.
40. Pratt P, Edwards E, Arora A, Tolley N, Darzi AW, Yang G-Z. Image-guided transoral robotic surgery for the treatment of oropharyngeal cancer. In: Hamlyn Symposium. 2012.
41. Liu WP, Azizian M, Sorger J, Taylor RH, Reilly BK, Cleary K, Preciado D. Cadaveric feasibility study of da Vinci Si-assisted cochlear implant with augmented visual navigation for otologic surgery. JAMA Otolaryngol: Head Neck Surg. 2014;140:208–14.
42. Wann JP, Rushton S, Mon-Williams M. Natural problems for stereoscopic depth perception in virtual environments. Vis Res. 1995;35:2731–6.
43. Bichlmeier C, Wimme F, Heining SM, Navab N. Contextual anatomic mimesis hybrid in-situ visualization method for improving multi-sensory depth perception in medical augmented reality. In: IEEE and ACM International Symposium on Mixed and Augmented Reality. 2007. p. 129–38.
44. Liu WP, Richmon JD, Sorger JM, Azizian M, Taylor RH. Augmented reality and cone beam CT guidance for transoral robotic surgery. J Robot Surg. 2015;9:223–33.
45. Hufner T, Citak M, Imrecke J, Krettek C, Stubig T. Handling modern imaging procedures in a high-tech operating room. Der Unfallchirurg. 2012;115:220–5.
46. Liu WP, Otake Y, Azizian M, Wagner OJ, Sorger JM, Armand M, Taylor RH. 2D-3D radiograph to cone-beam computed tomography (CBCT) registration for C-arm image-guided robotic surgery. Int J Comput Assist Radiol Surg. 2015;10(8):1239–52.
47. Goepfert RP, Liu C, Ryan WR. Trans-oral robotic surgery and surgeon-performed trans-oral ultrasound for intraoperative location and excision of an isolated retropharyngeal lymph node metastasis of papillary thyroid carcinoma. Am J Otolaryngol. 2015;36:710–4.
48. Clayburgh DR, Byrd JK, Bonfili J, Duvvuri U. Intraoperative ultrasonography during transoral robotic surgery. Ann Otol Rhinol Laryngol. 2015; 125(1):37–42.
49. Blanco RG, Califano J, Messing B, Richmon J, Liu J, Quon H, Neuner G, Saunders J, Ha PK, Sheth S, Gillison M, Fakhry C. Transcervical ultrasonography is feasible to visualize and evaluate base of tongue cancers. PLoS One. 2014;9:e87565.
50. Yokoyama J, Ooba S, Fujimaki M, Anzai T, Yoshii R, Kojima M, Ikeda K. Impact of indocyanine green fluorescent image-guided surgery for parapharyngeal space tumours. J Cranio-Maxillo-Facial Surg: Off Publ Eur Assoc Cranio-Maxillo-Facial Surg. 2014;42:835–8.
51. Nakamura Y, Fujisawa Y, Nakamura Y, Maruyama H, Furuta J, Kawachi Y, Otsuka F. Improvement of the sentinel lymph node detection rate of cervical sentinel lymph node biopsy using real-time fluorescence navigation with indocyanine green in head and neck skin cancer. J Dermatol. 2013;40:453–7.
52. Betz CS, Zhorzel S, Schachenmayr H, Stepp H, Havel M, Siedek V, Leunig A, Matthias C, Hopper C, Harreus U. Endoscopic measurements of free-flap perfusion in the head and neck region using red-excited indocyanine green: preliminary results. J plast Reconstr Aesth Surg: JPRAS. 2009;62:1602–8.
53. Lee LN, Smith DF, Boahene KD, Byrne PJ. Intraoperative laser-assisted indocyanine green imaging for objective measurement of the vascular delay technique in locoregional head and neck flaps. JAMA Facial Plast Surg. 2014;16:343–7.
54. Intuitive Surgical, I.: 510 (k) Summary (21 CFR 807.92(c)). 2013.
55. Candell L, Campbell MJ, Shen WT, Gosnell JE, Clark OH, Duh QY. Ultrasound-guided methylene blue dye injection for parathyroid localization in the reoperative neck. World J Surg. 2014;38:88–91.

21 Management of the Neck for Oropharyngeal Squamous Cell Carcinoma in the Era of Transoral Robotic-Assisted Surgery (TORS)

Rajarsi Mandal, Ian Ganly, and Snehal G. Patel

21.1 Introduction

In recent years, transoral robotic-assisted surgery (TORS) has revolutionized the surgical management of malignant tumors of the oropharynx that were once only accessible through open procedures such as mandibulotomy and pharyngotomy. TORS has facilitated the de-escalation of chemoradiation therapy in select patients, sparing them the morbidity of these therapies while not compromising oncologic outcome. However, the oncologic efficacy of TORS also relies on the appropriate management of the neck as this greatly influences locoregional and distant recurrence, as well as overall survival. Therefore, neck dissection is an important component of any TORS procedure performed for malignancy. This chapter will discuss the basic elements related to neck dissection for squamous cell carcinoma for oropharyngeal primary tumors resected by TORS and current controversies surrounding neck dissection such as the impact of HPV status on the behavior of nodal metastases. Additionally, relevant complications of neck dissection and preventative measures during neck dissection (i.e., prophylactic transcervical arterial ligation) to reduce the severity of complications of TORS will also be discussed.

R. Mandal, MD • I. Ganly, MD, PhD
Head and Neck Service, Department of Surgery, Memorial Sloan Kettering Cancer Center, 1275 York Ave, New York, NY 10021, USA

S.G. Patel, MD, FRCS (Glasg) (✉)
Head and Neck Service, Department of Surgery, Memorial Sloan Kettering Cancer Center, 1275 York Ave, New York, NY 10021, USA

Weill Medical College of Cornell University, New York, NY, USA
e-mail: patels@mskcc.org

Z. Gil et al. (eds.), *Atlas of Head and Neck Robotic Surgery*, DOI 10.1007/978-3-319-49578-1_21

21.2 Oropharyngeal Lymphatic Drainage and Nodal Metastasis

An understanding of oropharyngeal lymphatic drainage patterns is critical to the selection of appropriate cervical nodal dissection levels. Lymphatic drainage patterns of the neck have been extensively studied over several decades and are now well recognized. Based upon the predictive pathways of lymphatic drainage, the neck is typically divided into levels I–VI. Level I is divided into levels Ia (submental) and Ib (submandibular). Level Ia is bounded by the digastric muscles laterally, the mandible superiorly, and the hyoid bone inferiorly. Level Ib is bounded by the anterior and posterior bellies of the digastric muscle and the inferior border of the mandible and represents the submandibular triangle. Levels II–IV contain the internal jugular nodes. Level II (upper jugular) extends from the skull base to the level of the hyoid bone. It is posteriorly bounded by the posterior edge of the sternocleidomastoid muscle and anteriorly by the stylohyoid muscle. Level II is further subdivided into levels IIa and IIb which are separated by the spinal accessory nerve. Level IIa extends anterior to the nerve, while level IIb denotes the area posterior to the nerve. Level III (midjugular) extends from the inferior border of the hyoid to the inferior border of the cricoid cartilage. Its anterior border is the sternohyoid muscle, and its posterior border is the posterior edge of the sternocleidomastoid muscle. Level IV (lower jugular) extends from the cricoid cartilage to the clavicle. Level V (posterior triangle) is the zone bounded by the anterior border of the trapezius muscle and the posterior border of the sternocleidomastoid muscle. It extends inferiorly to the level of the clavicle. Level VI (anterior compartment) is found in the midline and extends from the hyoid to the suprasternal notch inferiorly. Its lateral boundary is the lateral border of the sternohyoid muscle or, as more recently proposed, the medial border of the common carotid artery [1].

Lymphatic drainage patterns vary significantly from patient to patient, but in general oropharyngeal tumors first drain to the retropharyngeal and internal jugular nodal basins. Lateral pharyngeal tumors tend to spread to the lateral neck nodes, whereas more posteriorly located tumors tend to first drain to the retropharyngeal nodes. A comprehensive analysis of nodal metastasis patterns of oropharyngeal and oral cavity squamous tumors was performed by Shah who reviewed 1,119 elective and therapeutic neck dissections for squamous cell carcinoma of the oral cavity, oropharynx, hypopharynx, and larynx (Table 21.1) [2]. Of elective neck dissections performed for oropharyngeal primaries, the percentages of metastatic nodes in levels II, III, and IV were 80 %, 60 %, and 27 %, respectively (Fig. 21.1), whereas the percentage of nodal metastasis in levels I and V was both only 7 % each. It should be noted that this pattern

Table 21.1 The percentage of identified cervical nodal metastases of squamous cell cancers of the head and neck stratified by primary site

Level of cervical nodal metastases	Oral cavity primary (elective ND)	Oral cavity primary (therapeutic ND)	Oropharyngeal primary (elective ND)	Oropharyngeal primary (therapeutic ND)	Hypopharyngeal primary (elective ND)	Hypopharyngeal primary (therapeutic ND)	Laryngeal primary (elective ND)	Laryngeal primary (therapeutic ND)
I	58	61	7	17	0	10	14	8
II	51	57	80	85	75	78	52	68
III	26	44	60	50	75	75	55	70
IV	9	20	27	33	0	47	24	35
V	2	4	7	11	0	11	7	5

Modified from Shah [2]

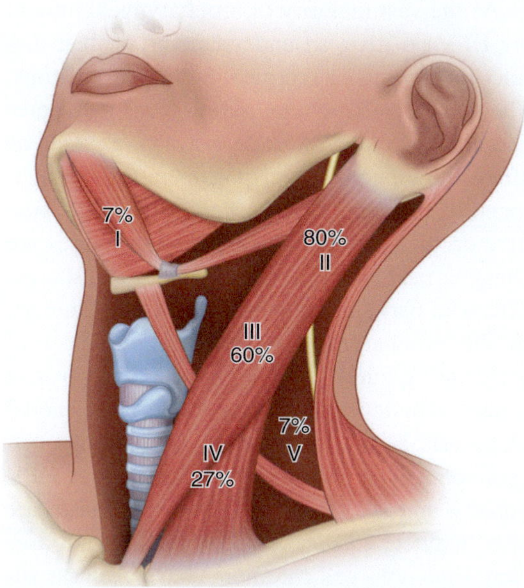

Fig. 21.1 Percentages of total occult cervical nodal metastases from oropharyngeal primaries identified after elective neck dissection

of metastasis is different from that of oral cavity squamous cell carcinoma which typically involves levels I–III. When nodal metastases occur outside of levels II–IV, it is typically associated with concurrent level II–IV metastasis. Isolated "skip" lesions are extremely rare; in a study of 333 patients with oropharyngeal/hypopharyngeal primaries, only one patient (0.3 %) was found to have an isolated skip metastasis outside of levels II–IV [3]. Recent studies have also confirmed that nodal metastases in the N0 neck from oropharyngeal primaries mainly occur at levels II–IV [4]. Therefore, in the elective management of the neck for oropharyngeal primaries, dissection of levels II–IV is generally performed as an initial approach for selective neck dissection in these patients. While retropharyngeal nodes are not routinely dissected electively for TORS, surgeons should be aware of the potential for metastasis to these nodes from cancers of the oropharynx. Larger retropharyngeal nodal metastasis may be accessible during TORS, but alternatively most retropharyngeal nodal metastases will need to be included in the fields of radiation therapy if adjuvant treatment is indicated.

21.3 Neck Dissection Classification

Neck dissection can be subclassified into comprehensive neck dissection and selective neck dissection based on the extent of surgical resection of key cervical structures.

21.3.1 Comprehensive Neck Dissection

The most extensive type of neck dissection is radical neck dissection which entails removal of the cervical nodes from levels I to V as well as the sternocleidomastoid muscle, spinal accessory nerve, and internal jugular vein. It is infrequently performed today; radical surgery is usually necessary for therapeutic neck dissection if key structures are involved with extensive nodal disease.

In contrast, modified radical neck dissection involves removal of cervical nodes located at levels I–V but with preservation of one or more of the following structures: the sternocleidomastoid muscle, spinal accessory nerve, and internal jugular vein. Modified radical neck dissection type I involves preservation of only the accessory nerve, while modified radical neck dissection type II involves preservation of the accessory nerve and the internal jugular vein. Type III modified radical neck dissection, also referred to as functional neck dissection, involves preservation of the internal jugular vein, accessory nerve, and sternocleidomastoid muscle. Sacrifice of these structures for TORS oropharyngeal primaries is appropriate only when these structures are clearly involved with disease. A clear surgical plane, not artificially created, should be present to ensure optimal oncologic outcome when preserving these structures but achieving gross total resection of all nodal disease.

21.3.2 Selective Neck Dissection

Selective neck dissection for elective management of the clinically negative neck entails removal of lymph nodes at nodal levels which are at the highest risk for metastatic spread with preservation of the internal jugular vein, sternocleidomastoid, and spinal accessory nerve. Nodal metastasis from oropharyngeal primaries occurs mainly to levels II–IV, and therefore selective neck dissection of the clinically negative neck in patients undergoing TORS for squamous cell carcinoma of the oropharynx should include these levels (also known as lateral neck dissection).

The need for dissection of level IIb, the nodal subdivision defined as the area posterior to the spinal accessory nerve in level II, for squamous cell carcinoma of the oral cavity and oropharynx is debated among surgeons. Recent analyses have shown that dissection of level IIb is beneficial particularly for squamous cell carcinoma of the tonsil and in all patients with oropharyngeal primaries who have clinically N+ disease (within and outside of level II) [5, 6]. In experienced hands, dissection of level IIb adds only minimally increased risk of accessory nerve dysfunction and can be safely performed for appropriate cases.

21.4 Clinicopathological Differences Between HPV Positive and HPV Negative Neck Disease

Recent work has genetically characterized HPV positive and HPV negative tumors as distinct entities in regard to the drivers of their oncogenesis [7]. Therefore, it is not surprising that nodal metastases from these two distinct cancer subtypes have different characteristics and behavior. The percentage of oropharyngeal tumors in the 1990s that were HPV positive is estimated to be approximately 50 %; however, recent analysis has shown that this percentage has dramatically increased to as high as 80 % currently in North America and Europe [8].

As the vast majority of oropharyngeal tumors are HPV positive, an understanding of their distinct characteristics is critical for TORS surgeons. These characteristics can aid surgeons in the preoperative workup of these patients as well as affect intraoperative and postoperative management. It is generally well accepted that HPV positive oropharyngeal squamous cell primaries are characterized by frequent and early nodal spread. This is in part due to the rich lymphatic drainage of the oropharynx. The prognostic impact of early and frequent nodal spread in HPV positive disease is believed to be not as important as nodal metastasis is for HPV negative squamous cell carcinoma. The physical characteristics of HPV positive and HPV negative nodal metastases are also distinct. Cystic cervical nodal metastases from squamous cell carcinoma have been associated with primary tumors which originate from Waldeyer's ring (which includes the base of the tongue, palatine tonsils, and nasopharynx) in 72–90 % of cases in which the primary tumor is detected [9, 10]. Furthermore, the cystic nature of oropharyngeal nodal metastases has also been linked to HPV positivity [10, 11]. The precise reasons for the occurrence of cystic metastases in oropharyngeal carcinoma are unclear but have been attributed to malignant salivary gland-type cells that metastasize from the oropharynx to cervical nodes and which subsequently express their parental property in these lymph nodes [12]. Alternative explanations involve the transformation of keratinocytes which have an inherent propensity for cyst formation after malignant conversion to a transitional type of squamous cell carcinoma [10]. Regardless of the precise mechanism of formation of cystic nodal metastases in HPV oropharyngeal tumors, surgeons should be aware of their frequent occurrence in the preoperative evaluation of these patients. It should be noted, however, that the presence of cystic cervical node metastases also occurs in other diseases processes as well, such as papillary thyroid carcinoma and hypopharyngeal carcinoma.

21.5 Management of the Neck in HPV Negative and HPV Positive Oropharyngeal Disease

As HPV positive and HPV negative tumors represent biologically distinct tumor entities, we advocate that the elective and therapeutic management strategy of the neck should differ between these two cancer subtypes. Here, we outline our clinical practice in regard to the surgical management of the neck for oropharyngeal squamous cell primaries in the context of HPV status (Fig. 21.2).

21.5.1 The N0 Neck in HPV Positive and HPV Negative Disease

21.5.1.1 Selective Neck Dissection (Levels II–IV)

Occult cervical nodal metastases occur in approximately 30 % of early-stage tumors in both oral cavity and oropharyngeal primaries [13, 14]. As a result, elective neck dissection is usually offered to patients with a clinically and radiographically negative neck. As previously discussed, the nodal basins most commonly involved by both HPV positive and HPV negative oropharyngeal squamous primaries are located at levels II–IV of the ipsilateral neck. Occult metastases outside of these levels are extremely uncommon, and true isolated skip metastases to levels I and V are even rarer. As a result, we advocate elective ipsilateral levels II–IV selective neck dissection for management of the clinically N0 neck in well-lateralized HPV positive and HPV negative oropharyngeal tumors. Bilateral elective neck dissection of levels II–IV needs to be considered

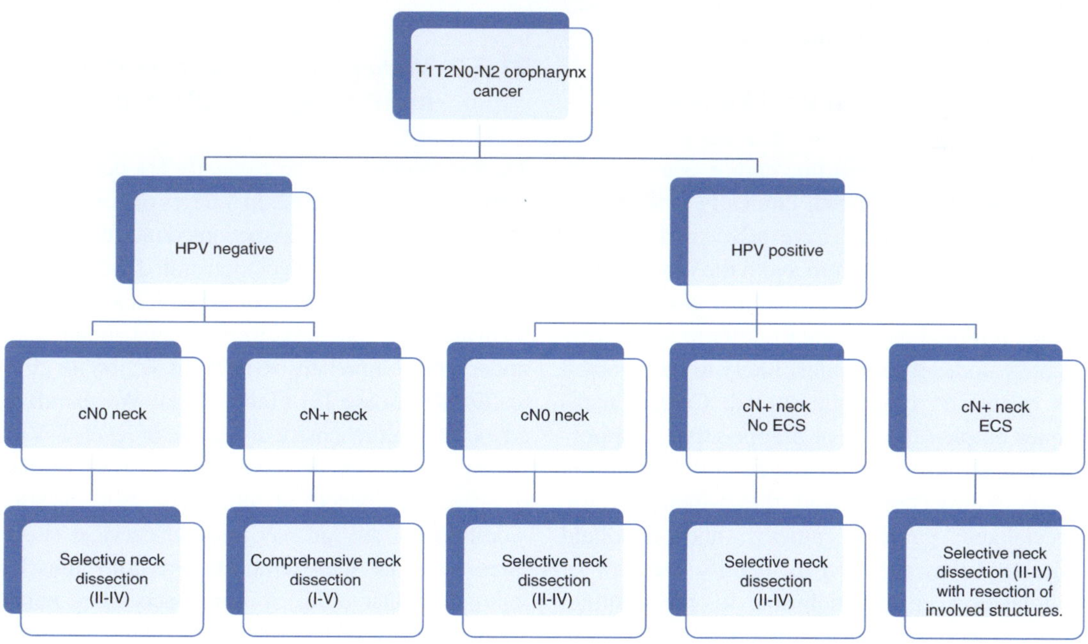

Fig. 21.2 Proposed treatment paradigm for the surgical management of the neck in HPV positive and HPV negative squamous cell primaries of the oropharynx

for base of tongue lesions that are centrally located or approaching the midline.

A recent publication reported an overall survival advantage for early-stage oral cavity cancer after elective neck dissection [15]. However, these results cannot be extrapolated meaningfully to the oropharynx because of the distinct biological behavior of HPV-related oropharynx cancer. On the other hand, the obvious utility of elective neck dissection in any head and neck cancer including oropharyngeal primaries is its ability to provide definitive histopathologic staging information that is otherwise not available from any other existing investigative modality including modern radiographic imaging. This information can then be used by the multidisciplinary team for designing an individualized therapeutic plan for the patient based on risk versus benefit rather than an empiric estimation of the possibility of nodal metastatic disease.

Elective radiation to the neck can be performed in select patients who have contraindications to or refuse elective neck dissection or whose primary tumor is amenable to treatment with radiation therapy alone. While generally outside of our treatment paradigm, close observation followed by surgical salvage if necessary may be an alternative option in these patients.

21.5.1.2 Role of Sentinel Node Biopsy

As the majority of patients with early-stage oropharyngeal cancer will not harbor occult nodal metastases when staged clinically and radiographically N0, some have advocated sentinel node biopsy in an effort to avoid the morbidity of elective neck dissection. Sentinel node biopsy entails lymphatic mapping in order to selectively identify nodes that are most likely to be involved via metastatic lymphatic spread. Current techniques employ the use of preoperative lymphoscintigraphy with a radiolabeled colloid solution which is injected around the primary tumor. Specialized gamma cameras and handheld gamma probes are used to identify the flow of radiolabeled colloid solution to the sentinel nodes. Once identified intraoperatively, these nodes are biopsied, and the need for subsequent treatment is determined based on the histological analysis of the biopsied sentinel node(s) as cancer metastases usually spread in a serial fashion and the first encountered nodes (sentinel nodes) will harbor cancer cells before progressive spread to subsequent nodal basins.

There is a paucity of data surrounding the accuracy of sentinel node biopsy for oropharyngeal cancer. Furthermore, logistic and technical difficulties exist with the injection radioactive tracer material preoperatively for hard to access areas within the oropharynx. A large multi-institutional trial specifically examining *oral cavity* squamous cancers demonstrated accurate prediction of the pathologically negative neck based on negative sentinel nodes as high as 96 % [16]. A recent trial evaluating the efficacy of sentinel node biopsy in oral cavity cancer (including oropharyngeal-bordering tumors) demonstrated a negative predictive value of 95 % [17]. It is unclear how well these results will translate to oropharyngeal primaries and sentinel node biopsy for oropharyngeal primaries is not currently recommended as standard-of-care outside of clinical trials.

21.5.2 Management of the N+ Neck in HPV Negative Disease

The management of the clinically N+ neck differs from that of the N0 neck. In a series of comprehensive therapeutic neck dissections done for oropharyngeal primaries, Shah demonstrated the presence of a significant number of level I and V nodal metastases as compared to those of patients who underwent comprehensive neck dissection for clinically N0 disease [2] (Table 21.1). We therefore advocate comprehensive dissection of levels I–V in patients with HPV negative oropharyngeal primaries with evidence of clinically N+ disease. Additionally, any grossly invaded cervical structures such as the sternocleidomastoid muscle, internal jugular vein, or spinal accessory nerve should be resected for optimal oncologic outcome.

21.5.3 Management of the N+ Neck in HPV Positive Disease

Previous studies examining the impact of nodal metastases on patient outcome did not take into account the effect of HPV status on tumor behavior and prognosis. As previously discussed, we now understand that HPV positive and HPV negative tumors are very different biological cancer subtypes that also have distinct clinical behavior. Given these inherent differences, questions have arisen regarding the ideal management of the clinically N+ neck in HPV positive oropharyngeal cancer and whether treatment paradigms should be the same as N+ disease in HPV negative cancers. A recent large retrospective analysis of 201 patients with surgically resected oropharyngeal cancer from our institution has provided significant insight regarding the differences in prognostic factors between HPV positive and HPV negative tumors [18]. Interestingly, pathologic nodal status had no impact on survival for HPV positive patients but showed a trend toward significance in HPV negative patients (Fig. 21.3). This suggests that nodal metastases in HPV positive patients are more indolent and generally do not portend worse clinical outcome as compared to HPV negative nodal metastases. As a result, our clinical practice for clinically N+ oropharyngeal HPV positive squamous cell primaries is to perform an ipsilateral selective neck dissection of levels II–IV (including any clinically involved neck levels). Some of these patients will go on to receive adjuvant postoperative radiation therapy based on their pathologic characteristics. Radiation therapy appears to be sufficient to address the rare occult nodal metastases in levels I and V that are not addressed surgically. The addition of postoperative radiation therapy in N1 disease remains at the discretion of the surgeon and multidisciplinary treatment team. N1 nodal disease that has been satisfactorily resected without adverse features such as extensive extracapsular nodal spread can be observed without the addition of postoperative radiation therapy. In contrast, N1 nodal disease that possesses adverse features such as extensive extracapsular spread may receive postoperative radiation at the discretion of the multidisciplinary treatment team. Further discussion of postoperative radiation therapy following neck dissection is detailed below.

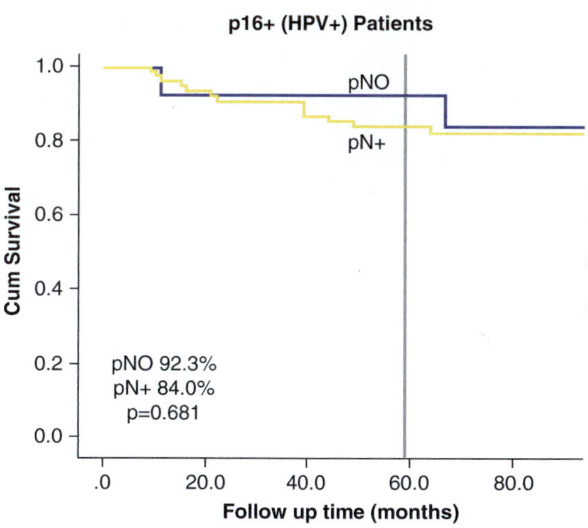

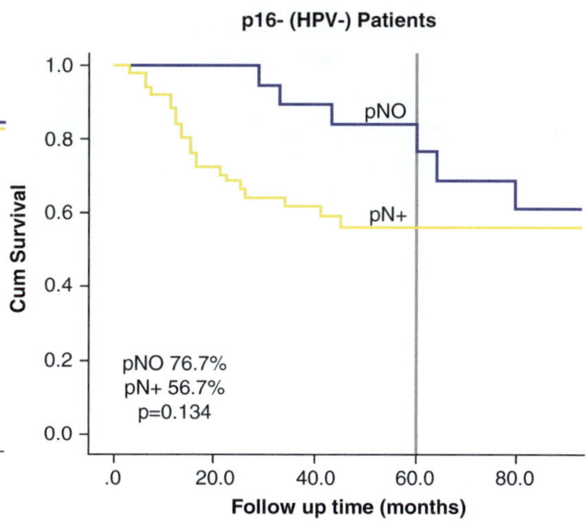

Fig. 21.3 Kaplan-Meier plots demonstrating the impact of pathologic cervical nodal status in HPV positive and HPV negative tumors of the oropharynx on patient survival (Reproduced with permission from Iyer et al. *Annals of Surgical Oncology*, 2015 [18])

21.6 Pharyngeal Defects Following Primary Tumor TORS and Neck Dissection

When neck dissection is carried out concurrently with TORS resection of the primary tumor, there is always the possibility that a full thickness defect can be created through the pharyngeal musculature into the neck. Because of this risk, some surgeons prefer to delay the neck dissection until 2–4 weeks after TORS of the primary. However, the majority of surgeons now carry out neck dissection in conjunction with TORS in order to facilitate adjuvant radiation treatment in a timely fashion. Surgeons must therefore be aware of the potential for pharyngeal defects to result from such combined surgeries and be prepared to repair such defects. TORS of a large oropharyngeal primary can have significant implications for neck dissection. Through-and-through defects can create an open communication between the neck and pharynx that must be addressed intraoperatively. The presence of a pharyngocervical salivary fistula in close proximity to an exposed carotid artery increases the risk of carotid rupture postoperatively. Thus large primary pharyngeal resection beds may require primary closure or coverage with local flaps or free tissue transfer if a salivary communication exists or is likely to develop. Recently, the Classification of Oropharyngeal Robotic Defects (CORD) has been proposed to help guide reconstruction defects following TORS [19, 20]. This classification characterizes the surgical defect in terms of size, location, extent of oropharyngeal resection, presence of pharyngocervical fistula, and exposure of the carotid artery. Reconstruction can proceed, primarily, with local flaps or free tissue transfer through combined transoral and open approaches through the neck. Clearly, prophylactic transcervical arterial ligation (discussed below) should be avoided when reconstruction with microvascular free tissue transfer is anticipated. As discussed elsewhere in this book, a number of free flap reconstructive options have been used to repair pharyngeal/hypopharyngeal defects following TORS including radial forearm, anterolateral thigh, and jejunal flaps. Pedicled flaps have also been used including pectoralis major and supraclavicular artery flaps. Primary closure techniques with musculomucosal advancement flap pharyngoplasty have been described in order to decrease fistula rates and improve functional outcome following surgery [21]. In many of these techniques, including free flap reconstruction, the surgical robot has been utilized in performing parts of the reconstruction, including the microvascular anastomosis [22]. If the defect is small, most surgeons will allow the resection bed to heal by secondary intention, and neck dissection can thus proceed without any additional considerations for reconstruction of the primary site. Large resection beds are subject to salivary secretions and continuous movement of the oropharynx during deglutition, making the resection bed vulnerable to wound breakdown. This may increase the risk for postoperative pharyngocervical fistula, cervical infection, and/or vascular breakdown resulting in oropharyngeal hemorrhage. For these reasons, proper selection of cases for TORS is crucial, and we recommend avoidance of leaving large areas of the oropharynx to heal by secondary intention. Local, pedicled, or free flaps can aid in providing healthy tissue to cover the resection bed and can be inset during the time of neck dissection through combined open and transoral techniques.

21.7 Extracapsular Nodal Extension in HPV+ Oropharyngeal HSNCC

Traditionally, extracapsular nodal extension of head and neck cancers portended worse outcomes and survival [23–25]. This has led to the recommendation for adjuvant chemoradiation therapy for patients with evidence of extracapsular spread (ECS) following surgery. Locoregional control and survival have indeed been shown to be improved after chemoradiation in these patients in several studies [26–28]. However, these studies group all head and neck squamous cancers together, including HPV positive and HPV negative oropharynx cancer, in their analyses. It is now clear that HPV positive and HPV negative tumors represent distinct oncologic entities, and a significant survival advantage is seen in HPV positive tumors as compared to HPV negative tumors [29]. This has led to recent speculation regarding the prognostic effects of ECS in head and neck squamous cell nodal metastases. In a recent study by Sinha et al., disease-free survival was no better in p16-positive (which serves a surrogate measure for HPV positivity) patients with ECS treated with adjuvant chemoradiation therapy as opposed to patients who were not treated with adjuvant chemoradiation therapy despite ECS [30]. A subsequent study from the University of Pittsburgh confirmed that ECS was not an independent predictor of worse survival in HPV positive tumors suggesting that ECS alone may be insufficient criteria to merit adjuvant chemoradiation [31]. More recently, Iyer et al. demonstrated by retrospective analysis that ECS was prognostic in HPV negative tumors but had no statistically significant effect on survival in HPV positive tumors (Fig. 21.4). These early studies suggest that HPV positive patients with ECS may possibly be able to be spared adjuvant chemotherapy; however, randomized prospective trials will be needed first before definitive recommendations can be made regarding the sparing of chemotherapy in these patients, and these trials are indeed underway [32].

These studies on the impact of nodal ECS are particularly important in patient selection for TORS surgery. Traditionally, if chemoradiation appeared inevitable despite surgical resection, then the additional morbidity of surgery was considered as an argument to favor chemoradiation therapy as primary treatment for these patients. However, if ECS proves not to be a worse prognostic factor for patient survival and locoregional recurrence, then perhaps select patients may be better served with TORS surgery or radiation alone in order to avoid the morbidity of upfront primary chemoradiation. In a study from the University of Pittsburgh, TORS was able to obviate or reduce the need for additional therapy in 76 % of stage I/II and 46 % of stage III/IV patients [33].

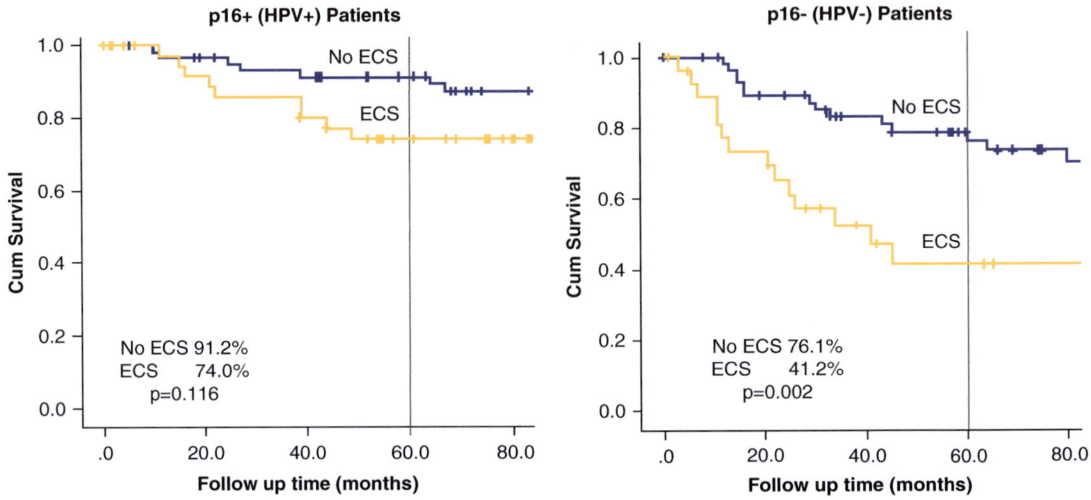

Fig. 21.4 Kaplan-Meier plots demonstrating the impact of extracapsular spread (ECS) of cervical nodal metastases in HPV positive and HPV negative tumors of the oropharynx on patient survival (Reproduced with permission from Iyer et al. *Annals of Surgical Oncology*, 2015 [18])

21.8 Adjuvant Radiation Therapy Following TORS/Neck Dissection

Clearly, avoidance and de-escalation of adjuvant therapy is a potential benefit of primary surgical treatment. As previously discussed, HPV positive HNSCC represents a biologically less aggressive subtype compared to HPV negative disease. Therefore, the need for conventional full-dose radiation therapy in patients with HPV positive tumors has fallen into question. It may be possible to de-escalate the total dose of radiation therapy in lower-risk HPV positive patients if surgically derived histopathologic information is used in rational decision-making. In an effort to more definitely answer this question, the Eastern Cooperative Group (ECOG) 3311 trial (NCT01898494) was designed to study the effect of radiation dose de-escalation in intermediate-risk HPV positive patients undergoing transoral surgery (Fig. 21.5). Low-risk patients are observed without any adjuvant therapy, whereas high-risk patients are treated with standard chemoradiation therapy. Here, low-risk patients are defined as those with T1–T2, N0–N1 disease with clear margins and no evidence of ECS, perineural invasion, or lymphovascular invasion. High-risk patients are defined as those with positive margins, extensive ECS, or greater than five positive metastatic lymph nodes. These treatment paradigms for low- and high-risk patients are in line with previous and current practice. Intermediate-risk patients are of particular interest in this study. Intermediate-risk patients are defined in this study as patients with either at least one close (<3 mm) margin, minimal (<1 mm) nodal ECS, two to four metastatic lymph nodes, perineural invasion, or lymphovascular invasion. Patients in the intermediate subgroup are randomized to receive either standard-dose radiation therapy at 60 Gy or de-escalated to receive 50 Gy. The trial is ongoing, and it will be important to see if de-escalation can offer equivalent survival and recurrence outcomes as full-dose radiation therapy. If oncologic outcomes are equivalent and functional results are superior, this may support the use of TORS in select "intermediate"-risk patients to decrease the toxicity of adjuvant treatment.

A recent retrospective analysis was performed on 175 patients with p16+ oropharyngeal SCC with ECS and/or close positive margins treated with either 66 Gy or 60 Gy postoperatively [34]. The authors found there was no difference in locoregional recurrence-free survival between the two groups. These data further suggest that HPV+ oropharyngeal nodal metastases represent a biologically less aggressive disease entity and may not require an aggressive adjuvant therapy as compared to HPV negative disease.

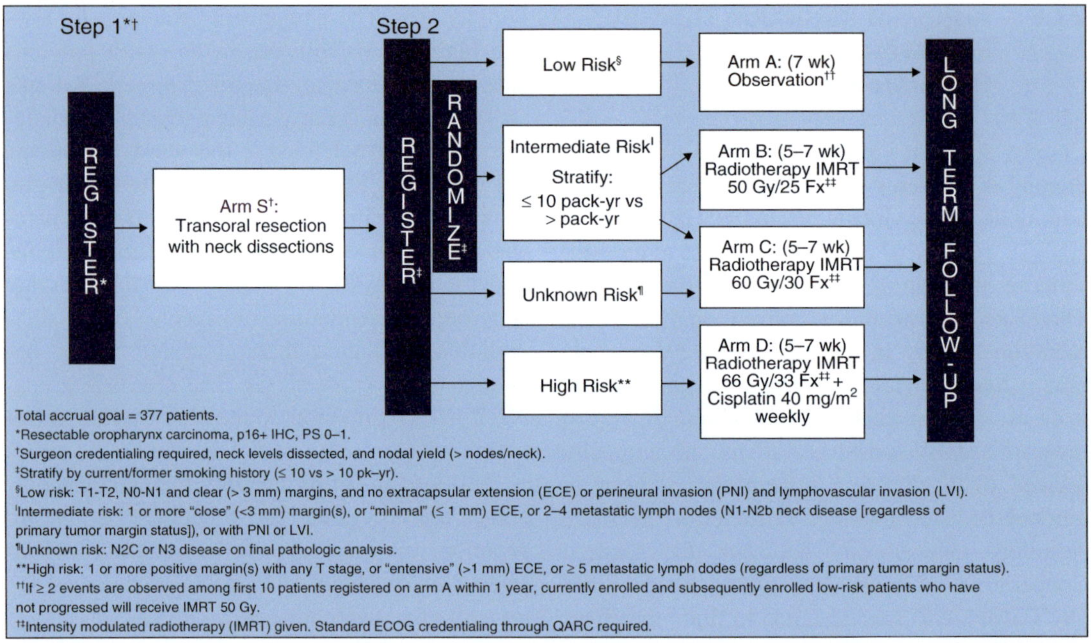

Fig. 21.5 Eastern Cooperative Oncology Group (ECOG) 3311 protocol for the evaluation of de-escalation of intermediate-risk patients following TORS. Low-risk patients receive observation postoperatively, and high-risk patients receive chemoradiotherapy (Reproduced with permission from: http://ecog-acrin.org/clinical-trials/e3311-educational-materials)

21.9 Transcervical Arterial Ligation During Neck Dissection for the Prevention of TORS-Related Hemorrhage

A particularly relevant concern for TORS is the risk of severe postoperative hemorrhage. This risk, albeit small, can lead to life-threatening complications secondary to the aspiration of large-volume blood loss. The reported frequency of postoperative hemorrhage varies widely in the literature and ranges from 1.5 % to 11.5 % with severe or life-threatening bleeds occurring only rarely [35–42]. The average time to postoperative hemorrhage is roughly 1 week, when most patients are no longer in the inpatient setting [39]. Severe complications in patients who suffer from life-threatening hemorrhage tend to occur in patients who are unable to protect their airway at the time of hemorrhage which underscores the need for appropriate patient selection for TORS [39].

Prophylactic transcervical arterial ligation performed at the time of neck dissection has been proposed as a means to mitigate the severity of postoperative hemorrhage following TORS in patients who experience such events. Evidence from high-volume TORS centers supports the use of prophylactic transcervical arterial ligation as a means to potentially decrease the overall severity of post-TORS hemorrhage [39, 40]. Consequently, many institutions, including our own, routinely perform prophylactic transcervical arterial ligation at the time of neck dissection to reduce the risk of postoperative hemorrhage in high-risk patients. We advocate distal vessel ligation of the superior thyroid, ascending pharyngeal, facial, and lingual arteries on the ipsilateral side of tumor resection. Bilateral vessel ligation should not be performed as this may significantly compromise end-organ blood flow.

It has been suggested that external carotid artery ligation may contribute to the development of first bite syndrome postoperatively through selective denervation of the cervical sympathetic plexus that accompanies the external carotid and ultimately innervates the parotid gland [43]. However, these events are exceedingly rare, and a clear association has yet to be established. The potential benefits of transcervical arterial ligation in preventing potentially life-threatening oropharyngeal hemorrhage greatly outweigh the small risk of developing first bite syndrome from ligation. Nevertheless, we advocate distal selective vessel ligation of the branches of external carotid supplying the oropharynx (e.g., ascending pharyngeal, lingual, facial arteries) rather than the main external carotid to minimize disruption of the sympathetic plexus. Additionally, preliminary functional cadaveric studies from our institution suggest that distal vessel ligation of external carotid artery branches may be more efficacious than external carotid artery ligation alone in the prevention of severe post-TORS hemorrhage given the extensive collateral flow from the contralateral carotid system as well as the ipsilateral internal carotid arterial system.

Prophylactic ligation is one method to help potentially reduce the adverse impact of postoperative hemorrhage following TORS. Other means include placing a temporary tracheostomy (<2 weeks) in high-risk patients at the time of neck dissection (or primary tumor resection) to assist airway protection in the event of a postoperative bleed. In the future more sophisticated technologies may allow for the closure of the tumor resection bed either primarily or with local flaps transorally. These interventions may help to eliminate the occurrence of severe postoperative hemorrhage in these patients.

21.10 Chylous Fistula

Chylous fistula following neck dissection can be distressing to the patient and prolong hospital stay following surgery. Its reported incidence is low and is approximately 1–2 % following neck dissection. During neck dissection, the thoracic duct is found in the left neck and can have a highly variable branching pattern. Two or more branches are seen in up to 40 % of patients. The duct typically terminates in the internal jugular vein and is vulnerable to injury at this location (particularly along the medial wall of the vein) as this region is highly accessible during surgery. Intraoperative measures taken during neck dissection can facilitate prevention. Particular attention to the extravasation of chyle during dissection of level IV is critical in preventing postoperative fistula. Prophylactic clamping and tying of adipose tissue in level IV as the nodal packet is dissected close to the jugular vein can reduce the occurrence of thoracic duct fistula. Surgeons should be aware of the location of the phrenic and vagus nerves during this process to avoid inadvertent injury to these structures. The thoracic duct or its branches are often not visualized during neck dissection, and meticulous ligation in level IV is therefore crucial. Intraoperative Valsalva maneuver can be used to aid in the visualization of extravasated chyle from an injured lymphatic duct. Any visualized extravasation should be immediately addressed intraoperatively with suture ligation.

Chylous fistulas that develop postoperatively may be initially managed conservatively if patients are asymptomatic and chylous drain output is less than 600 mL in a 24 h period. Chylous drain output greater than 300 mL per day for 3 days is unlikely to resolve with conservative measures alone [44]. Conservative management of chylous fistula involves dietary measures including a nonfat or low-fat diet which decreases the flow/production of lymphatic fluid/chyle. In more severe cases, oral intake can be entirely restricted, and nutritional support is provided parenterally until chyle leakage is controlled. If patients are receiving nutritional tube feedings, formulations with medium-chain triglycerides are recommended as medium-chain triglycerides bypass the lymphatic system via the portal vein and are thus transferred directly to the liver. Somatostatin analogs such as octreotide are also useful in the conservative management of chylous fistula. These agents decrease chyle production and are often used in the management of low-output chyle leaks. In fact, some evidence suggests that octreotide may be useful in the treatment of high-flow chyle leaks as well [45]. Compressive dressings may also be useful in the conservative management of chylous fistula, particularly if accumulation of fluid is observed under intact skin flaps.

If chyle output exceeds the abovementioned thresholds or remains persistent despite conservative management, surgical intervention should be considered. Exploration and suture ligation in the operative room can be technically challenging but is an effective means to address persistent or high-volume chylous fistula. Thoracic duct embolization and transthoracic endoscopic thoracic duct ligation have also been described as minimally invasive alternatives to surgical exploration. While highly successful in some cases, the overall reported success rates are highly variable, and the procedure is not without its potential complications.

21.11 Contraindications and Patient Selection

The advent of TORS with neck dissection has significantly expanded the treatment options for cancers of the oropharynx. It has provided surgical access to the oropharynx that was once only accessible via more invasive open procedures. However, as other treatment modalities such as radiation and chemoradiation therapy are also effective, appropriate selection of patients is critical to provide the most efficacious and safe treatment for the patient. While an exhaustive discussion of relative and absolute contradictions for TORS is not presented here, key contraindications as they relate specifically to neck dissection are presented.

Frank involvement of carotid artery by tumor or tumor nodal metastases can present a challenge to successful neck dissection. Patients who have tumor encasing the carotid artery are best treated nonsurgically because complete surgical resection is not feasible or safe even with carotid artery resection and grafting, especially in those who have extensive disease at the skull base. Other contraindications include invasion of the prevertebral fascia, paraspinal muscles, and brachial plexus.

21.12 Summary

Management of the regional lymphatics is a critical component of treatment selection and surgical planning in management of patients with squamous cell carcinoma of the oropharynx. The patterns of nodal metastases from the oropharynx have been well recognized for several decades, but we now know that nodal metastases have different characteristics and behavior depending on HPV status of the tumor. Improved understanding of these differences has led to an evolution of management strategies of not only the primary tumor but also of cervical nodal metastases. Individualized patient selection balancing risk versus benefit based on multidisciplinary interaction is crucial for successful outcome after surgical treatment of oropharyngeal squamous cell carcinoma.

References

1. Robbins KT, Shaha AR, Medina JE, Califano JA, Wolf GT, Ferlito A, et al. Consensus statement on the classification and terminology of neck dissection. Arch Otolaryngol Head Neck Surg. 2008;134(5):536–8.
2. Shah JP. Patterns of cervical lymph node metastasis from squamous carcinomas of the upper aerodigestive tract. Am J Surg. 1990;160(4):405–9.
3. Candela FC, Kothari K, Shah JP. Patterns of cervical node metastases from squamous carcinoma of the oropharynx and hypopharynx. Head Neck. 1990;12(3):197–203.
4. Lim YC, Koo BS, Lee JS, Lim JY, Choi EC. Distributions of cervical lymph node metastases in oropharyngeal carcinoma: therapeutic implications for the N0 neck. Laryngoscope. 2006;116(7):1148–52.
5. Corlette TH, Cole IE, Albsoul N, Ayyash M. Neck dissection of level IIb: is it really necessary? Laryngoscope. 2005;115(9):1624–6.
6. Seethala RR. Current state of neck dissection in the United States. Head Neck Pathol. 2009;3(3):238–45.
7. Cancer Genome Atlas N. Comprehensive genomic characterization of head and neck squamous cell carcinomas. Nature. 2015;517(7536):576–82.
8. O'Sullivan B, Huang SH, Su J, Garden AS, Sturgis EM, Dahlstrom K, et al. Development and validation of a staging system for HPV-related oropharyngeal cancer by the International Collaboration on Oropharyngeal cancer Network for Staging (ICON-S): a multicentre cohort study. Lancet Oncol. 2016;17(4):440–51.
9. Gourin CG, Johnson JT. Incidence of unsuspected metastases in lateral cervical cysts. Laryngoscope. 2000;110(10 Pt 1):1637–41.
10. Thompson LD, Heffner DK. The clinical importance of cystic squamous cell carcinomas in the neck: a study of 136 cases. Cancer. 1998;82(5):944–56.
11. Stelow EB, Jo VY, Stoler MH, Mills SE. Human papillomavirus-associated squamous cell carcinoma of the upper aerodigestive tract. Am J Surg Pathol. 2010;34(7):e15–24.
12. Regauer S, Beham A, Mannweiler S. CK7 expression in carcinomas of the Waldeyer's ring area. Hum Pathol. 2000;31(9):1096–101.
13. van den Brekel MW, Stel HV, Castelijns JA, Nauta JJ, van der Waal I, Valk J, et al. Cervical lymph node metastasis: assessment of radiologic criteria. Radiology. 1990;177(2):379–84.
14. Ross GL, Soutar DS, MacDonald DG, Shoaib T, Camilleri IG, Robertson AG. Improved staging of cervical metastases in clinically node-negative patients with head and neck squamous cell carcinoma. Ann Surg Oncol. 2004;11(2):213–8.
15. D'Cruz AK, Vaish R, Kapre N, Dandekar M, Gupta S, Hawaldar R, et al. Elective versus therapeutic neck dissection in node-negative oral cancer. N Engl J Med. 2015;373(6):521–9.
16. Civantos FJ, Zitsch RP, Schuller DE, Agrawal A, Smith RB, Nason R, et al. Sentinel lymph node biopsy accurately stages the regional lymph nodes for T1-T2 oral squamous cell carcinomas: results of a prospective multi-institutional trial. J Clin Oncol Off J Am Soc Clin Oncol. 2010;28(8):1395–400.
17. Schilling C, Stoeckli SJ, Haerle SK, Broglie MA, Huber GF, Sorensen JA, et al. Sentinel European Node Trial (SENT): 3-year results of sentinel node biopsy in oral cancer. Eur J Cancer. 2015;51(18):2777–84.
18. Iyer NG, Dogan S, Palmer F, Rahmati R, Nixon IJ, Lee N, et al. Detailed analysis of clinicopathologic factors demonstrate distinct difference in outcome and prognostic factors between surgically treated HPV-positive and negative oropharyngeal cancer. Ann Surg Oncol. 2015;22(13):4411–21.
19. de Almeida JR, Genden EM. Robotic assisted reconstruction of the oropharynx. Curr Opin Otolaryngol Head Neck Surg. 2012;20(4):237–45.
20. de Almeida JR, Park RC, Genden EM. Reconstruction of transoral robotic surgery defects: principles and techniques. J Reconstr Microsurg. 2012;28(7):465–72.
21. Genden EM, Park R, Smith C, Kotz T. The role of reconstruction for transoral robotic pharyngectomy and concomitant neck dissection. Arch Otolaryngol Head Neck Surg. 2011;137(2):151–6.
22. Selber JC. Transoral robotic reconstruction of oropharyngeal defects: a case series. Plast Reconstr Surg. 2010;126(6):1978–87.
23. Snow GB, Annyas AA, van Slooten EA, Bartelink H, Hart AA. Prognostic factors of neck node metastasis. Clin Otolaryngol Allied Sci. 1982;7(3):185–92.

24. Johnson JT, Myers EN, Bedetti CD, Barnes EL, Schramm Jr VL, Thearle PB. Cervical lymph node metastases. Incidence and implications of extracapsular carcinoma. Arch Otolaryngol. 1985;111(8):534–7.
25. Ferlito A, Robbins KT, Shaha AR, Pellitteri PK, Kowalski LP, Gavilan J, et al. Current considerations in neck dissection. Acta Otolaryngol. 2002;122(3):323–9.
26. Johnson JT, Wagner RL, Myers EN. A long-term assessment of adjuvant chemotherapy on outcome of patients with extracapsular spread of cervical metastases from squamous carcinoma of the head and neck. Cancer. 1996;77(1):181–5.
27. Cooper JS, Pajak TF, Forastiere AA, Jacobs J, Campbell BH, Saxman SB, et al. Postoperative concurrent radiotherapy and chemotherapy for high-risk squamous-cell carcinoma of the head and neck. N Engl J Med. 2004;350(19):1937–44.
28. Bernier J, Domenge C, Ozsahin M, Matuszewska K, Lefebvre JL, Greiner RH, et al. Postoperative irradiation with or without concomitant chemotherapy for locally advanced head and neck cancer. N Engl J Med. 2004;350(19):1945–52.
29. Ang KK, Harris J, Wheeler R, Weber R, Rosenthal DI, Nguyen-Tan PF, et al. Human papillomavirus and survival of patients with oropharyngeal cancer. N Engl J Med. 2010;363(1):24–35.
30. Sinha P, Lewis Jr JS, Piccirillo JF, Kallogjeri D, Haughey BH. Extracapsular spread and adjuvant therapy in human papillomavirus-related, p16-positive oropharyngeal carcinoma. Cancer. 2012;118(14):3519–30.
31. Maxwell JH, Mehta V, Wang H, Cunningham D, Duvvuri U, Kim S, et al. Quality of life in head and neck cancer patients: impact of HPV and primary treatment modality. Laryngoscope. 2014;124(7):1592–7.
32. Washington University School of Medicine. Post operative adjuvant therapy de-intensification trial for human papillomavirus-related, p16+ oropharynx cancer (ADEPT). ClinicalTrialsgov [Internet] Bethesda: National Library of Medicine (US) 2000- [6/2016] Available from: https://clinicaltrials.gov/ct2/show/study/NCT01687413 NLM Identifier: NCT01687413. 2016.
33. Gildener-Leapman N, Kim J, Abberbock S, Choby GW, Mandal R, Duvvuri U, et al. Utility of up-front transoral robotic surgery in tailoring adjuvant therapy. Head Neck. 2016;38:1201–7.
34. Chin RI, Spencer CR, DeWees T, Hwang MY, Patel P, Sinha P, et al. Reevaluation of postoperative radiation dose in the management of human papillomavirus-positive oropharyngeal cancer. Head Neck. 2016;38:1643–9.
35. Asher SA, White HN, Kejner AE, Rosenthal EL, Carroll WR, Magnuson JS. Hemorrhage after transoral robotic-assisted surgery. Otolaryngol Head Neck Surg: Off J Am Acad Otolaryngol Head Neck Surg. 2013;149(1):112–7.
36. Chia SH, Gross ND, Richmon JD. Surgeon experience and complications with Transoral Robotic Surgery (TORS). Otolaryngol Head Neck Surg: Off J Am Acad Otolaryngol Head Neck Surg. 2013;149(6):885–92.
37. Hurtuk A, Agrawal A, Old M, Teknos TN, Ozer E. Outcomes of transoral robotic surgery: a preliminary clinical experience. Otolaryngol Head Neck Surg: Off J Am Acad Otolaryngol Head Neck Surg. 2011;145(2):248–53.
38. Lorincz BB, Mockelmann N, Busch CJ, Knecht R. Functional outcomes, feasibility, and safety of resection of transoral robotic surgery: single-institution series of 35 consecutive cases of transoral robotic surgery for oropharyngeal squamous cell carcinoma. Head Neck. 2015;37(11):1618–24.
39. Mandal R, Duvvuri U, Ferris RL, Kaffenberger TM, Choby GW, Kim S. Analysis of post-transoral robotic-assisted surgery hemorrhage: frequency, outcomes, and prevention. Head Neck. 2016;38(1):E776–82. doi: 10.1002/hed.24101. Epub 2015 Jul 15.
40. Pollei TR, Hinni ML, Moore EJ, Hayden RE, Olsen KD, Casler JD, et al. Analysis of postoperative bleeding and risk factors in transoral surgery of the oropharynx. JAMA Otolaryngol Head Neck Surg. 2013;139(11):1212–8.
41. Richmon JD, Feng AL, Yang W, Starmer H, Quon H, Gourin CG. Feasibility of rapid discharge after transoral robotic surgery of the oropharynx. Laryngoscope. 2014;124(11):2518–25.
42. Vergez S, Lallemant B, Ceruse P, Moriniere S, Aubry K, De Mones E, et al. Initial multi-institutional experience with transoral robotic surgery. Otolaryngol Head Neck Surg: Off J Am Acad Otolaryngol Head Neck Surg. 2012;147(3):475–81.
43. Chiu AG, Cohen JI, Burningham AR, Andersen PE, Davidson BJ. First bite syndrome: a complication of surgery involving the parapharyngeal space. Head Neck. 2002;24(11):996–9.
44. Scorza LB, Goldstein BJ, Mahraj RP. Modern management of chylous leak following head and neck surgery: a discussion of percutaneous lymphangiography-guided cannulation and embolization of the thoracic duct. Otolaryngol Clin N Am. 2008;41(6):1231–40. xi
45. Barili F, Polvani G, Topkara VK, Dainese L, Roberto M, Aljaber E, et al. Administration of octreotide for management of postoperative high-flow chylothorax. Ann Vasc Surg. 2007;21(1):90–2.

Erratum to: Transoral Robotic Resection of Parapharyngeal Space Tumors

Moran Amit, Irit Duek, and Ziv Gil

Erratum to:
Chapter 13 in: Z. Gil et al. (eds.), *Atlas of Head and Neck Robotic Surgery*,
DOI 10.1007/978-3-319-49578-1_13

The second author's name had been incorrectly spelt and the same has been corrected. The author's full name is Irit Duek.

The updated online version of this chapter can be found at
DOI 10.1007/978-3-319-49578-1_13

M. Amit, MD, PhD
The Laboratory for Applied Cancer Research, Department of Otolaryngology Head and Neck Surgery, the Head and Neck Center, Rambam Healthcare Campus, Clinical Research Institute at Rambam, Rappaport Institute of Medicine and Research, The Technion, Israel Institute of Technology, Haifa, Israel

I. Duek, MD
Department of Otolaryngology Head and Neck Surgery, the Head and Neck Center, Rambam Healthcare Campus, Clinical Research Institute at Rambam, Rappaport Institute of Medicine and Research, The Technion, Israel Institute of Technology, Haifa, Israel

Z. Gil, MD, PhD (✉)
The Laboratory for Applied Cancer Research, Department of Otolaryngology Head and Neck Surgery, the Head and Neck Center, Rambam Healthcare Campus, Clinical Research Institute at Rambam, Rappaport Institute of Medicine and Research, The Technion, Israel Institute of Technology, Haifa, Israel

Department of Otolaryngology, Rambam Medical Center, The Technion, Israel Institute of Technology, Haifa 66036, Israel
e-mail: ziv@baseofskull.org

Z. Gil et al. (eds.), *Atlas of Head and Neck Robotic Surgery*, DOI 10.1007/978-3-319-49578-1_22

MIX
Papier aus verantwortungsvollen Quellen
Paper from responsible sources
FSC® C105338

If you have any concerns about our products,
you can contact us on
ProductSafety@springernature.com

In case Publisher is established outside the EU,
the EU authorized representative is:
Springer Nature Customer Service Center GmbH
Europaplatz 3, 69115 Heidelberg, Germany

Printed by Libri Plureos GmbH
in Hamburg, Germany